PROBIOTICS 3

PROBIOTICS 3

Immunomodulation by the Gut Microflora and Probiotics

Edited by

R. FULLER

Freelance Consultant in Gut Microecology,
Reading, U.K.

and

G. PERDIGON

Professor of Immunology,
Tucumán University, Argentina

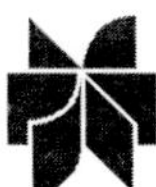

KLUWER ACADEMIC PUBLISHERS
DORDRECHT / BOSTON / LONDON

Library of Congress Cataloging-in-Publication Data

ISBN 0-7923-6244-6

Published by Kluwer Academic Publishers,
P.O. Box 17, 3300 AA Dordrecht, The Netherlands.

Sold and distributed in North, Central and South America
by Kluwer Academic Publishers,
101 Philip Drive, Norwell, MA 02061, U.S.A.

In all other countries, sold and distributed
by Kluwer Academic Publishers,
P.O. Box 322, 3300 AH Dordrecht, The Netherlands.

Printed on acid-free paper

Printed in the Netherlands.

This book is dedicated with gratitude to Professor Ricardo Margni for his inspiration as a teacher and his support and encouragement in my subsequent career in immunology.

Gabriela Perdigón

Table of contents

Preface

The way in which probiotics work is still not clearly defined, but it is becoming more and more apparent that immune stimulation is an important feature in some of the observed effects.

In the previous two books in this series the scientific basis and the practical applications were considered. It seemed that the immunogenic potential of probiotics merited a book of its own with experts from all over the world covering the general effect of the gut microflora on immunity as well as the particular response that probiotic microorganisms generate.

The importance of immune stimulation by probiotic organisms cannot be overemphasised. It opens up the technique for use, not only as a treatment for intestinal diseases, but also as a treatment that could be effective against infections outside the gastrointestinal tract.

This book considers how the body reacts to the presence of orally administered microorganisms (normally lactic acid bacteria). The responses may be in the form of antibodies (IgA, IgG, IgM), cytokines, killer cells or macrophage activity. Do these responses result in antagonism of the stimulating bacteria, do they affect the composition of the indigenous gut microflora and are they sufficienty strong to kill bacterial pathogens or tumour cells? Where we have answers these will be reported and discussed; where there are no answers there will be speculation and prediction. What we hope this book will achieve is a reasonable and objective assessment of the information currently available and a stimulation of interest in the immune properties of probiotic organisms.

We are extremely grateful to the authors for their expert contribution and we trust that with their help we have provided a critical survey of the work being done in this field of immunomodulation by probiotic organisms. The present use of probiotics is limited but rapidly increasing. It is hoped that by drawing attention to a property directly related to infection and health, that we can aid the spread of the probiotic concept amongs scientists and throughout the health industry generally.

We are grateful to all the contributors and hope that the book serves a useful purpose in promoting a deeper understanding of the science of probiotics.

Roy Fuller
Gabriela Perdigón

Contributors & Editors

R Bernier
BioAtlantech, Fredericton, NB, Canada E3B 5A6.

W Boersma
Institute for Animal Science and Health ID-DLO, PO Box 65, 8200 AB Lelystad, The Netherlands.

E Brochu
Institut Rossell, Montreal, QC, Canada H2P 2M6.

E Claassen
Department Immunology, Pathobiology and Epidemiology, Institut for Animal Science and Health ID-DLO, PO Box 65, 8200 AB Lelystad, The Netherlands.

A Florin-Christensen
Department of Medicine, CEMIC, Buenos Aires, Argentine.

R Fuller
59 Ryeish Green, Three Mile Cross, Reading RG7 1ES, U.K.

V Gaboriau-Routhiau
Unité d'Ecologie et de Physiologie du Système Digestif, Batiment 440, INRA, 78350 Jouy en Josas, France.

J Goulet
Université Laval, Quebec, QC., Canada G1K 7P4.

B Guy
Pasteur Mérieux Connaught, 1541, Avenue Marcel Mérieux, 69280 Marcy L'Etoile, France.

E Isolauri
Department of Pediatrics, University of Turku, 20520 Turku, Finland.

I Kato
Yakult Central Institute for Microbiological Research, 1796 Yaho, Kunitachi, Tokyo, Japan 186-8650.

JD Laman
Department Immunology, Pathobiology and Epidemiology, Institute for Animal Science and Health ID-DLO, PO Box 65, 8200 AB Lelystad, The Netherlands.

M del C Lopez
Division of Cellular Pathology, University of Cambridge, Cambridge, U.K.

CBM Maassen
TNO Prevention and Health, Division of Immunological and Infectious Disease, Leiden, The Netherlands.

C Matar
Université de Moncton, Moncton, NB, Canada, E1A 3E9.

MC Moreau
Unité d'Ecologie et de Physiologie du Système Digestif, Batiment 440, INRA, 78350 Jouy en Josas, France.

G Oliver
Centro de Referencias para Lactobacilos (CERELA), Chacabuco 145, 4000 Tucumán, Argentina.

G Perdigón
Instituto de Microbiología. Facultad de Bioquímica, Química y Farmacia de la Universidad Nacional de Tucumán. CERELA. Chacabuco 145, 4000, Tucumán, Argentina.

A Pesce de Ruiz Holgado
Centro de Referencias para Lactobacilos (CERELA), Chacabuco 145, 4000, Tucumán, Argentina.

J Ronco
Pasteur Mérieux Connaught, 1541, Avenue Marcel Mérieux, 69280 Marcy L'Etoile, France.

ME Roux
Laboratory of Cellular Immunology, CONICET. Department of Biological Sciences, Faculty of Pharmacy and Biochemistry, University of Buenos Aires, Argentine.

M Shaw
TNO Prevention and Health, Division of Immunological and Infectious Disease, Leiden, The Netherlands.

CHAPTER 1

Mucosal Immunity

M E Roux, M del C Lopez and A Florin-Christensen

1.1 Introduction

Mucosal surfaces represent the interface between the host and the environment and are the most common portal of entry for antigens.

Mucosal surfaces are in contact with the environment and are constantly exposed to antigens of microbial origin; the intestinal mucosa is exposed to antigens derived from food and the respiratory mucosa is exposed to inhaled antigens. Therefore, the mucosal lymphoid tissues fulfill several functions necessary for immunological protection.

The total surface area of the mucosa is much greater than that of the skin and their moist nutrient- rich secretions provide an ideal milieu for the proliferation of many potentially pathogenic micro-organisms. Moreover, the total mucosal surface in the adult human gastrointestinal tract extends to 200-300 m², the largest area of the body in contact with the external environment (Brandtzaeg, 1995 a, b, Lamm, 1976).

1.2 Mucosa associated lymphoid tissues

The presence of organised collections of lymphoid tissues, which have been termed MALT (mucosa-associated lymphoid tissues), is a characteristic of mucosal surfaces. The term MALT arose from the realisation that not only did mucosal surfaces share organisational similarities in their lymphoid elements, but also functional ones (Bienenstock *et al.*, 1978, Mc Dermott and Bienenstock , 1979). MALT is characterised by the predominance of local IgA production and by the finding that activated lymphocytes derived from one mucosal surface can recirculate and localise selectively in other mucosal surfaces. This connection between different mucosal surfaces permits immunity initiated at one anatomical site to protect other mucosal sites. The tissues that are part of the MALT include the middle ear, parts of the urogenital tract, the mammary gland, the conjuctivae, the salivary glands and the tonsils which are also part of the nasopharingeal lymphoid tissue

R. Fuller and G. Perdigon (eds.), Probiotics 3, 12–28.

(NALT) as well as BALT (bronchus-associated lymphoid tissue) and GALT (gut-associated lymphoid tissue) that is represented by the Peyer's patches, the caecal appendix, mesenteric lymphoid nodes (MLN) and solitary lymphoid nodules (Croitoru and Bienenstock,, 1994). Fig.1.1, Fig.1.2.

1.3 Mucosal lymphoid cells

The mucosal immune system comprises three basic kinds of lymphoid tissue that are compartmentalised and, to a large degree, functionally distinct:

1. central or organised lymphoid tissues constitute the Peyer's patches and related aggregates in other organs such as in the lung, tonsils and caecal appendix (Croitoru and Bienenstock, 1994, Cebra and Shroff, 1994, Phillips- Quagliata and Lamm, 1988, Bienenstock, 1982, Bienenstock and Clancy, 1994, Pabst, 1990, Sminia *et al.*, 1989);
2. the second kind of tissue is located diffusely in the various lamina propria of the mucosal system; after receiving B cells from the centralised aggregates which are already precommitted to IgA they undergo further differentiation and give rise to IgA plasma cells (Brandtzaeg, 1995 a, b, Cebra *et al.*, 1999, Roux *et al.*, 1981);

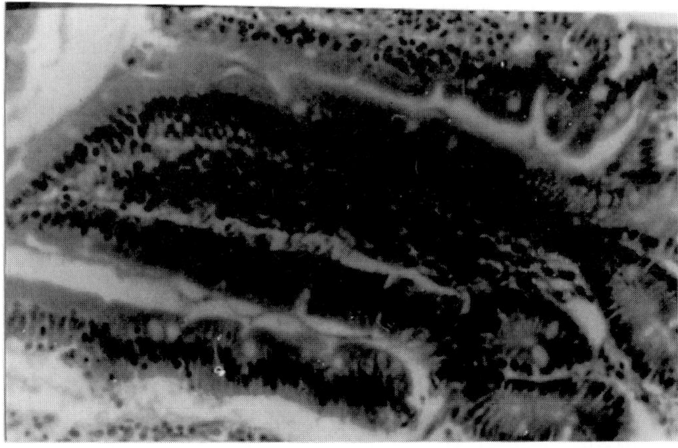

Figure 1.1. Hematoxilin/Eosin-stained tissue section of small intestine from 60 days old rats. A) gut ×200.

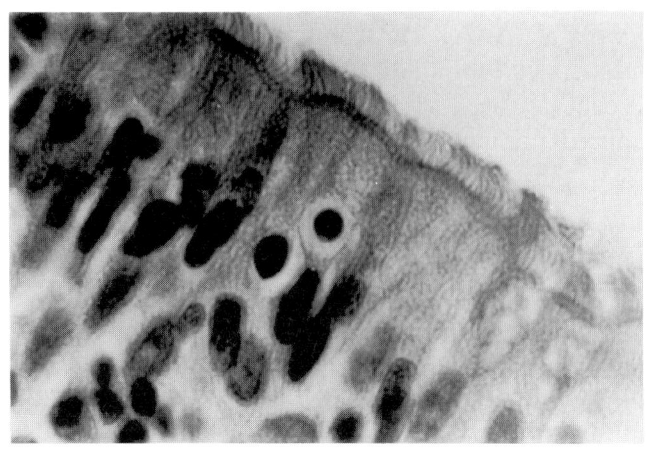

Figure 1.2. Localisation of BALT in the Hematoxilin/Eosin-stained tissue section from the lower respiratory tract from 60 days old rats. A) BALT ×1000.

3. the third type of lymphoid mucosal tissue consists of cells that lie between the epithelial cells of the various membranes, the so called intraepithelial lymphocytes (IEL) (Lefrançois, 1994, Lefrançois and Puddington, 1999).

The mucosal immune system in higher mammals, and a related form in other phyla, consists of an integrated network of tissues, lymphoid and mucus membrane-associated cells, and effector molecules for host protection. Major effector molecules include antibodies, largely of the immunoglobulin A (IgA) isotype as well as cytokines, chemokines, and their receptors, which appear to function in synergy with innate host factors such as defensins inducing immunity (Brandtzaeg, 1995 a, b, Lamm, 1976).

The mucosal immune system is anatomically divided into sites where foreign antigens are encountered and selectively taken up for initiation of immune responses, and the more diffuse collections of B and T lymphocytes, differentiated plasma cells, macrophages and other antigen-presenting cells (APCs) as well as eosinophils, basophils, and especially mast cells, which comprise the effector cells for mucosal immunity (Cebra *et al.*, 1999)

1.3.1 Origin of IgA plasma cells

The route by which GALT-derived IgA-committed B lymphocytes travel in the course of their normal maturation and migration from the GALT nodules back to the lamina propria of the gut forms an almost complete circle and hence has been called the IgA cell cycle (Lamm, 1976). A similar cyclic route is apparently followed by BALT-derived IgA-committed B lymphocytes in their migration to mucosal sites in the respiratory tract (Mc Dermott and Bienenstock, 1979).

Three features of mucosal B lymphocyte populations distinguish them from the B cells of the systemic immune system:

1. their ability, during their resting stages, to traffic through mucosal lymphoid follicles where they can be stimulated by antigens penetrating the specialised epithelium;
2. their ability as plasmablasts to migrate to the lamina propria and
3. their tendency to become committed to IgA production. Mucosal T cells, evidently share with mucosal B cells the ability to traffic through mucosal follicles and, at the effector cell stage, to migrate to the lamina propria. There, by cytokine production they may induce IgA plasma cells and IgA secretions. Their tendency to be expressed together in mucosal B lymphocyte populations could be the outcome of responses to either inductive or selective influences (Phillips-Quagliata, *et al.*, 1983).

   Proliferation and commitment to IgA production appear to take place in the lymphoid nodules of GALT and BALT.

1. B cells coming from the circulating pool or bone marrow arrive in the Peyer's patch by chance or selection at the level of high endothelial venules;
2. the B cells blast there, switch from IgM to IgA B cell blasts by the ability of switch T cells to induce IgA switch differentiation, leave the PP and are transported by lymph into the mesenteric lymph node where they mature into IgA B plasmablast in the case of GALT (Mc Williams *et al.*, 1977, Guy-Grand *et al.*, 1974), and into the bronchial (mediastinal) lymph nodes in the case of BALT (Mc Dermott and Bienenstock, 1979) and
3. they leave the efferent lymph, passing into the thoracic duct (Gowans and Knight, 1964) and from there into the blood circulation by which the lymphoid cells (blasts, plasmablasts) are delivered to the lamina propria at various sites of the gut where they become IgA plasmacells and memory cells recirculate through the HEV of the nodules (Rott *et al*, 1996.);
4. under hormonal influence (oestrogens, progesterone and prolactin) from blood circulation, the immature mucosa-committed B lymphoblasts migrate to an exocrine gland such as the mammary gland where they also

mature into plasma cells (Roux *et al.*, 1977). There also, T cells are found and probably have a similar life cycle to that of the B cells and the predominance of the T-helper cell subset suggest that T cells regulate also B cell development within the mammary gland (Parmely and Manning, 1983).

Moreover, evidence derived from studies of the ontogeny of the immune system in humans and animals, the phenotypes of B cells in different lymphoid compartments, immune responses generated by various routes of immunisation and adoptive transfer of B cells obtained from the peritoneum into immunodeficient mice favour the possibility that IgA-secreting plasma cells in mucosal tissue are derived not only from the Peyer's patches but also from the peritoneum (Kroese *et al.*, 1989). Several authors propose that the human fetal omentum contains more $CD5^+$ B cells than the liver and therefore should be considered a primary lymphoid organ and a site of B-cell generation, in addition to the foetal liver and the bone marrow (Solvasson and Keamy, 1992).

Studies on protein depleted rats have shown an impaired differentiation of IgA-B cell precursors in the Peyer's patches with the appearance of a pre-B cell population that is found in bone marrow (Lopez and Roux, 1989). Once IgA is secreted by the plasma cells it is taken up by an overlying epithelial cell, transported across the cell and released into external secretions. This system transports only polymeric immunoglobulin and the receptor that transports the IgA and also the IgM is known as the polymeric immunoglobulin receptor (pIgR). The receptor is synthesised in the endoplasmic reticulum of the epithelial cell and is then transported to the Golgi apparatus. The pIgR is delivered to the basolateral surface of the epithelial cell where it can bind IgA and can be subsequently endocytosed. The receptor is packaged into transcytotic vesicles and transported to the apical surface of the epithelial cell where the extracellular, ligand portion of the pIgR is removed. This cleared fragment is known as secretory component (sc) and remains associated with the IgA in the extracellular secretions (Mostov, 1994, Mazanec *et al.*, 1993).

1.4 Common Mucosal Immune System

The exposure of IgA precursor cells to environmental antigens and their subsequent migration to remote mucosal tissues and glands results in dissemination of SIgA (mediated specific immune responses). The physiological importance of these findings is considerable (Mazanec *et al.*, 1993). Stimulation of an IgA-inductive site (e.g. GALT) is likely to lead to the generalised protection of remote sites such as nasopharynx and genital tract; S-IgA antibodies in milk of orally immunised mothers may protect the gastrointestinal and possibly upper respiratory tract of breast-fed neonates.

In addition to gut and bronchus associated lymphoid tissues, IgA inductive sites in the Waldeyers ring of oropharyngeal lymphoid tissue (nasal, palatinal and lingual tonsils) or rectum also may contribute to the pool of precursor cells that preferentially populate upper respiratory or bowel-intestinal and genital tract.

The existence of this common mucosal immune system can be exploited in the design of novel types of vaccines that, given orally, result in protection at mucosal surfaces and glands (e.g. mammary gland) that are less accessible to local immunisation (Mestecky *et al.*, 1994, Quiding-Jarbrink *et al.*, 1996).

Several experiments in animals and humans led to the evidence that the stimulation of GALT by oral immunisation can be exploited for the induction of a secretor immune response to several microbial agents that infect mucosal surfaces distant from the gastrointestinal tract.

1.5 Antigen uptake

1.5.1 Role of epithelial and dendritic cells

In the gastrointestinal and upper respiratory tracts, nose, middle ear, gall bladder, uterine mucosa, as well as in the salivary, lactating mammary gland, lachrymal glands, the number of plasma cells producing IgA greatly exceed those producing other isotypes, emphasising the importance of IgA in their defence and, in the defence of the whole body.

Data from several laboratories (Brandtzaeg, 1995 a, b, Lamm, 1976, Bienenstock *et al.*, 1978) indicate that 5×10^{10} IgA- producing immunocytes populate the adult human small bowel alone, and if estimates of the numbers of IgA plasma cells in other mucosal sites are added, approximately 75% of all the Ig- producing immunocytes in the body make IgA.

Humans have two subclasses of IgA: IgA_1, and IgA_2. Cells producing these subclasses show regional differences in distribution. IgA_1 cells predominate over IgA_2 in the spleen, peripheral and mesenteric lymph modes, tonsils, stomach and duodenum, the numbers of cells producing the two subclasses are nearly equivalent in the lachrymal and salivary glands, and IgA_2-producing cells predominate in the large intestine.

Antigen uptake by M cells occurs in MALT (GALT, BALT and NALT) and results in the initial induction of the immune response. Antigen-sensitised, precursor surface IgA^+ B cells, $CD4^+$ Th cells and $CD8^+$ CTL5 in PP (GALT) leave *via* efferent lymphatics and migrate to mesenteric lymph nodes (MLN) and then into the thoracic duct (TD) to reach the blood stream. These migrating cells enter mucosal effector sites such as the lamina propria of the gastrointestinal tract or the upper respiratory tract or glands (hormone requirement), salivary or lachrymal glands. There, terminal differentiation, synthesis and transport of secretory IgA occurs . This induction in MALT and exodus to effector sites is termed the common mucosal immune system (CMIS), (Mestecky *et al.*, 1994, Quiding-Jarbrink *et al.*, 1996).

Therefore, we think that antigen crosses the epithelium of the MALT nodule through the M cells (found in the Peyer's Patch dome region to sample antigen) and makes contact with dendritic cells (interdigitating dendritic cells) resulting in 1) B and T cells that have entered the nodule through its HEV in the presence of integrins such as α4ß7; cytokines, such as TGF-β available in the nodule, promote switching (Tsw) of IgA B cells in the germinal centre; TGF-β induces Tsw that in the presence of follicular dendritic cells and other cytokines such as IL-4, IL-5, IL-10 promote the switching of IgM^+ B cell to IgA^+ B cell in the germinal centre, 2) a mixed population of cells coming both from the nodule and the lamina propria is carried with antigen in the lymph to the regional mucosa-associated lymph node, 3) in the mucosa-associated lymph node, unprimed B cells are primed and memory B cells are boosted. Some primed B cells mature into IgM-bearing plasmablasts capable of seeding the lamina propria, some into memory B cells capable of recirculating through HEV (α4β7 integrins). B cells derived from memory cells that were boosted by antigen in the MALT nodule mature into IgA plasmablasts, 4) mature plasmablasts and memory cells leave in efferent lymph and are carried by the blood to the mucosa and exocrine glands as well as to other lymphnodes, 5) plasmablasts capable of extravasating in lamina propria at mucosal sites and in exocrine glands do so and settle down to become plasma cells, which are mostly IgA producers, 6) memory cells with appropriate HEV-binding receptors (α4ß7 integrins) enter the MALT nodule or mucosa-associated lymph mode, where they encounter their specific antigen again and the population is expanded. MALT nodular influences (such as cytokines i.e. IL-4, IL-5, IL-10) that promote IgA production drive the population toward a major commitment. Therefore, the terminal differentiation synthesis (IL-6 cytokine influence) and transport of secretory IgA occurs (Fig.1.3).

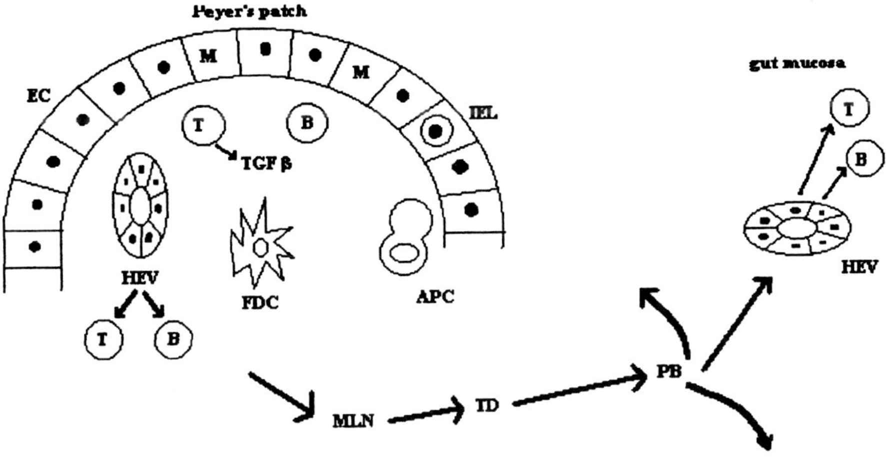

Fig. 1.3. Antigen Uptake

EC, epithelial cell; M, M cell; IEL, intraepitelial lymphocytes; HEV, high endothelial venule; FDC, follicular dendritic cell; ML, mesenteric lymph node; TD, thoracic duct; PB, periferal blood; APC, antigen presenting cell.

Oral tolerance (OT) has been defined as an antigen specific hyporesponsiveness after prior oral encounter of the antigen.

The administration of exogenous antigen *via* the intestinal tract and GALT to the peripheral immune system leads to OT which is, by definition, an antigen-driven peripheral immune tolerance. This form of immunological tolerance is not programmed into the germline but is acquired during post natal maturation. In this context, it is interesting to remember that the epithelium of the gut develops, as does the thymus, from the endoderm and may also play an important role in the peripheral (post thymic) tolerance induction. The development of immunogenic responses, i.e. responses generally elicited by antigens associated with mucosal pathogens and that result in immune effector elements with the potential of mediating host defence relative to the latter, are the exception rather than the rule in the mucosal immune system. More frequently, mucosal responses are marked by the development of tolerogenic responses i.e., by responses elicited by a far more common class of mucosal antigen, those associated with the resident microbial flora or the proteins in the food stream that result in partially or completely immunologic silence on subsequent exposure to the antigen. Three basic immunological mechanisms are implicated in peripheral tolerance induction: a) antigen-driven suppression, b) clonal anergy and c) clonal deletion (Chen and Weiner, 1996). The relative role of these three mechanisms in oral tolerance is primarily determined by the dose of antigen fed. The regulatory events after the oral antigen administration in the GALT consists in the passage through the mucosa and processing by the GALT (including enterocytes) antigen and presentation in connection with class1 or class 2 molecules. Preferential presentation in association with class 1 antigen may lead to activation of specific $CD8^+$ T suppressor cells, and more rarely presentation in association with class 2 antigens will activate $CD4^+$ T cells and lead to memory induction (Chen and Weiner, 1996).

Therefore, oral tolerance may follow either of two pathways. A low dose of antigen results in the generation of antigen-regulatory cells, and their generation involves presentation of antigen by gut-associated presenting cells. Such presentation induces regulatory cells (Th3 cells) that secrete the suppressive cytokine TGF-β and Th2 (IL4/IL10) upon recognition of the antigen *in vivo*. These antigen specific regulatory cells migrate to lymphoid organs and suppress immune responses by inhibiting the generation of effector cells and to the target organ suppressing diseases by releasing antigen non-specific cytokines (bystander suppression). High doses of antigen induce unresponsiveness of Th1 function *via* clonal anergy and or clonal deletion.

Two major mechanisms of oral tolerance have been described extensively, tolerance due to mucosa-derived suppressor T cells and tolerance due to clonal anergy and clonal deletion. Both initially and in recent studies, it was shown that suppressor T-cells that mediate oral tolerance are mainly $CD8^+$ T cells, even though in certain studies $CD4^+$ but not $CD8^+$ T cells were required for the induction of oral tolerance, involving cell transfer techniques. The suppressor cell was shown to be an antigen specific cell and it was generally assumed that the antigen specificity characterised both the inductive phase and the effector phase of the T cell response. Recently, it has been shown that oral antigen-induced suppressor T cells are indeed antigen-specific but such specificity applies to their induction, not to their effector function. The latter is mediated by antigen non-specific suppressor factors. Proof that oral tolerance induces antigen-non-specific suppressor function comes from observations that oral antigen-induced suppressor cells manifest "bystander" suppression, i.e., suppression of responses induced to antigens that are totally unrelated to the fed antigen inducing the suppressor cells.

Another mechanism of oral tolerance is mediated by suppressor T cells related to $CD8^+$ suppressor T cells that bear γδ T-cell receptors. A number of studies have provided evidence that $CD8^+$ T cells are the main suppressor T cells in models of oral tolerance in which the end point is the lack of responsiveness to subsequent parenteral administration of antigen

(Chen and Weiner, 1996). These investigators have shown that the CD8+ T cells are nearly exclusively γδ T cells (Mc Ghee *et al.*, 1999) and other studies showed that oral tolerance can be transferred with γδ TCR-bearing T cells (Marquez *et al.*, 1999 b). The mechanism by which oral antigen induced suppressor- cells exert their antigen non-specific suppression is through the secretion of a suppressor cytokine such as TGF-β that is produced by Th3 cells and is a suppressor cytokine. Certain studies (Chen and Weiner, 1996) showed that the suppressor T cells induced by oral antigen and inhibiting experimental autoimmune encephalitis (EAE) were, in fact, T cells producing TGF-β and it could be demonstrated in the lesional tissue of EAE, indicating that the suppressor cells, once induced, migrate to other tissues.

Nonallergic food hypersensitivities and inflammatory bowel diseases (Crohn's disease and ulcerative colitis) could be considered as a product of defects in the process by which the body controls responses to environmental antigens, resulting in enhanced responses that lead to disease. Both diseases are due to failure of oral tolerance.

Studies in animal models of autoimmunity and in human disease states, seem to indicate that orally administered autoantigens may find a place in the treatment of human organ-specific autoimmune diseases. For instance, oral administration of myelin basic protein (MBP) suppresses acute experimental autoimmunencephalomyelitis (EAE), and chronic relapsing EAE can be suppressed after the onset of disease by oral administration of MBP or myelin. Moreover, oral tolerance is effective in suppressing other experimental autoimmune diseases such as arthritis, uveitis, diabetes mellitus and multiple sclerosis. Oral antigen administration coupled with procedures that minimise Th_1 responses and maximise Th2 responses would lead to optimal oral tolerance, at least the form of tolerance that depends on the induction of TGF-β producing suppressor T cells.

1. 7 Vaccines

1.7.1 Mucosal vaccines

The development of mucosal vaccines has been given less attention when compared to their parental counterparts, perhaps due to the lack of understanding concerning the relative efficacy of various immunisation routes (e.g., oral, rectal or nasal) in humans. As it was described at the beginning of this chapter, in the mucosal immune system major effector molecules, including antibodies, especially of the secretory immunoglobulin A (S-IgA) isotype, cytokines, chemokines and chemokine receptors, appear to function in synergy with innate factors as defensins (α and β). All these factors, as well as other which are less well characterised, are contained in external secretions and display antiviral, antibacterial and antiparasitic activities that may be further potentiated by antibodies or by cell-mediated immunity (CMI). Also very important to the mucosal immune system is its immunological unresponsiveness (tolerance) which is elicited by natural or deliberate mucosal exposure to antigen.

Since specific humoral defence is provided both by serum and by secretory antibodies predominantly of the IgA class which are transported by a receptor-mediated mechanism into external secretions, most vaccines are required to induce both systemic and mucosal responses. Therefore, the advantage of mucosal vaccine development is to induce both mucosal and systemic immune responses. Thus, the possibility of manipulating the mucosal immune system toward positive immunity or tolerance appears extremely attractive when considering strategies aimed at protecting the host from colonisation or invasion by microbial pathogens and also presenting and/or modulating the development of harmful systemic immunological reactions.

Since Jenner introduced vaccination over 200 years ago with the use of Vaccinia virus to prevent smallpox fewer than 50 vaccines have been approved for human use, and some of these are improved versions of earlier forms. All but four of the current vaccines, two of which (the oral rotavirus and the nasal live attenuated influenza virus) which are just now in phase III testing (influenza) or have completed testing (rotavirus), are administered parenterally and as such do not induce significant mucosal immunity. The present status is unfortunate since almost viral and bacterial pathogens for which vaccines are desirable, invade mucosal tissues where CMI and antibody-mediated immunity would be most effective.

One of the best studied viral vaccines is the polio vaccine. The introduction of inactivated (Salk) polio vaccine (IPV) in 1955 followed by the trivalent oral polio virus vaccine (OPV) in 1963, has resulted in the elimination of an endogenously transmitted paralytic disease caused by wild poliovirus. Experimental studies with OPV and IPV administered to children have shown that OPV elicits development of S-IgA antibody to poliovirus in the nasopharynx and intestine one to three weeks after immunisation that persists over a period of as long as five to six years. Immunisation with IP fails to induce a secretory antibody response in the nasopharynx or intestines.

In the respiratory syncitial virus (RSV) infection that causes a severe lower respiratory tract infection in early childhood, a combined immunisation with both enteric and intranasal routes may afford better antiviral immunity. In addition to live or inactivated vaccines, subunit vaccines prepared from fusion proteins are useful as well as immunostimulating complex (ISCOM) vaccine, made from fusion protein and nucleoprotein of human RSV, that induces circulating neutralising antibody when given by the mucosal intranasal route.

Moreover, in rotavirus infection, the oral administration of reassortant vaccines has been found to be effective in inducing antibody seroconversion in over 70% of vaccines.

When designing vaccines one has to remember the regulation of mucosal immunity. T cells are required whether it develops as inflammation, as tolerance or as help for specific S-IgA antibodies to protein-based vaccines, viral and bacterial pathogens, allergens or autoantigens. T cells include $CD4^+$ T helper cell subsets, $CD8^+$ suppressor/cytotoxic T lymphocytes and their subsets for induction of mucosal tolerance. B cell commitment ($\mu \rightarrow \alpha$ switching) and B-T interactions resulting in the induction of plasma cells producing polymeric IgA (pIgA) are of central importance to mucosal immunity. Cytokines and chemokines produced by $CD4^+$ and $CD8^+$ T cell subsets and by classical APCs (dendritic cells and B cells) as well as by nonclassical APCs (e.g., epithelial cells) contribute to all aspects of normal mucosal immunity, tolerance and inflammation in the immune response.

One of the major reasons to use the mucosal immune system in vaccine development is the realisation that more of 80% of current HIV infections occur through sexual transmission where mucosal immunity is of utmost importance (McGhee *et al.*, 1999).

1.7.2 Bacterial vaccines

Vaccines designed for treatment of salmonellosis, cholera, shigellosis, *Haemophillus influenzae* infections used as components of oral vaccines given to human volunteers as a protective measure against infections and the use of formalin-killed *Streptococcus mutans*, for oral immunisation of humans to induce enzyme neutralising antibodies in saliva and reduce *S. mutans* counts in dental plaque, are the most common bacterial vaccines used till now.

1.8 Immunomodulators

Immunomodulators are immunostimulant substances that provoke non-specific activation. Some of them, such as bacterial extracts, have been in use for a long time and it is known that ingestion of microbial antigens induces the appearance of secretory IgA in external secretion. However, the effectiveness of the oral or inhalator use of immunomodulators in humans is still the subject of discussion. Previously, it was described that bacterial immunomodulators administered during the protein deprivation period to suckling rats promotes cellular differentiation and maturation in GALT and a good repopulation of gut lamina propria with IgA B cells and $CD5^+$ T cells when rats were refed a 20% casein diet (Gonzalez Ariki *et al.*, 1993). Recently, another bacterial immunomodulator (RN-301) given by the oral route to suckling Wistar rats during the protein deprivation period improves the repopulation of bronchus-associated lymphoid tissue (BALT) with IgA^+ B and $CD5^+$ T cells (Marquez *et al.*, 1997, Marquez, 1999 a).

More detailed studies on the use of bacterial immunomodulators will be discussed in a following chapter.

The usefulness of the oral administration of thymomodulin (TmB: thymic peptide extract Bagó, Argentina) during the protein refeeding as a therapeutic agent has been studied (Roux. *et al.*, 1998).

Table 1.1. Number of cells from gut LP in 30 fields per section

	$\bar{X}$±SE				
	IgA B cells	T cells			
		CD5	CD4	TCRα/β	TCRγ/δ
Control	230.95±19.2	218.1±15.6	161.6±7.7	275.2±15.8	107.4±9.07
R21	94.5±13.2*	179±19.3*	131.6±4.2*	238.0±13.08*	184.0±12.9*
R21 TmB	266.4±20.8	262.4±8.8	163.2±14.3	121.5±5.18	115.9±24.6

* p<0.001

Table 1.1 describes the phenotype from gut LP cells that are significantly decreased in R21 (IgA B cells and CD5, CD4, TCRα/β and TCRγ/δ T cells, p<0,001) and returns to control values with TmB. CD8α/α, CD8α/β and CD25 T cells were not altered.

Table 1.2. Number of T cells from gut IE in 30 fields per section

	X±SE				
	CD5	CD25	CD8α/α	TCRα/β	TCRγ/δ
Control	17.6±0.9*	31.4±6.4	28.6±1.8	26.6±3.8	15.8±1.7
R21	17.4±1.0*	68.2±4.1*	61.8±5.5*	39.8±6.5*	24.2±1.96*
R21 TmB	29.6±2.8	39.4±1.3	36.4±2.4	16.6±1.1	16.9±2.19

* p< 0,001

In Table 1.2, the phenotype from gut IE lymphocytes that are altered in R21 (CD5, CD25, CD8α/α, TCRα/β and TCRγ/δ T cells, p< 0,001) and returns to control value when rats are orally fed with TmB is described. TmB breaks unresponsiveness to dextrin even though Table 1.3 shows that this reactivity to dextrin is better that in the R21 group but decreased with respect to the control. The positive DTH to another carbohydrate such as levan seen in the control as well as in R21 and R21-TmB indicates the specificity of the suppression to dextrin. The immunohistochemistry results seen in the intraepithelium are in agreement with flow cytometry analysis.

Table 1.3. DTH to dextrin. Increment in foot pad thickness (mm)

	X±ES	n
Control	0.7277±0.1649	(5)
R21	0.1068±0.0112*	(5)
R21- Tm B	0.35±0.07	(6)

* $p< 0.01$ (n)= number of rats

Recently, the triggering of γ/δ cells by mycobaterial antigens during the early and progressive stages of infection and an immune protection and control of inflammatory tissue necrosis by this population have been described. The above circumstance may explain their increase in the R21 group. The immunomodulator TmB is able to down-regulate not only the CD8α/α+, CD25$^+$ but also γ/δ+ T cells that have been early stimulated by TNF-α, perhaps by promoting the production of IL10 that is known to inhibit the inflammatory cytokine such as TNF-α (Lanh *et al.*, 1998). TmB may be acting in this way and our next goal is to study the production of these cytokines.

1.9 Summary

The mucosal immune system is unique in that it provides both positive and negative signals for the induction and regulation of immune responses in both mucosal and systemic compartments. The diverse compartments located in the gastrointestinal tracts, pulmonary and genitourinary tracts, and exocrine glands are connected in the mucosal immune system through intertissue communication such as the migration of lymphocytes *via* adhesion molecules that recognise integrins expressed on HEV cells. These properties distinguish the mucosal from the systemic immune system. Moreover, the induction of peripheral immune responses by parenteral antigen does not result in significant mucosal immunity, whereas mucosal immunisation, e.g. oral, nasal or possibly rectal administration of vaccine, can induce antigen-specific S-IgA and CTL responses in distant mucosa-associated tissues.

Mucosal administration of antigens may theoretically result in the concomitant expression of S-IgA antibody responses in various mucosal tissues and secretions, and under appropriate conditions, in the simultaneous down regulation of CMI reactivity at mucosal and systemic sites.

Acknowledgements

This research was supported by grants from CONICET PIP 4147.

References

Bienenstock, J. (1982) Gut and bronchus associated lymphoid tissue: An overview. *Ad. Exp. Med. Biol.* **149**, 471-477.

Bienenstock, J., Clancy, R (1994) Bronchial mucosal lymphoid tissue, in *Handbook of Mucosal Immunology,* (eds. P.L. Ogra, J. Mestecky, M.E. Lamm, W. Strober, J.R. McGhee., J. Bienenstock) Orlando Florida Academic Press, pp. 529-538.

Bienenstock, J., McDermott, M.R., Befus, D. and O'Neill, M. (1978) A Common mucosal immunologic system involving the bronchus, breast and bowel. *Adv. Exp. Med. Biol..* **107**, 53-58.

Brandtzaeg, Per. (1995 a) Basic Mechanisms of Mucosal Immunity, A mayor adaptive defence system. *The Immunologist* **3**, 89-96.

Brandtzaeg, Per. (1995 b) Mucosal Immunology , A long way to the surface. *The Immunologist* **3**, 75-77.

Cebra, J.J., Jiang, Hang-Ging, Sterzl, J., Tlaskalova-Hogenova, H. (1999) The role of mucosal microbiota in the development and maintenance of the mucosal immune system. In *Mucosal Immunology* (eds. P.L. Ogra,, J. Mestecky, M.E. Lamm,, W. Strober, J.R. McGhee, J. Bienenstock), Academic Press Orlando Florida, pp. 267-280.

Cebra, J.J., Shroff, E.S. (1994) Peyer's patches as inductive sites for commitment. In *Handbook of Mucosal Immunology,* (eds. P.L. Ogra, J. Mestecky, M.E. Lamm, W. Strober, J.R. McGhee, , J. Bienenstock). *A*cademic Press Orlando Florida, pp. 151-158.

Chen, Y. H., and Weiner, H. L (1996). Dose dependent activation and deletion of antigen-specific T cells following oral tolerance. In Oral tolerance: *Mechanisms and applications.* (eds. H.L. Wienel, L.F. Mayer,). N.Y. Acad. Sci. 778: 111-121.

Croitoru, K., Bienenstock, J. (1994) Characteristics and functions of mucosa associated lymphoid tissue. In *Handbook of Mucosal Immunology,* (eds. P.L. Ogra,, J. Mestecky, M.E. Lamm, W. Strober, J.R. McGhee, J. Bienenstock) Academic Press Orlando Florida, pp. 144-149.

Gonzalez Ariki, S., Florin-Christensen, A., Roux, M.E. (1993) Efecto del immunomodulador IM-104 sobre la poblacion linfocitaria de la mucosa intestinal de ratas immunodeficientes. *Immunologia,* **12**, 59-63.

Gowans, J.L. and Knight, E.J. (1964) The route of recirculation of lymphocytes in the rat *Proc. R. Soc. London B* **159**, 1427-1451.

Guy-Grand, D., Griscelli, C. And Vassalli, P. (1974) The gut associated lymphoid system: Nature and properties of the large dividing cells. *Eur. J. Immunol.* **4**, 435-443.

Kroese, H.G.M., Butcher, E.C., Stall, A.M., Lalor, P.A., Adams, S. and Herzemberg, L.A. (1989) Many of the IgA producing plasma cells in murine gut are derived from self-replenishing precursors in the peritoneal cavity. *Int. Immunol.* **1**, 75-84.

Lamm, M.E. (1976) Cellular aspects of immunoglobulin A, *Adv. Immunol.* **22**, 223-290.

Lanh, M., Kalataradi, H., Mittelstadt, P., Pnum, E., Vollner, M., Cady, C., Mukasa, A., Mukasa, A.T., Vella, A.T., Ikle, D., Harbeck, R., O'Brien, R. And Born, W. (1998) Early preferential stimulation of γ/δ T cells by TNF-α. *J. Immunol.* **160**, 5221-5230.

Lefrançois, L. (1994) Basic aspects of intraepithelial lymphocyte immunobiology. In *Handbook of Mucosal Immunology* (eds. P.L.Ogra, J. Mestecky, M.E. Lamm, W. Strober, J.R. McGhee, J. Bienenstock), Academic Press Orlando Florida, pp. 287-297.

Lefrançois, L., Puddington, L. (1999) Basic aspects of intraepithelial lymphocyte immunobiology In *Handbook of Mucosal Immunology*,(eds. P.L. Ogra, J. Mestecky, M.E. Lamm, W. Strober, J.R. McGhee, J. Bienenstock,) Academic Press Orlando Florida, pp. 413-428.

Lopez, M.C., Roux, M.E. (1989) Impaired differentiation of IgA-B cell precursors in the Peyer's patches of protein depleted rats. *Dev. Comp. Immunol.* **13**, 253-262.

Marquez, M.G. (1999 a) Common mucosal immune system: bronchial and intestinal mucosa. Subcompartmentalisation studies in a model of secondary immunodeficiency. Thesis, Faculty of Pharmacy and Biochemistry, University of Buenos Aires Argentina.

Marquez, M.G., Galeano, A., Roux, M.E. (1999 b) Functional studies of TCR$\gamma\delta$ and TCRα/β intestinal epithelial lymphocytes (iIEL) from immunoreactive rats. In *The Faseb Journal.*, Exp. Biol. 99, Washington vol. 13, April 17-2.

Marquez, M.G., Sosa, G.A., Slobodianik, N.H., Florin-Christensen, A., Roux, M.E. (1997) Effect of RN-301 immunomodulator on bronchus-associated lymphoid tissue (BALT) in protein depleted rats at weaning. *Medicina,* **57**, 428-432.

Mazenec, M.B., Nedrun, J.G., Kaetzel, Ch.S. and Lamm, M. (1993) A three-tiered view of IgA in mucosal defence. *Immunol. Today* **14**, 430-435.

McDermott, M.R. and Bienenstock, J. (1979) Evidence for a common mucosal immunologic system, I migration of B immunoblasts into intestinal, respiratory and genital tissues. *J. Immunol.* **!22**, 1892-1897.

McGhee, J.R., Czerkinsky, C., Mestecky (1999) Mucosal vaccines: An overview. In *Handbook of Mucosal Immunology* (eds. P.L. Ogra, J. Mestecky, M.E. Lamm, W. Strober, J.R. McGhee, J. Bienenstock), Academic Press Orlando Florida, pp. 413-428.

McGhee, J.R., Lamm, M.E., Strober, W. (1999) Mucosal Immune Responses: An overview. In *Handbook of Mucosal Immunology* (eds. P.L. Ogra, J. Mestecky, M.E. Lamm, W. Strober, J.R. McGhee, J. Bienenstock.) Academic Press Orlando Florida, pp. 485-506.

McWilliams, M., Phillips-Quagliata, J.M. and Lamm, M.E. (1977) Mesenteric lymph node B lymphoblasts which home to the small intestine are precommitted to IgA synthesis. *J. Exp. Med,* 866-875.

Mestecky, J., Abraham, R., Ogra, P.L. (1994) Common mucosal immune system and strategies for the development of vaccines effective at the mucosal surfaces. In *Handbook of Mucosal Immunology,* (eds. P.L. Ogra, J. Mestecky, M.E. Lamm, W. Strober, J.R. McGhee, J. Bienenstock) Academic Press Orlando Florida, pp. 357-372.

Mostov, K.E. (1994) Transepithelial transport of immunoglobulins. *Ann. Rev. Immunol.* **12**, 63-84.

Pabst, R. (1990) Compartmentalisation and kinetics of lymphoid cells in the lung. *Reg. Immunol.* **3**, 62-71.

Parmely, M.J. and Manning, L.S. (1983) Cellular determinants of mammary cell-mediated immunity in the rat: Kinetics of lymphocyte subset accumulation in the rat mammary gland during pregnancy and lactation. In *The Secretory Immune System*, (eds. J.R. McGhee and J. Mestecky) Ann. N.Y. Ac. Sc. 409, pp. 517-532.

Phillips-Quagliata, J.M. and Lamm, M.E. (1988) Migration of lymphocytes in the mucosal immune system. In *Migration and homecoming of lymphoid cells*, (ed. A.J. Husband), CRC Press Boca Raton Florida, **2**, 53-75.

Phillips-Quagliata, J.M., Roux, M.E., Arny, M., Kelly-Hatfield, P., McWilliams, M., Lamm, M.E. (1983) Migration and regulation of B cells in the mucosal immune system. In *The secretory Immune System*, (eds. J.R. McGhee, J. Mestecky) Ann. N.Y. Acad. Sci 409, pp. 194-202.

Quiding-Jarbrink, M., Eriksson, K., Lakew, M., Butcher, E., Bauchereau, J., Lazarovits, A., Holmgren, J., Czerkinsky, C. (1996) Generalised and compartmentalised mucosal immune responses in humans: Cellular and molecular aspects. *Essentials of Mucosal Immunology*, pp. 477-487.

Rott, L.S., Briskin, M.J., Andrew, D.P., Berg, E.L., Butcher, E.C.(1996) A fundamental subdivision of circulating lymphocytes defined by adhesion to mucosal addressin cell adhesion molecule-1. Comparison with vascular cell adhesion molecule-1 and correlation with β7 integrins and memory differentiation. *J. Immunol.* **156**, 3727-3736.

Roux, M.E., McWilliams, M., Phillips-Quagliata, J.M. and Lamm, M.E. (1981) Differentiation pathway of Peyer's patch precursors of IgA plasma cells in the secretory immune system.. *Cell. Immunol.* **161**, 141-153.

Roux, M.E., McWilliams, M., Phillips-Quagliata, J.M., Weisz-Carrington, P. and Lamm, M.E. (1977) Origin of IgA-secreting plasma cells in the mammary gland. *J. Exp. Med.* **146**, 1311-1322.

Roux, M.E.B., Marquez, G.A., Sosa, G. And Florin-Christensen, A. (1998) Intestinal mucosae T cells and delayed-type hypersensitivity (DTH) to dextrin in immunodeficient rats orally treated with thymomodulin (TmB). In *Proceedings International Congress of Immunology*, (eds. G.P. Talnar, I. Nalt, N.K.Ganguli, K.V.S. Rao) Monduzzi Editore Bologna (Italy), pp. 1461-1464.

Sminia, T., Van der Brugge-Gamelkoorn, G.J., Jeurissen, S.H.M. (1989) Structure and function of bronchus-associated lymphoid tissue (BALT). *Crit.Rev. Immunol.* **9**, 119-150.

Solvasson, N. and Kearny, J.F. (1992) The human fetal omentum: A site of B cell generation . *J. Exp. Med.* **175**, 397-404.

CHAPTER 2

Adjuvants for Mucosal Vaccines

J. Ronco and B. Guy

PART 2.I - General Features

2.I.1 Introduction

The term 'adjuvant' (Latin: adjuvare, to help), as was first defined by Ramon (1926), has been used in many ways in biology and medicine. Most commonly, adjuvants are immunostimulatory compounds or associations of compounds that potentiate or modulate the immune system against an antigen or vaccine beyond the level achieved by administration of the immunogen alone. These compounds with immunostimulatory properties will generally act in a non-specific manner on one or many of the steps of the immune system, resulting in an improvement of the specific immunity to an antigen.

Adjuvants have been extensively used in order to increase the immune response in experimental immunology, as well as in practical vaccination, for more than six decades. A series of simple but elegant experiments performed by Ramon (1925) showed that the antitoxin response to tetanus and diphtheria was increased when these vaccines were injected together with other compounds, such as metal salts, oil, tapioca, pyogenic bacteria or saponins. Those experiments indicated for the first time that components of a vaccine formulation other than the antigen itself are important for a successful biological response and started a search that is still ongoing for vaccine adjuvants.

Traditional vaccines currently available contain antigen preparations that are frequently impure and poorly characterised; however, these preparations are capable of eliciting protective immunity and have been proven to be safe. In some cases, such as with killed bacterial vaccines, the contaminants themselves may act as immuno-potentiating agents boosting the immune response against the vaccine, as adjuvants do; however these same contaminants may also be responsible for most of the side-effects induced by the vaccine (Munoz, 1964, Stewart, 1985, Griffith, 1989).

R. Fuller and G. Perdigon (eds.), Probiotics 3, 29–68.

Advances in DNA technology and biochemistry have led to the production of increasingly pure antigens allowing an induction of more specific immune responses, this progress culminating in the introduction of the first recombinant subunit vaccine based on the Hepatitis B surface antigen (HbsAg) in the 1980's (Valenzuela *et al.*, 1982; Michel *et al.*, 1984). Unfortunately, many of these highly purified protein preparations have also been shown to be relatively weak immunogens; nevertheless this major difficulty encountered during development of modern vaccines can be overcome by the use of adjuvants. Aluminum salts as hydroxides and phosphates are the only adjuvants widely approved for use in humans. These compounds, however, are not active with all immunogens and stimulate mainly humoral responses. Consequently the availability of a new generation of improved adjuvants is crucial for the development of new vaccines. Fortunately, the considerable progress in the fields of adjuvants, antigen formulations and delivery systems made in recent years should help to find ways to increase the immunogenicity of subunit vaccines, to modulate the balance between T-cell responses of Th1 and Th2 types, and to induce local immunity, opening new routes such as mucosal vaccine administration for prevention of infection.

The different fields within the domain of vaccinology are growing, and active immunisation is now being applied to distinct pathologies not only involving infectious agents. Cancer, autoimmune disorders, and other afflictions are also being attacked by different new approaches to vaccination, involving the concept of modulating the immune responses to specific antigens.

2.I.2 Adjuvants

2.I.2.1 What are adjuvants?

Adjuvants are a group of structurally heterogeneous comounds that have the property of overall adjuvanticity as the only functional characteristic in common. However, the ways in which they affect the immune system and their toxicity profiles are variable, and must probably depend on their individual chemical and biological properties. Indeed, the hyper-activation of the immune response by adjuvants may be accompanied by adverse reactions that implicate distinct mechanisms involving the immune system, or physiological parameters outside the immune system. For many years, research has been focused on finding adjuvants with the ability to potentiate the immune response but with minimal or no toxicity.

Table 2.I.1 lists examples of adjuvants undergoing development and testing for use with human vaccines. Vaccine adjuvants commonly used or considered for human or veterinary vaccines mainly include mineral salts, emulsions, compounds from bacterial cell walls, saponins and other synthetic products (Cox and Coulter, 1992, 1997; Stewart-Tull, 1994; Vogel and Powell, 1995). The use of cytokines, which can also act as modulators through the natural pathway of the immune response, may be also considered as promising compounds, especially for human vaccines.

2.1.2.2 Strategies for improving vaccines

Even though adjuvants, as described above, correspond to a group of compounds with immunomodulatory characteristics, the term “adjuvant effect” is frequently used to describe an improved action on the immune response (either by modulation or enhancement) elicited by a compound or a vaccine strategy. Therefore, adjuvants can be included as a topic in a list of the different strategies developed to enhance the immune response to weak immunogens. These strategies have been the subject of several reviews (Edelman, 1986; Bomford, 1990; Del Giudice, 1992; Gupta and Siber, 1995a) and are briefly described here. To improve immunity, an antigen can be administered: (a) together with an adjuvant, such as those listed in Table 1, which can, in itself, promote certain host defence mechanisms (as described later in this chapter); (b) in a delivery system such as biodegradable microparticles (Morris *et al.*, 1994) which have no intrinsic adjuvant activity; (c) by direct targeting to the immune system by fusion with a cytokine (Hazama *et al.*, 1993), a monoclonal antibody specific for class II MHC determinants (Carayanniotis and Barber, 1987) or with a complement fragment (Dempsey *et al.*, 1996); (d) as part of an attenuated, defective or non-replicating microbial vector such as vaccinia virus (Smith *et al.*, 1983) or Salmonella species (Bowen *et al.*, 1990).

Table 2.I.1. Vaccine adjuvants

Adjuvant	References
Minerals salts	Alum (aluminum hydroxide and phosphate) (Glenny et al., 1926; Gupta and Siber, 1994),
	Calcium phosphate (Relyveld, 1986; Gupta and Siber, 1994)
Synthetic	Polyphosphazene (Payne et al., 1995, 1998)
	Non-ionic block copolymers (Johnson, 1994; Hunter et al., 1991)
	Muramyl dipeptide analogues (Allison and Byars, 1991; Kahn et al., 1994; Azuma, 1992; Chedid et al. 1986, Audibert et al., 1985)
	Oligodinucleotides (ODN) (Moldoveanu et al., 1998)
Bacterial	E. coli heat labile toxin (LT) (Clements et al. 1988)
	Monophosphoryy lipid A (MPLA) (Baker et al., 1988; Johnson, 1994)
	Cholera toxin (CT) (Holmgren *et al.*, 1993)
Emulsion-based	Lipomes (Gregoriadis and Panagiotidi, 1989; Gregoriadis, 1990; Wassef et al., 1994; Shahum and Therien, 1995)
	MF59 (Valensi et al., 1994; Kahn et al., 1994; Ott et al., 1995a, 1995b)
	Syntex (SAF) (Allison and Byars, 1991)
	Freund's incomplete adjuvant (IFA) (Stuart-Harris, 1969; Putkonen et al., 1994)
	Montanide (Seppic) (Scalzo et al., 1995)
Others	Saponins (QS21) (Soltysik et al., 1995; Kensil, 1996; Newman et al., 1992)
	Immunostimulating complexes (ISCOMs) (Morein, 1988; Villacres-Eriksson, 1995; Barr and Mitchel, 1996)
	DC-Chol lipid 3α-[N-(N',N'-dimethylaminoethane) arbamoyl]cholesterol
	(Haensler et al., 1996; Brunel et al., 1999) interleukin-12 (Bliss et al., 1996)

2.1.2.3 Mode of action of adjuvants

- *Major mechanisms*

Some distinct mechanisms by which adjuvants can act are summarised as follows:

a)depot effect for slow release of antigen from the site of injection. This effect causes antigen to persist for a longer period at the site of injection or in the draining lymph nodes, improving its uptake by antigen-presenting cells (APCs);

b) effects on APCs by targeting the antigen to APCs (i.e. carbohydrate adjuvants can target lectin receptors on macrophages and dendritic cells), activation and/or recruitment of APCs and others lymphoid cells;
c) improvement of antigen presentation, for example by enabling B cells to be exposed to epitopes involved in pathogen neutralisation;
d) activation of complement;
e) stimulation of APCs expression of costimulatory molecules and prodution of immuno-regulatory substances such as cytokines (immunomodulating action that modifies the cytokine network);
f) facilitation of the phagolysosome entry pathway (MHC class II presentation) in APCs for $CD4^+$ T-lymphocyte mediated responses (T helper effector cells), enhancing antibody production;
g) delivery of antigen to the cytoplasmic pathway (MHC class I presentation) in APCs, favouring induction of $CD8^+$ cytotoxic T lymphocytes (CTL) .

For soluble antigens, at least two additional mechanisms can explain the immunopotentiating activity when aluminum salts and many other adjuvants (emulsions in general, liposomes, ISCOMs, etc.) are used.. By physical association, these adjuvants are able to transform partially or completely a soluble antigen into a particulate one (i.e. antigen adsorbed in the aluminum precipitate, or included in the oil microdroplets of emulsions), and as a result there is a shift from soluble antigen uptake by B cells to particulate uptake by macrophages or dendritic cells. We know that B cells internalise antigens via specific binding to their cell surface immunoglobulins (Abbas *et al.*, 1985) and can present soluble antigens in concentrations as low as 1 ng/ml (Malynn *et al.*, 1985). On the other hand, APCs like macrophages and dendritic cells internalise antigens by non-specific phagocytosis and pinocytosis (Unanue, 1985), and present these as peptides in association with major histocompatibility complex (MHC) class II molecules to T cells. Consequently we can conclude that particulate forms of antigens, which may be employed herein, effectively mediate the complete accessory cell activation of naive T cells, while a soluble form of antigen best mediates B cell interaction with helper T cells (Paul and Seder, 1994).

We can conclude that adjuvants influence the immune response in one or more ways by the above mechanisms, and, consequently, adjuvanticity can be defined as follows: "adjuvanticity is the resultant of the addition of several modes of action, shared more or less by most of adjuvants. However, the proportion and the contribution of each of these mechanisms on the whole adjuvanticity are particular to each adjuvant".

Through the distinct mechanisms mentioned above, major benefits that can be expected by the use of vaccine adjuvants should be: a) enhancement of the speed (kinetics), strength, and persistence (long lasting immunity) of the immune response to a given immunogen, and b) modulation of the humoral or the cell-mediated immunity, or both.

2.I.3 Development of new adjuvants

2.I.3.1 Introduction

To date our knowledge about the events involved in the generation of protective immunity, and the ways that adjuvants can modulate or influence so many parameters of the immune response is not sufficient to allow us to be capable of tailoring adjuvants to the requirements of a particular vaccine. Indeed, most of research on vaccine adjuvants has been empirical, in that, an antigen preparation was given with and without an adjuvant and the specific immune responses were compared by assessing humoral and/or cellular mediated immunity. Selection was then based on the balance between toxicity and adjuvanticity in an animal model. The advent of improved biochemical techniques has allowed the purification or construction of new and well characterised adjuvants, but these have been generally based upon the older empirical experiments. As our knowledge of the cell types and cytokines interacting in the immune responses increases, so does our understanding of the mode of action of adjuvants, as well as the way in which they produce side-effects. Nevertheless, it has now become possible to address many of the factors that must be considered in the rational design of new adjuvants for use in vaccines (and the side-effects to be avoided). Moreover, a clear understanding of the latter may facilitate regulatory approval and all these points taken together have rejuvenated adjuvant research so that it is once again at the forefront of biomedical sciences.

2.I.3.2 Criteria

It is most likely that there is no such thing as an "universal" adjuvant since the immunity elicited by adjuvanted vaccines is modulated strongly by many different factors, such as the nature and dose of the immunogens, the nature of the adjuvant, the final vaccine formulation and its stability, the immunisation schedule, the route of administration, and the animal species. Nevertheless, the following general characteristics should be considered for the development of new adjuvanted vaccines:

(I) The adjuvant should be produced or be made available according to GMP (Good Manufacturing Practices), and defined chemically and biologically, allowing for stability and lot-to-lot variation studies in the manufactured product, thereby assuring safety and consistent responses in vaccinees over time.

(II) The adjuvant combined with immunogens should elicit a stronger protective immunity than the same immunogens without adjuvant.

(III) The safety of the adjuvant must be assured, including immediate and long-term studies of side effects.

(IV) The adjuvant should be intrinsically non-immunogenic, biodegradable and biocompatible.

2.1.3.3 State of the art

Adjuvants are often effective with some antigens and not with others. For example, aluminum compounds work successfully for vaccines against diphtheria (Aprile and Wardlaw, 1966), polio (Drescher et al., 1967), rabies (Wiktor et al., 1978), and hepatitis B (Scolnick et al., 1984), but fail to augment the response to vaccines against whooping cough (Butler et al., 1962), typhoid fever (Cvjetanovic and Uemura, 1965), trachoma (Woolridge et al., 1967), adenovirus hexon antigens (Kasel et al., 1971), influenza haemagglutinin (Davenport et al., 1968), and Haemophilus influenzae type b (Hib) capsular polysaccharide conjugated to tetanus toxoid (Claesson et al., 1988).

It is not always possible to predict compatible and incompatible adjuvant-vaccine combinations before the late stages of preclinical or early clinical development. The predictability concerning adjuvantation in human is especially difficult because, very often, there are no reliable animal models. For this reason, when the selected adjuvant reaches the development stage, it is recommended that at least two strains of mice are utilised (inbred and outbred strains), and other species such as rabbits or monkeys included in further immunogenicity studies. These additional experiments will allow us not only to better predict adjuvanticity in humans but also to calculate the adjuvant dose and frequency of immunisation for use in clinical trials. Furthermore, vaccine alone, adjuvant, and vaccine adjuvant combinations should be studied for toxicity and immunogenicity, and their concentrations should mimic and exceed the calculated human doses (Gupta and Siber, 1995[a]; Goldenthal *et al.*, 1993).

Although preclinical studies should be done with the antigen that will be used in clinical studies (Gupta and Siber, 1995[a]; Goldenthal *et al.*, 1993), the use of antigen models for adjuvant screening may be helpful to carry out comparative experiments among distinct adjuvant formulations. This may help to study their mechanisms of action and capability to induce protection in well-known animal models.

Aluminum hydroxide can be used as a reference for the evaluation of new adjuvants for human vaccines. Therefore, it is important that aluminum adjuvants be used optimally to allow correct evaluation of the experimental adjuvant (Edelman and Tacket, 1990; Gupta and Siber, 1995a, 1995b). Thus, during the adsorption of antigens on aluminum adjuvants, attention must be paid to the chemical and physical characteristics of the antigen, type of aluminum salt, conditions of adsorption, and concentration of adjuvant (Gupta and Siber, 1995a, 1995b).

2.1.3.4 Safety

The most important feature of any adjuvanted vaccine is that it is more efficacious than the non-adjuvanted vaccine and that this benefit outweighs its risk. During the past, several vaccines adjuvanted with mineral salts have been developed, and their immediate and delayed toxicity has been evaluated. Today, the potential use of some new strong adjuvants revealed in animal models, some of them being real immunomodulatory drugs, makes it necessary to review and update the traditional toxicological studies carried out in the field of vaccinology. In fact, some of these immunomodulory compounds should not be considered as vaccine excipients but instead as pharmacologically active drugs.

The current attitude regarding risk-benefits of vaccination favours safety over efficacy when a vaccine is given to the healthy population. In high-risk groups, including, for example, patients with cancer or acquired immunodeficiency syndrome (AIDS), and for some therapeutic vaccines, an additional level of toxicity may be acceptable if the benefit of the vaccine is substantial. Unfortunately, the absolute safety of adjuvanted vaccines, or any vaccine, cannot be guaranteed, so we must minimize the risks. The real and potential risks of administering vaccine adjuvants have been discussed in detail (Edelman and Tacket., 1990; Goldenthal *et al.*, 1993; Bussiere *et al.*, 1995).

Safety of new adjuvants is a major concern. In particular, one has to look for those rare reactions that may only occur once in several thousand doses, and thus may not be detected until late in the development program. At present, no specific guidelines exist for assessing the safety of adjuvant preparations for use in humans. The only guidelines issued by health authorities refer to tests on the final container lot of all biological products, which includes adjuvanted vaccines. These standard tests include: potency (by in vitro or in vivo tests), general safety (in two different animal species), sterility, purity (including a pyrogenicity assay in rabbits), and identity. In addition, for each vaccine, the adjuvant is tested for safety on a case-by-case basis, often with the help and guidance of the health authorities.

Therefore, even though separate and extensive preclinical toxicity studies have been performed on both the adjuvant and the final vaccine formulation, the preliminary safety evaluation of the human candidate formulation may only be first conducted in a Phase I clinical trial. It arises from what was dicussed above that decades of expensive and time-consuming follow-up are required to identify potential low-incidence reactions, and, at present, proceedings for the systematic, active follow-up of vaccinees given experimental adjuvants is not available.

2.I.4 Adjuvants for human use

The number of clinical trials using adjuvants has increased dramatically in recent years, even though the knowledge related to their mechanisms of action remains limited. The empirical approach that has guided the development of early vaccines, still plays a key role in the development of the « new technology adjuvanted vaccines » (Leclerc and Ronco, 1998). Adjuvanticity is usually judged in terms of levels, duration and localisation of the antibody responses. Nevertheless, some adjuvants display the ability to fine-tune cellular immune responses upon vaccination, including CTLs, a key driver of modern vaccine strategies.

The number of vaccine adjuvants tested in animals is too large to be reviewed in this chapter. Instead, a smaller number of novel adjuvants or adjuvant formulations used to enhance a variety of experimental vaccines in humans are considered in Table 2.I.2 and some of the more encouraging ones described below.

In many instances, several adjuvants have been combined in one adjuvant formulation in the hope of obtaining a synergistic or additive effect. The majority of these adjuvants are being developed and tested by the pharmaceutical industry.

Table 2.I.2. Clinical trials with new adjuvants

Trial adjuvant		References
MF-59		HIV (Kahn et al., 1994), Flu (Ott et al., 1995a, 1995b; Martin, 1997), Herpes (Ott et al., 1995; Straus et al., 1997)
SAF (Syntex)		HIV (McElrath, 1994)
QS21		HIV (McElrath, 1994; Keefer et al., 1997), Flu (Van Hoecke et al., 1995; Bouveret Le Cam et al., 1998), Cancer (Livingston et al., 1994)
MDP (Murabutide)		Tetanus toxoid (Telzak et al., 1986), S. pyogenes (Olberling et al., 1983), Leishmania (Monjour et al., 1986)
Nor-MDP		Cancer (Triozzi et al., 1993)
MTP-PE		Flu (Glück et al., 1994)
Polyphosphazene (PCPP)		Flu (Bouveret Le Cam et al., 1998)
Liposomes		Flu (Powers et al., 1995)
Virosomes		Flu (Glück et al., 1994)
Montanide		HIV (Trauger et al., 1994; Turner et al., 1992)
Montanide ISA 720		Malaria (Lawrence et al., 1997)
IFA		Flu (Stuart-Harris, 1969; Beebe et al., 1972), Polio (Salk and Salk, 1977)
Cytokines	IL-12	HIV (Jacobson et al., 1996), Cancer (Del Vecchio and Bajetta, 1997)
	IFN-γ	HBV (Quiroga et al., 1990; Patou et al., 1989), Malaria (Stürchler et al., 1989)
	IFN-α	Malaria (Stürchler et al., 1989, 1990), HBV (Grob et al., 1984)
	IL-2	HBV (Meuer et al., 1989; Jungers et al., 1994)
	GM-CSF	HBV (Lin et al., 1995
Adjuvant combinations		
QS21+MPLA+O/Wemulsion		Malaria (Stoute et al. 1997)
MPL®+Aluminum		HBV (Leroux-Roels et al., 1993, 1994; Koutsoukos et al., 1994; Thoelen et al., 1998), Malaria (Gordon et al., 1995)
MF59+MTP-PE		HIV (Kahn et al., 1994; Keefer et al., 1996)
Liposome+ MPL®+Aluminum		Malaria (Fries et al., 1992), HIV (McElrath, 1994),
DETOXTM		Malaria (Hoffman et al., 1994; Rickman et al., 1991 Cancer (MacLean et al., 1992; 1993; Mitchell et al., 1988, 1990; Elliott et al., 1993; Schultz et al., 1995)

PART 2.II - Mucosal Immunity/Adjuvants and Techniques

2.II.1 Introduction

In general, mucosal immunisation can be used to reach two different goals : the induction of a mucosal response against a mucosal pathogen (or a pathogen penetrating through mucosae), and/or the induction through mucosal route of a systemic response against a non-mucosal pathogen. The latter objective would be to replace injectable vaccines by needle-free ones while the former objective would be to target mucosal pathogens more specifically. The use of a mucosal route is considered to be required in that case; however, targeting systemic immunisation may also work, and we will discuss this point. One may also aim to induce both systemic local and immune responses, and actually the means used in mucosal immunisation (adjuvants/formulation) are usually able to do so. However, some adjuvants and/or formulations may orientate the response towards being predominantly or even only mucosal, while other adjuvants will enhance simultaneously both mucosal and systemic responses. The definition of an adjuvant, and the distinction between immunostimulatory and antigen-delivery capacities has already been addressed. These terms and concepts also apply to the field of mucosal immunisation.

Immunising through mucosae often requires specific formulations and adjuvants, of which the choice and development is guided by the knowledge acquired on the structure and the role of the mucosa-associated lymphoid tissue (MALT), which is described in other chapters of this book. Various reviews have addressed in details the different characteristics of the mucosal immune system and their implications in vaccine development (Walker, 1994; Staats *et al.*, 1994; Gupta *et al.*, 1993). The present review will focus on two aspects : adjuvants/formulations used in mucosal immunisation, and techniques used to measure at the mucosal level immune responses induced by a pathogen or by immunisation.

Briefly, the gastrointestinal immune system and the related mucosae (nasal, rectal) present some specific features. From place to place along the mucosal epithelium are found some specialized structures – the most characteristic being the intestinal Peyer's patches – which are responsible for the uptake of pathogens and/or antigens, and subsequent initiation of the immune response (Brandtzaeg *et al.*, 1989). Some cells are specialised in the uptake of pathogens and antigen, called M cells in the intestinal Peyer's patches, and M-like cells are also found in other mucosal lymphoid structures, such as the nasopharyngeal tonsils for instance (Kuper *et al.*, 1992; Hopkins *et al.*, 1998; Lemoine *et al.*, 1998).

In theory, an optimal formulation should be able to target these M cells and inductive sites in order to initiate an optimal mucosal response. For instance, M cells preferentially handle particulate antigens, therefore particulate formulations could be used to target these cells (Jones et al., 1995; Giannasca et al., 1994). However, the epithelium itself plays a role in the induction of mucosal – and systemic – immune responses and other formulations/adjuvants able to target and eventually penetrate and cross epithelial cells would also do the job. We can try to summarize this in Fig. 2.II.1. An adjuvant/formulation should ideally have at least two properties, the first one being to target and bind M cells and/or epithelial cells. However, targeting and binding these cells are not sufficient to induce the desired immune response, and may even result in the induction of tolerance if the appropriate signals are not delivered at the same time (Waldo *et al.*, 1994). Therefore the second property of a mucosal adjuvant/formulation should be to activate the immune system in the desired direction to obtain a mucosal/systemic response. We can then arbitrarily divide adjuvants in different categories. The first category would comprise adjuvants just mixed with antigen that would in turn benefit from a bystander effect due to the activation of the immune system at the very time when it is delivered. These adjuvants could be toxins (the cholera toxin is the prototype), cytokines, or non proteic compounds. The second category comprises adjuvants/formulations that would specifically target the antigen towards inductive sites. In this case, antigen can be within and/or presented on the surface of such formulations. Liposomes and microspheres are the most representative of this second group; however, these formulations often require the addition of an immunostimulant in order to properly activate the immune sytem. Finally, antigen can be expressed by live vectors (bacteria or viruses) (see chapter) that naturally target the mucosae, and these vectors would constitute a third group; this aspect will not be developed extensively here, although we will mention the more representative vectors used in the research area. An alternative approach would be to use systemic immunisation – and systemic adjuvants – to induce immune responses in the mucosae, and we will also address this point.

In the third part of this chapter, we will describe the techniques used to measure the immune responses in the secretions or in the mucosae themselves.

Before addressing all these points, it is important to point out that most studies published in this field have been done in laboratory animals, mice in particular. We have to stress that important differences exist in the mucosal immune systems, between mice and human beings in particular, and that many promising adjuvants and formulations selected in animals go on to fail in clinical trials. For instance, particular attention has to be paid when analysing results obtained by nasal route in mice, regarding the volume administered and the use of anaesthetised or unanaesthetised animals. A large volume (> 5 -10 μl) administered in anaesthetised mice will reach the lungs where a very strong response will be induced. This is clearly different from what will be called « nasal immunisation » in man. In addition the dose/weight ratio has to be considered when one tries to extrapolate animal experiments to the human situation. We have to keep this in mind, and human studies will be mentionned as often as possible in this review.

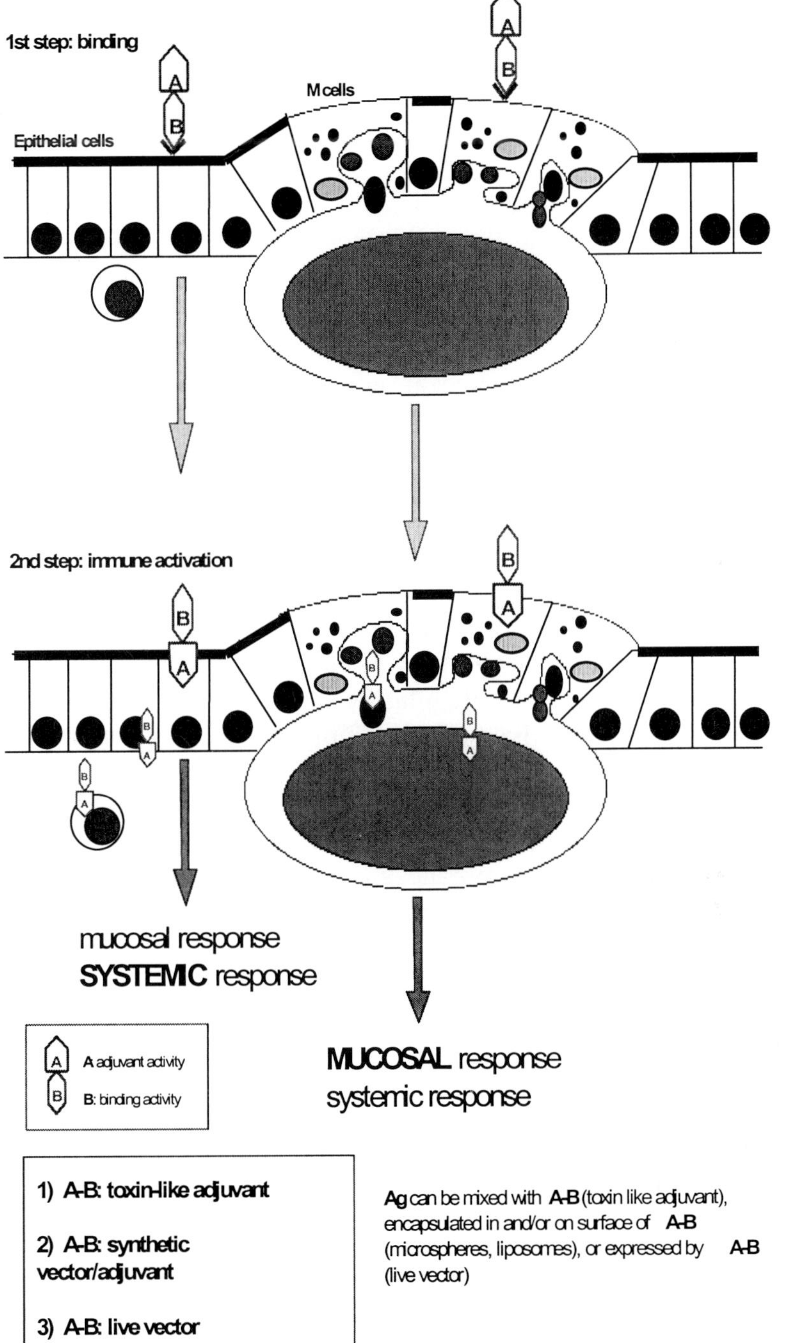

Figure 2.II.1. Properties required for mucosal adjuvantation

2.II.2 Adjuvants

2.II.2.1 Soluble adjuvants mixed with antigens

2.II.2.1.1 Toxins

- *Cholera Toxin*

Cholera toxin (CT, from Vibrio cholerae) is the prototype « gold standard » mucosal adjuvant, and so far the most widely used and studied, along with the related heat labile toxin from E. coli (LT). These two toxins are very potent mucosal adjuvants and have been tested in combination with a large number of antigens in different animal species. CT (and LT) are composed of two subunits : a monomeric, enzymatically active A subunit (CTA) and a pentameric, non-toxic, B subunit (CTB) that binds GM1 ganglioside at the surface of eukaryotic cells (Elson et al., 1989). As proposed in Fig. 2.II.1 in the introduction, an adjuvant should bind to cells and activate the immune system. CT and LT almost perfectly fulfill these two criteria : CTB first binds to the widely expressed GM1 ganglioside, and, in a second step, CTA activates the cell by catalysing the ADP ribosylation of the regulatory protein Gsα of adenylate cyclase, which in turn increases the synthesis of the intracellular second messenger 3', 5' cyclic AMP (cAMP) (Lycke and Strober, 1989). An important signalling reaction occuring in CT-treated eukaryotic cells is an increased synthesis of prostaglandins, which results from CT-mediated release of arachidonic acid from membrane phospholipids (Peterson *et al.*, 1996). From an immunological point of view, feeding animals with antigen and CT results in the break of oral tolerance and the induction of a strong immune response (with a long-lasting memory) towards CT itself and the co-administered antigen (Elson *et al.*, 1984). The immune response induced in the presence of CT by the mucosal route is mostly of the Th2 type, resulting in particular in the synthesis of local sIgA, but also in high circulating antibody titres (mainly IgG1 in mice, representative of the Th2 type) (Xu Amano *et al.*, 1994). The adjuvant effect is most likely linked to the activity of CTA, although some studies have demonstrated an adjuvant effect of CTB itself, and we will discuss this point below.

Different authors have looked more precisely at the consequences of cell activation induced by CT : the observed effects include synthesis of pro-inflammatory cytokines IL-1 and IL-6 (Mc Gee *et al.*, 1993), B cell isotype differentiation (Lycke and Strober, 1989), alteration of T cell function (Elson *et al.*, 1995), and upregulation of costimulatory molecule B7-2 (Cong *et al.*, 1997). However, the magnitude of the adjuvant effect depends on the genetic background of the animal and is controlled by different genes, including H-2 and lps genes (Elson and Ealding, 1987).

The major problem linked to CT is its high toxicity in man, while this is not the case in mice. Therefore different authors have investigated if CTB alone could have an adjuvant effect. Although some initial studies carried out with purified CTB demonstrated some adjuvant effect, this was linked to minute amounts of residual CTA. Using recombinant CTB (rCTB), different authors were not able to find any adjuvant effect, at least when administered by the oral route (Blanchard *et al.*, 1998). However, several studies did show an adjuvant effect of rCTB when using nasal route (De Gens *et al.*, 1997). Other authors intentionally mixed small amounts of CTA with CTB and found that the doses of CTA required for adjuvantation were dramatically reduced, which would enable a potential use in humans (Tamura *et al.*, 1994). Alternatively, the use of CTB as a carrier has been investigated by some authors, and this will be discussed below. Nevertheless, CTB by itself is a very potent immunogen and has indeed been included in vaccine formulations against cholera in human trials, inducing significant immune responses (Begue *et al.*, 1995).

Another way to use CT in humans more safely is to genetically construct non-toxic mutants retaining some adjuvanticity. Several mutants have been constructed by different groups, targeting different sites of the molecule. Although it seems that some ADP-ribosylating activity should be maintained, some mutants completely devoid of such activity in vitro were still active as adjuvant, although still only by the nasal route (Yamamoto *et al.*, 1998).

Recently, the construction and use of a CTA-protein A fusion as an adjuvant was reported to exhibit the same adjuvanticity as CT, without any toxicity. This chimeric adjuvant targets B cells and potentially other APCs in which ADP ribosylation and subsequent activation takes place. It seems to work both mucosally or parenterally but it is unclear why the formulation reaches preferentially mucosal inductive sites where APCs are located (Agren *et al.*, 1995).

- *E. coli heat labile toxin (LT)*

Most of the characteristics of CT, including toxicity in man, are shared by its counterpart from E. coli, LT (Clements *et al.*, 1988; Walker and Clements, 1993). However, one potentially important difference is the report that they induce different Th profiles. While CT induces a Th2 biased response by mucosal route, it seems that LT induces a more balanced Th1/Th2 response (Takahashi *et al.*, 1996); this would be important if one aims to induce one or the other type of immune response against one defined pathogen. Despite its toxicity, LT has been used in human clinical trials, with modest adjuvant effect by oral route (Baquar *et al.*, 1995). Less-toxic or non-toxic mutants of LT have also been constructed by different groups, which appear active when given by oral, nasal or intravaginal routes in mice (Douce *et al.*, 1995; Chong *et al.*, 1998; De Magistris *et al.*, 1998). However, adjuvanticity of these mutants is still to be confirmed in humans, in particular by oral route.

- *Other toxins*

Other toxins have been tested for their adjuvant effect, including the ADP-ribosylating toxin from B. pertussis (PTX). Similar to CT and LT, mutants of this toxin have been constructed, one of them -PT 9K/129G– still acting as a potent adjuvant when co-administered by nasal route in mice (Roberts *et al.*, 1995).

2.II.2.1.2 Lipoproteins

It had been observed that the adjuvanticity of CT was linked to its very high immunogenicity and its ability to induce proinflammatory cytokines. It was tempting to investigate if other proteins presenting the same properties were able to similarly adjuvant co-administered proteins. The outer membrane lipidated protein from Borrelia burdogferi (OspA) had been demonstrated to induce pro-inflammatory cytokines, and in our laboratory we have observed that it was a potent mucosal immunogen. We also showed that it was –by nasal route in mice – as potent as CT as a mucosal ADJUVANT with different co-administered antigens (Erdile and Guy, 1997). The same strategy could be applied to a number of potent mucosal immunogens. However, in the case of OspA for instance, it is unclear if a real targeting of mucosal inductive sites is achieved; adjuvanticity rather resulting from a broad local immune activation.

2.II.2.1.3 Cytokines

Apart from toxins, other biologically active proteins could act as adjuvants, and in the first place cytokines themselves. Actually, several authors have explored this approach to enhance and/or modulate the efficacy of mucosal immunisation (Rollwagen *et al.*, 1996). Indeed, mucosal inductive sites generally present a Th2 biased environment which may be required according to the considered pathogen to reorientate the immune response. IL-12 or IFN-γ cytokines have been successfully used by the oral route to shift the Th2 response towards a more balanced Th1/Th2 profile, as measured by cytokine levels and antibody isotypes (IgG2a/IgG1 balance in mice) (Marinaro *et al.*, 1997). In addition, it seems that the sIgA local response is not affected by such an administration of rIL-12. However, in contrast, according to a different study, nasal administration of the same cytokine did suppress IgA responses (Arulanandam *et al.*, 1998). Other authors have used vectors, such as herpes simplex virus, to express cytokines such as IL-4 or IFN-γ and observed results are consistent with their respected and expected biological activities (Kuklin *et al.*, 1998).

Finally, plasmids encoding cytokines such as IL-12 or GM-CSF have been administered by the nasal route in mice to enhance the immune response to DNA vaccines encoding HIV proteins (Okada *et al.*, 1997). All these different works illustrate the potential of cytokines to modulate mucosal responses, as previously observed for systemic responses.

2.II.2.1.4 Non proteic adjuvants

Beside proteic mucosal adjuvants, non proteic formulations can be mixed with antigens in order to increase their immunogenicity. They can include polysaccharidic compounds such as Chitosan (Jabbal-Gill *et al.*, 1998), lipophilic preparations having mucoadhesive properties (Gizurarson *et al.*, 1995), lipopeptides such as MAP-P3C (Nardelli *et al.*, 1994), saponins (Estrada *et al.*, 1998), or even the widely used alum (Isaka *et al.*, 1998). Most of these adjuvants have been tested by nasal route in mice, as oral immunisation was in most cases unsuccessful, probably due to large dilution or antigen degradation. These adjuvants most likely do not selectively target mucosal inductive sites, and dilution of both adjuvant and antigen is clearly a limiting factor which has to be taken in consideration in humans, even when the nasal route is used.

Nevertheless, Chitosan enhances immune reponses against PTX by the nasal route in mice (Jabbal Gill *et al.*, 1998), while saponins (QS21) potentiate the response not only against co-administered antigens (ovalbumin or CT), but also against proteins expressed by co-administered plasmids, such as plamids encoding HIV antigens (Sasaki *et al.*, 1998). It is interesting to notice that aluminum hydroxide, which is so far almost the only accepted adjuvant for human use, is also able to act as a mucosal adjuvant by the nasal route in mice (Isaka *et al.*, 1998).

Finally, in the growing area of CpG oligonucleotides used as adjuvants, and besides their use in parenteral immunisation, recent reports demonstrate some adjuvanticity of these compounds, again when given by the nasal route in mice (Mc Cluskie *et al.*, 1998; Moldoveanu *et al.*, 1998).

This further illustrates that a potentially large number of systemic adjuvants tested so far may also work by the nasal route. Actually, nasal immunisation not only enables antigens to be presented at a mucosal surface (where they may induce a local response), but also the antigen (and the adjuvant) may reach the circulatory system via the extensive submucosal blood supply in the nasal cavity and stimulate a systemic response too. This is probably the reason why the use of the nasal route in mice is so popular when one aims to demonstrate a mucosal adjuvanticity for any given compound, although, unfortunately, efficacy is not always achieved when the same experiment is performed in humans.

2.II.3 Particulate adjuvants/vectors/carriers

2.II.3.1 Liposomes

In order to protect and target antigen in the case of mucosal immunisation, in theory, particulate formulations such as liposomes constitute a promising vehicle. These structures are commonly made of phospholipids constituting cell membranes and can be filled or coated with a large variety of antigens. The composition and the size of liposomes may be adapted to specific needs, may include lipids having an adjuvant effect by themselves, or may alternatively co-encapsulate antigens with selected adjuvants. Depending on their composition, liposomes are usually non-toxic and protect their loads from being diluted or degraded in biological fluids,– but may not resist biliary salts for instance. Liposomes have been widely used to encapsulate drugs, and their potential for vaccination by the systemic or mucosal routes has also been extensively investigated.

One of their major potential targets is antigen presenting cells (APCs), but they may also target M cells in the mucosae, due to their particulate structure. However, liposomes themselves may be extensively diluted in the digestive tract, and most likely no real targeting occurs after oral administration. Once again the nasal route appears more promising (De Haan *et al.*, 1994), but such formulations have also been given by other routes in mice with some success (Zhou *et al.*, 1995).

As mentioned above, the nature of the lipid that can be used to prepare the liposomes is fairly flexible; it can be neutral, negatively or positively charged. The lipids used may also act in some cases as adjuvants. In our research department, we have had good results with cationic liposomes made of DC Chol in inducing systemic and mucosal responses against mixed flu antigens administered by nasal route in non-anaesthetised mice; using equivalent doses, the nasal route in mice induced systemic responses comparable to those induced by systemic route, as well as a much better mucosal response. Interestingly, some authors have observed that neutral liposomes may act not only as carriers, but also as immunostimulants, as administration of empty liposomes (negatively charged) 48 hours prior antigen administration also enhanced the immune response (De Haan *et al.*, 1994). Good responses were also obtained when immunising with liposomes in the lower respiratory tract (De Haan *et al.*, 1995). Theses responses were not restricted to the respiratory tract, but were also induced in distant mucosae such as the uro-genital tract. However, as we pointed out in the introduction, immunisation in the lungs is not likely to be routinely applied in the field.

Liposomes acting as carriers may also be simply mixed with adjuvants, as has been done with CT administered by the rectal route (Zhou *et al.*, 1995). An interesting point from this study is the potential use of IgA-coated liposomes that would enhance the uptake of the liposomes by M cells.

Other modified liposomes have been used, some of them been tested in clinical trials, such as Virosomes TM which carry the two glycoproteins of influenza virus on their surface (Mengiardi *et al.*, 1995). Clinical trials have been conducted with these carriers administered by parenteral route, but also by nasal route with the flu antigens, that have now reached phase II. Significant increases of pre-existing titres were observed, but it is unclear if results were really different from those observed in other studies with non-formulated antigens.

Although administration of vaccines by the oral route in humans is difficult, liposomes have been used with some success when encapsulating Streptococcus mutans carbohydrates, at least for inducing local immune responses (Childers *et al.*, 1991).

One potential and major limitation of the use of liposomes is the scale-up of such vectors in conditions allowing human immunisation, and this will also apply to microspheres; if non-sterilisable or non-filtrable, these compounds would have to be prepared under sterile conditions during the whole process. However, small liposomes may be filtrable and further progresses is likely to be achieved in that respect in the coming years.

2.II.3.2 Microspheres

Beside liposomes, microspheres constitute another type of particulate carrier that has been undergoing tests for a long time, for both parenteral and mucosal administration. Indeed, the concept of antigen encapsulation in biodegradable microspheres for immunising animals or humans has been considered very early on as an attractive delivery system (for a review see Eldridge *et al.*, 1991). Encapsulated antigen is protected from degradation, and depending on the microsphere composition, antigen release can be controlled over time. In addition, the size and hydrophilicity/hydrophobicity ratio of microspheres can be adapted to the route of immunisation. For instance, uptake by M cells appears to depend on both hydrophobicity and size (micron range), but varies with different animal species. Oral immunisation with flu antigens encapsulated in microspheres gave promising results in mice (Moldoveanu *et al.*, 1993), but this has not been confirmed in humans. Once again, the use of the nasal route avoids too a large a dilution and induces both systemic and mucosal immunity. This may constitute a more viable alternative, and has been demonstrated as an efficient way to enhance immune responses.

However, several limitations are linked to the use of microspheres. Some are the same as those encountered with liposomes used by mucosal routes (inter-species differences, no real targeting of inductive sites, large dilution in mucosal fluids, potential problems of scaling-up), and some are specific to the preparation of microspheres. For instance, in most cases, the use of organic solvents is required, which may be a critical limitation for some antigens if appropriate conformation and folding are absolutely required. However, as for liposomes, significant progresses are likely to be made in the future to make these vectors suitable for human use.

2.II.3.3 Other particulate carriers

Apart from liposomes and microspheres, many different carriers have been tested for mucosal immunisation. The goals are usually the same when using such compounds : allowing delivery of antigens in a particulate form, together with an adjuvant, and if possible in a vehicle protecting antigen from degradation in the mucosal fluids.

We can mention ISCOMS, for which strong adjuvanticity had already been observed in parenteral immunisation, and that appear to constitute an appropriate delivery system for mucosal immunisation by the nasal route (Morein *et al.*, 1998). More recently, a new family of carriers (BiovectorsTM) has been developed. These are nanoparticles of polymerised polysaccharides substituted with phosphate residues and surrounded by covalently bound palmitic acid (Castignolles *et al.*, 1996). In collaboration with Biovector Therapeutics, we have tested these carriers in mice with flu vaccine given by the nasal route, and observed good systemic and local responses (unpublished results). A phase I clinical trial with these formulations has recently been carried out, using the nasal route and flu antigens, and immune responses have been induced at significant levels in some volunteers, but again it is unclear whether the carrier was critical in the induction of such responses.

Proteosomes have also been tested by the nasal route, as were recombinant Norwalk virus-like particles by the oral route (Ball *et al.*, 1998), alone or in combination with adjuvants like CT, and induced good levels of systemic and local antibodies in mice (Lowell *et al.*, 1997).

2.II.3.4 Carrier proteins

Proteins presenting an affinity for mucosal surfaces may constitute carriers for other antigens. In that respect, CTB and LTB are among the most attractive ones, due to their high affinity to GM1 gangliosides (for a review see Nashar *et al.*, 1993). When coupling antigens to CTB or LTB - genetically or chemically-, the binding capacity of the carrier has to be conserved, and many constructions have been tested by different groups. However, one has to be aware of what kind of response is desired, in particular if one aims to induce systemic responses by the mucosal route using this approach. It has been reported that coupling CTB to different antigens may enhance peripheral tolerance to these antigens, when administered by mucosal (oral or nasal) routes (Sun *et al.*, 1994). A selective tolerisation of Th1-like cells plays a role in this process (Mc Sorley *et al.*, 1998), and this strategy is considered to have potential for the prevention or cure of some auto-immune disorders.

2.II.4 Live vectors

Although we will not develop this section in detail since it is addressed elsewhere in this book, it is important to mention some vectors used to express and deliver foreign antigens to mucosal inductive sites. Among these vectors, those having a particular tropism for M cells are particularly attractive, e.g. attenuated *Shigella* and *Salmonella* vectors (Tacket *et al.*, 1997; Nardelli-Haefliger *et al.*, 1996). These vectors can express foreign proteins or deliver plasmids bearing the corresponding genes for expression in eukaryotic cells (Sizemore *et al.*, 1995). Other bacterial vectors can be used, including Listeria (Paglia *et al.*, 1997), BCG (Kremer *et al.*, 1998) or *Vibrio cholerae* (Ryan *et al.*, 1997) that have been used to express foreign antigens. Viruses are also good candidates and their natural tropism for different mucosae is a strong advantage for some of them, adenoviruses in particular with regard to respiratory mucosae (for a review see Imler, 1995). Even plant viruses have been used as vectors by nasal route, inducing significant immune responses (Durrani *et al.*, 1998). Another advantage of live vectors is often their capacity to induce both Th1 and Th2 responses, balancing the natural Th2 bias generally inherent to mucosal inductive sites in the case of immunisation with purified antigens.

On the other hand, one potential limitation of these vectors is their residual toxicity that may prevent their use in immunocompromised hosts (Sinha *et al.*, 1997). In addition, instability of the vectors and their capacity for inducing an immune response against themselves is another drawback that may prevent repeated use.

Moreover, the efficacy of these vectors, although well demonstrated in animals, may not be the same in humans. In recent clinical trials using Salmonella vectors, it has been observed that although some response was effectively raised against the vector, none was expressed against the antigen (Tacket *et al.*, 1997).

Beside these vectors for which residual toxicity may be a problem, commensal micro-organisms such as Gram-positive bacteria (e.g. lactic acid bacteria) have been used as immunostimulants (Miettinen *et al.*, 1998), and also to express foreign antigens (Medaglini *et al.*, 1995; Di Fabio *et al.*, 1998). Although expression and mucosal targeting of these antigens is usually achieved by such vectors, it has to be demonstrated that appropriate immune activation takes place in a second step, leading to significant immune responses. This seems to be the case in mice (Medaglini *et al.*, 1997, 1998) as well as a recent monkey study conducted with recombinant *Streptococcus gordonii* (Di Fabio *et al.*, 1998). On the other hand, these vectors may be used to induce oral tolerance in order to prevent auto-immune disorders, as recently proposed in the case of multiple sclerosis (Maassen *et al.*, 1999). Another potential application of lactic bacteria is their ability to compete with pathogenic bacteria for colonization of mucosae. This has been shown in the case for H. pylori gastric colonization in mice or in humans, directly, and/or through soluble mediators (Coconnier *et al.*, 1998; Aiba *et al.*, 1998; Michetti *et al.*, 1999).

This area will be explored and discussed much more extensively in other chapters of this book.

2.II.5 Enhancement of mucosal responses by targeted systemic immunisation

The fields of mucosal immunity and mucosal immunisation have been extensively explored only relatively recently, and in comparison more knowledge has been acquired in the past decades on systemic immunity and the adjuvants required to boost it. Moreover, some authors have stated that any sufficiently strong and appropriate systemic immunisation would effectively prevent any infection, wherever it takes place and data obtained after a long-standing and extensive use of the currently marketed vaccines to some extent uphold this point of view. However, a more selective alternative to mucosal immunisation would be to direct systemic immunisation to induce local responses in the desired mucosae (Coffin *et al.*, 1995; Lehner *et al.*, 1996). This would enable the use of adjuvants that have been shown to be efficient in systemic immunisation and to provide a broader choice of compounds with which to orientate the immune response in the desired direction. This concept has been widely explored and validated by the group of T. Lehner, in particular in monkeys with the SIV model (Lehner *et al.*, 1996). The choice of the systemic immunisation site is dictated by the lymphatic drainage of the injection site and of the target mucosa (Barone, 1996), which should be the same. Targeting any lymph node draining a mucosal surface would, in theory, favour a mucosal response, due to the particular environment in these lymph nodes, which would favour the expression on lymphoid cells of mucosal integrins, such as $\alpha4\beta7$.

We have in our laboratory explored this concept and demonstrated the importance of the site of systemic immunisation using different antigens (flu or Helicobacter antigens) in different animal species (mice and monkeys) (Guy *et al.*,1998 a, b, c,1999). In these studies we compared « parenteral » adjuvants such as QS21, cationic lipid DC Chol, Bay synthetic glycolipopeptides or phosphopolymers such as polyphosphazene (PCPP), and observed that targeted immunisation with an appropriate adjuvant could induce the desired local response in the target mucosa, and a significant protection in the case of *H. pylori* (Guy *et al.*, 1998 a, b, e, 1999). In addition, we also used mucosal adjuvants such as CT or LT by the parenteral route, and again observed good protective efficacy in an *H. pylori* challenge model when such adjuvants were given by systemic route. However, the high local toxicity of CT or LT at the injection site requires a dramatic reduction of the doses used; this can be achieved by combining CTB or LTB with minute amounts of CT or LT, as we described above. Alternatively, a new concept has recently been explored by G. Glenn and coworkers uses CT as an adjuvant for transcutaneous immunisation, without inducing any local reaction (Glenn *et al.*, 1998). Although the doses needed both for adjuvant and antigen are very high compared to subcutaneous immunisation, latitude for improvement exists and such a way to immunise against systemic and mucosal diseases is interesting and sufficiently challenging to justify further studies and sustained efforts, both in animals and humans.

Finally, another way to exploit the potency of systemic immunisation with chosen adjuvants is to combine mucosal and parenteral vaccination. Many different combinations have since long been tested, and show the effectiveness of such a strategy (Keren *et al.*, 1988). From an immunological point of view, antigen would be processed by different APCs, present in mucosal and systemic inductive sites, resulting in presentation of different peptides (Todryck *et al.*, 1998). The feasibility of such protocols in the field remains, however, an important issue.

2.II.6 Techniques

Measurement of mucosal responses is required if one aims to look at natural immune responses against a mucosal pathogen, or to analyse the quality and the level of responses induced after mucosal immunisation.

Although most immunological techniques used to measure systemic immunity apply quite well to the overall domain of mucosal immunity, some specific tools exist to investigate immune responses at the mucosal level.

2.II.6.1 Measurement of humoral responses

Routine ELISA techniques can be used to measure antibody or other immune mediator levels in various mucosal secretions (saliva, intestinal or vaginal secretions, tears, broncho-alveolar and nasal lavages...). However, the first step, namely the collection of fluids or mucosal cells, often constitutes some limitation, the quality and the quantity of obtained secretions being sometimes limited.

In laboratory animals, some techniques have been described to collect and store secretions in vivo, and allow repeated measurements of antibodies (Elson, 1984). Alternatively, or in addition, the collection of secretions can take place after sacrifice by using absorbent wicks which may allow a better quantitative recovery and measurement of responses (Haneberg *et al.*, 1994). These can also be measured in easily collected and air-dried samples of faeces and saliva, allowing an easier storage not always requiring refrigeration (Vetvik *et al.*, 1998).

In humans, different tools exist to collect a large number of secretions, for instance tears and saliva (Laufer *et al.*, 1995), and different companies market specific devices to collect and store individual samples. These devices are now being used routinely in clinical trials. Rectal and vaginal secretions can also be collected, using marketed rectal absorbent wicks for instance (Kozlowski *et al.*, 1997; Kantela *et al.*, 1998).

Once collected, centrifuged, filtrated and diluted in appropriate buffers, samples are then analysed by conventional techniques. All isotypes can be measured in secretions, but the most commonly analysed is the IgA isotype. Due to the highly variable dilution of the collected secretions according to different experiments, it is often necessary to normalise the level of specific Ig to the total level of the corresponding isotype present in the same sample. In addition, detecting the presence of the secretory component (SC) may help to confirm the nature of IgA detected (monomeric or dimeric), as only the secreted dimeric form (SIgA) bears this peptide. Alternatively or in addition, HPLC techniques may allow the discrimination between monomeric and polymeric IgA.

It is to be noted that some secretions (bronchoalveolar lavages for instance) may be a source of immune cells, and once obtained, they can also be analysed by conventionnal techniques used for measuring cellular immunity.

2.II.6.2 *Measurement of cellular responses*

ELISPOT (antibodies and cytokines)

The quantification of antibodies or other soluble mediators accumulated in secretions has some limitations: it brings little information on the dynamic aspects of immune responses and in particular is unable to yield information concerning the precise anatomical location(s) of antibody or cytokine formation. The analysis of secretions at the cellular level is more informative in that respect. Since its original description (Czerkinsky *et al.*, 1983), the ELISPOT technique (or ELISA plaque assay) has been employed as an alternative to the conventional plaque-forming cell assay to enumerate specific, as well as total, immunoglobulin secreting-cells and also to detect a variety of cells (lymphoid or non lymphoid) that secrete factors with immunological properties such as cytokines (Mega *et al.*, 1992). Antigen (against which antibodies are directed) or capture antibodies (directed against a cytokine for instance) are adsorbed onto a solid surface and, in a second step, cells to be analysed for secretion are added into the wells. After a variable time of incubation depending on the experiment, cells are removed by the use of a detergent (Tween for instance), and subsequent steps are similar to those followed in ELISA tests, except for the final revelation step. The secreting cells are then visualised as spots that are then counted under a dissecting microscope. The spots appear distinct from the background, and counting them is usually not difficult for someone with some experience. However, it is often time consuming, and some companies now propose devices for automated counting.

The method can be employed to detect secreting cells in suspensions prepared from a variety of animal species (for which reagents exist) and from different anatomic compartments. As for the collection of secretions, the limiting factor here is the source of cells and the recovery yields. When working on animals, collection of different organs can be made after sacrifice, and this usually allows recovery of substancial numbers of cells after appropriate digestion. However, the digestion step is a critical one, in particular with organs with a low number of lymphoid cells. The enzymes and conditions used have to keep cells in a physiological state, not damage them, and not activate them non-specifically. Dispase and/or collagenase are among the most popular enzymes used (Mega *et al.*, 1992), but digestion is often preceded by a chopping step that can be done manually or with automated tissue choppers marketed by different companies. After digestion, a final purification step may be required using Ficoll or equivalent reagents. This is recommanded in the case of crude preparations that may induce too high a background signal after revelation of the spots, and thus prevent an accurate quantification, although one has to be aware that such steps often result in a high loss of cells. This can be a problem when the number of cells is initially very low, and a compromise has to be found.

In humans, the source of cells usually comprises biopsies or samples obtained after surgery, and in the former case the yields are usually low whatever the technique used to obtain the cells, which may constitute some limitation.

A considerable number of studies have used this technique to measure in particular IgA secretory cells in murine nasal tissue, salivary glands, Peyer's patches, lamina propria, lymph nodes or spleen (Asanuma *et al.*, 1998). Similarly, cytokine-secreting cells have been detected in different mucosal inductive and effector sites (Taguchi *et al.*, 1990; Mega *et al.*, 1992). The ELISPOT technique can be used with different revelation systems in order to visualise different cells secreting, for instance, different isotypes in the same well (Czerkinsky *et al.*, 1988). It can also be combined with specific purification steps (immunobeads) before incubation (Lakew *et al.*, 1997).

Apart from mice, it has been used in a large variety of animals, including monkeys (Van Cott *et al.*, 1993; Van Besouw *et al.*, 1994), and in humans, for IgE to IFNγ detection (Shinomyia *et al.* 1993; Hanke *et al.*, 1998). Due to the sometimes limited availability of biopsies, some authors have correlated the detection of antibody secreting cells in the blood circulation with the level of mucosal antibody responses (Nieminen *et al.*, 1998). When stimulated in inductive sites, cells bearing a mucosal adressin will, over a short time window (usually about 1 week after induction in mucosal sites), transit through the blood circulation where they can be picked up and quantified. This may constitute a convenient alternative to the use of biopsies when schedules of immunisation and sampling are well defined, and when correlation between local and peripheral detection has been clearly demonstrated within this interval of time.

Expansion of T cell clones from biopsies

Although the amount of lymphocytes in human biopsies is usually small, some T cell expansion can be carried out to allow subsequent analysis using conventionnal T cell immunology techniques. Actually, techniques used to generate clones from PBLs (Del Prete *et al.*, 1991) have been applied to biopsies from bronchial and nasal mucosae, or gastric mucosa respectively (Del Prete *et al.*, 1993; D'Elios *et al.*, 1997). Once obtained, clones can be characterised, and their antigenic specificity, phenotype and cytokine profile determined. One drawback of these techniques is the use of clones that usually result from non-specific polyclonal activation which constitutes, in most cases, the first step of the cloning procedure. This may preferentially select the more resistant or activatable clones, regardless of their Th profile or antigenic specificity.

Immunohistochemistry/FACS analysis, and more...

Techniques used to analyse immune responses in tissue sections apply quite well to the analysis of mucosal immunity. Although the ELISPOT technique is often preferred for the detection of antibodies or cytokines, immunohistochemistry can be used to analyse different cell markers in situ for instance (Elitsur *et al.*, 1998; Trajman *et al.*, 1997). This can be combined with FACS analysis.

There areas many different techniques as there are different subjects and laboratories, and we do not pretend to have described, or even listed, all of them here. Each technique has to be selected and developed according to the specific model and antigen(s) used. The current chapter has only described the most widely used techniques and compounds, and constitutes a source of references rather than a detailed description of each adjuvant and/or protocol.

References

Abbas, A.K., Haber S, and Rock, K.L. (1985) Antigen presentation by hapten-specific B lymphocytes, *J. Immun.* **135**, 1661-1667.

Agren L, Lowenadler B, Lycke N. A novel concept in mucosal adjuvanticity: the CTA1-DD adjuvant is a B cell-targeted fusion protein that incorporates the enzymatically active cholera toxin A1 subunit. *Immunol Cell Biol* 1998, **76**, 280.

Aiba Y, Suzuki N, Kabir AM, Takagi A, Koga Y. Lactic acid-mediated suppression of Helicobacter pylori by the oral administration of Lactobacillus salivarius as a probiotic in a gnotobiotic murine model. *Am J Gastroenterol* 1998, **93**, 2097-101.

Allison, A.C., Byars, N.E. (1991) Immunological adjuvants: Desirable properties and side-effects, *Mol Immunol*; **28**, 279-284.

Aprile, M.A. and Wardlaw, A.C. (1966) Aluminum compounds as adjuvants for vaccines and toxoids in man: a review, *Canadian Journal of Public Health* **57**, 343-360.

Arulanandam BP., and DW. Metzger. Modulation of mucosal and systemic immunity by intranasal IL-12 delivery. *Vaccine* 1998, **17** : 252

Asanuma H., C. Aizawa, T. Kurata and S. Tamura. (1998) IgA antibody forming cell responses in the NALT of mice vaccinated by intranasal, intravenous and/or subcutaneous administration. *Vaccine*, **16**, 1257.

Audibert, F., Leclerc, C., and Chedid, L. (1985) Muramyl peptides as immunopharmacological response modifiers, in P.F. Torrence, (eds), *Biological Response Modifiers. New Approaches to Disease Prevention*, Academic Press, Orlando, pp. 307-327.

Azuma, I. (1992) Synthetic immunoadjuvants: application to non-specific host stimulation and potentiation of vaccine immunogenicity, *Vaccine* **10**, 1000-1006.

Baker, P.J., Hiernaux, J.R., Fauntleroy, M.B., Stashak, P.W., Prescott B., Cantrell, J.L., and Rudbach, J.A. (1988) Ability of monophosphoryl lipid A to augment the antibody response of young mice. *Infect Immun* **565**, 3064-3066.

Ball JM., ME. Hardy, RL. Atmar, ME. Conner and MK. (1998) Estes. Oral immunisation with recombinant Norwalk virus like particles induces a systemic and mucosal immune response in mice. *J. Virol*, **72**, 1345.

Baquar S., AL Bourgeois, PJ. Schultheiss, RI Walker, DM. Rollins, DL Haberberger and OR. Pavlovskis (1995). Safety and immunogenicity of a prototype oral whole-cell killed campylobacter vaccine administered with a mucosal adjuvant in non-human primates. *Vaccine*, **13**, 22

Barone R. Anatomie comparée des mammifères domestiques. Tome 5. *Angiologie*, pp. 667-864. Vigot eds. Paris.1996.

Barr, I.G., and Mitchell, G.F.(1996) ISCOMS (Immunostimulating Complexes) The first decade, *Immunol and Cell Biol.* **74**, 8-25.

Beebe, G.W., Simon, A.H., and Vivona, S. (1972) Long-term mortality follow-up of army recruits who received adjuvant influenza virus vaccine in 1951-1953, *Am J Epidemiol* **95**, 337-346.

Begue RE., G. Castellares, C. Bezas, JL. Sanchez, R. Meza, DM. Watts and DN. Taylor. (1995) Immunogenicity in peruvian volunteers of a booster dose of oral cholera vaccine consisting of whole cells plus recombinant B subunit. *Infect. Immun.* **63**, 3726

Blanchard TG., N. Lycke, SJ. Czinn and JG Nedrud. (1998) Recombinant cholera toxin B subunit is not an effective mucosal adjuvant for oral immunisation of mice against *Helicobacter felis*. *Immunology*, **93**, 22.

Bliss, J.R., Maylor, K., Stokes, K.S., Murray, M.A., Ketchum, and Wolf, S.F. (1996) Interleukin-12 as vaccine adjuvant: characteristics of primary, recall, and long-term responses, *Annals of the New York Academy of Sciences* **795**, 26-35.

Bomford, R. (1990) Immunomodulation by adjuvants, in N.J. Dimmock.,P.D. Griffiths and C.R. Madeley (eds.), *Control of Virus Diseases. 45th Symposium of the Society for General Microbiology*. Cambridge University Press, pp. 143-154.

Bomford, R., Stapleton, M., Winsor, S., McKnight, A., and Andronova, T. (1992) The control of antibody isotype response to recombinant human immunodeficiency virus gpl20 antigen by adjuvants, *AIDS Res Human Retrovir* **8**, 1765-1771.

Bouveret Le Cam, N.N., Ronco, J., Françon, A., Blondeau, C., and Fanget, B. (1998) Adjuvants for influenza vaccine, *Res Immunol* **149**, 19-23.

Bowen, J.C., Alpar, O., Phillpotts, R., Roberts, I.S., and Brown, M.R.W. (1990) Preliminary studies on infection by attenuated Salmonella in guinea-pigs and on expression on Herpes simplex virus, *Res Microbial* **141**, 873-877.

Brandtzaeg P., TS. Halstensen, K. Kett, P. Krajcl, D. Kvale, O. Rognum, H. Scott, and LM. Sollid. (1989) Immunobiology and immunopathology of human gut mucosa: humoral immunity and intraepithelial lymphocytes *Gastroenterology*, **97**, 1562

Brunel, F., Darbouret, A., and Ronco, J. (1999) Cationic lipid induces an improved and balanced immunity able to overcome the unresponsiveness to the hepatitis B vaccine. *Vaccine*, in press.

Bussiere, I.L., McCormick, G.C., and Green, I.D. (1995) Preclinical safety assessment considerations in vaccine development, in M.F. Powell and M.I. Newman (eds.) Vaccine Design: *The Subunit and Adjuvant Approach*. New York, Plenum Press, pp. 61-79.

Butler, N.R., Wison, B.D.R., Benson, P.F., *et al.* (1962) Response of infants to pertussis vaccine at one week and to poliomyelitis, diptheria, and tetanus vaccine at six months, *Lancet* **2**, 112-114.

Carayanniotis, G., and Barber, B.H. (1987) Adjuvant-free IgG responses induced with antigen coupled to antibodies against class II MHC. *Nature* **327**, 59-61.

Castignolles N., S. Morgeaux, C. Gontier-Jallet, D. Samain, D. Betbeder and P. Perrin. (1996) A new family of carriers (biovectors) enhances the immunogenicity of rabies antigens. *Vaccine*, **14**, 1353

Chedid, L,. Audibert, F,. and Jolivet, M. (1986) Role of muramyl peptides for the enhancement of synthetic vaccines. *Dev Biol Stand* **63**, 133-140.

Childers NK., SM. Michalek, DG Pritchard and J. McGhee. (1991) Mucosal and systemic responses to an oral liposome-Streptococcus mutans carbohydrate vaccine in humans. *Regional Immunol.* **3**, 289

Chong C, M. Friberg and JD. Clements. LT (1998) (R192G), a non-toxic mutant of the heat-labile enterotoxin of Escherichia coli, elicits enhanced humoral and cellular immune responses associated with protection against lethal oral challenge with salmonella spp. *Vaccine*, **16**, 732.

Claesson, B.A., Trollfors, B., Lagergard, T., *et al.* (1988) Clinical and immunological responses to the capsular polysaccharide of Haemophilus influenzae type b alone or conjugated to tetanus toxoid in 18- to 23-month-old children, *J Pediatr* **112**, 695-702.

Clements JD., NM. Hartzog and FL. Lyon. (1988) Adjuvant activity of Escherichia coli heat labile enterotoxin and effect on the induction of oral tolerance in mice to unrelated protein antigens. *Vaccine*, **6**, 269

Coconnier MH, Lievin V, Hemery E, Servin AL. (1998) Antagonistic activity against Helicobacter infection in vitro and in vivo by the human Lactobacillus acidophilus strain LB. *Appl Environ Microbiol,* **64**, 4573-80.

Coffin SE, M. Klinek, and PO. Ofit. (1995) Induction of virus specific antibody production by lamina propria lymphocytes following intramuscular inoculation with rotavirus. *J. Infect. Dis.* **172**, 874.

Cong Y., CT. Weaver and CO. Elson. (1997) The mucosal adjuvanticity of Cholera toxin involves enhancement of costimulatory activity by selective up regulation of B7.2 expression. *J. Immunol*, **159**, 5301

Cox, J.C. and Coulter, A.R. (1992) Advances in adjuvant technology and application, in W.K. Yong (ed.), *Animal Parasite Control Utilizing Biotechnology*, CRC Press, Boca Raton, pp. 49-112.

Cox, J.C. and Coulter, A.R. (1997) Adjuvants - a classification and review of their modes of action, *Vaccine* **15**, 248-256.

Cvjetanovic, B. and Uemura, K. (1965) The present status of field and laboratory studies of typhoid and paratyphoid vaccines with special reference to studies sponsored by the World Health Organization, *Bull WHO* **32**, 29-36.

Czerkinsky C., C. Nilsson, H. Nygren, Ö. Ouchterlony and A. Tarkowsky. (1983) A solid phase enzymz-linked immunospot (ELISPOT) assay for enumeration of antibody secreting cells. *J. Immunol. Methods*, **65**, 109

Czerkinsky C., Z. Moldoveanu, J. Mestecky, LA. Nilsson and Ö. Ouchterlony. (1988) A novel two colour ELISPOT assay. *J. Immunol. Methods*, **115**, 31

D'Elios MM., M. Manghetti, F. Almerigognia, A. Amedei, F. Costa, D. Burroni, CT. Baldari, S. Romagnani, JL. Telford and GF., Dal Monte P., and FC. Szoka Jr. (1988) Effect of liposome encapsulation on antigen presentation in vitro. *J. Immunol*, **142**, 1437

Davenport, F.M., Hennessy, A.V., and Askin, F.B. (1968) Lack of adjuvant effect of $AlPO_4$ on purified influenza virus haemagglutinins in man, *J Immuno.l* **100**, 1139-1140.

De Haan A., Geerligs HJ., JP. Huchshorn, GJM. Van Scharrenburg, AM. Palache and J. Wilschut. (1994) Mucosal immunoadjuvant activity of liposomes : induction of systemic IgG and secretory IgA responses in mice by intranasal immunisation with an influenza subunit vaccine and coadministered liposomes. *Vaccine*, **13**, 155

De Haan A., KB. Renagar, P. Small Jr., J. Wilschut. (1995)Induction of scretory IgA response in the murine female urogenital tract by immunisation of the lungs with liposome-supplemented viral subunit antigen. *Vaccine*, **3**, 613

De Magistris MT., M. Pizza, G. Douce, P. Ghiara, G. Dougan and R. Rappuoli. (1998) Adjuvant effect of non toxic mutants of E. coli heat labile enterotoxin following intranasal, oral and intravaginal immunisation. *Dev. Biol. Stand.* **92**, 123

Del Giudice, G. (1992) New carriers and adjuvants in the development of vaccines, *Curr Opinion in Immunol.* **4**, 454-459.

Del Prete GF., M. De Carli, C. Mastromauro, R. Biagiotti, D. Macchia, P. Falagiani, M. Ricci and S. Romagnani. (1991) Purified protein derivative of Mycobacterium tuberculosis and excretory-secretory antigen(s) of Toxocara canis expand in vitro human T cells with stable and opposite (Th1 and Th2) profile of cytokine production. *J. Clin. Invest.* **88**, 346

Del Prete GF., M. De Carli, MM.D'Elios, P. Maestrelli, M. Ricci, L. Fabbri and S. Romagnani. (1993) Allergen exposure induces the activation of allergen specific Th2 cells in the airway mucosa of patients with allergic respiratory disorders. *Eur. J. Immunol.* **23**, 1445

Del Prete. (1997) Different cytokine profile and antigen specificity repertoire in Helicobacter pylori-specific T cell clones from the antrum of chronic gastritis patients with or without peptic ulcer. *Eur J Immunol.* **27**, 1751

Del Vecchio, M., and Bajetta, E. (1997) Results of the treatment with IL-12 in patients with malignant melanoma, *Melanoma Research* **7**, 159-161

Dempsey, P.W., Allison, M.E.D., Akkaraju, S., Goodnow, C.C., and Fearon, D.T. (1996) C3d of complement as a molecular adjuvant: Bridging innate and acquired immunity. *Science* **271**, 348-350.

Di Fabio S., D. Medaglini, CM. Rush, F. Corrias, GL. Panzini, M. Pace, P. Verani, G. Pozzi and F. Titti. (1998) Vaginal immunisation of Cynomolgus monkeys with Streptococcus gordonii expressing HIV1 and HPV16 antigens. *Vaccine*, **16**, 485

Douce G., C. Turcotte, I. Cropley, M. Roberts, M. Pizza, M. Domenghini, R. Rappuoli and G. Dougan. (1995) Mutants of Escherichia coli heat-labile toxin lacking ADP-ribosyltransferase activity, mucosal adjuvants. *Proc. Natl. Acad. Sci. USA*. **92**, 1644

Drescher, J., Grutzner, L., and Godgluck, G. (1967) Further investigations on the immunogenic activity of aqueous and aluminum oxide adsorbed inactivated poliovirus vaccines in Macaca mulatta, *Am. J. Epidemiology* **85**, 413-423.

Durrani Z., TL McInerney, L. McLain, T. Jones, T. Bellaby, FR. Brennan, NJ. Dimmock. (1998) Intranasal immunisation with a plant virus expressing a peptide from HIV1 gp41 stimulates better mucosal and systemic HIV1 specific IgA and IgG than oral immunisation. *J. Immunol. Meths*. **220**, 93

Edelman, R., and Tacket, C.O. (1990) Adjuvants, *Int Rev Immunol.* **7**, 1-66.

Eldridge JH., JK. Staas, JA. Meulbroek, JR Mc Ghee, TR. Tice, RM. Gilley. (1991) Biodegradable microspheres as a vaccine delivery system. *Molecular Immunology*, **28**, 287

Elitsur Y, S. Jackman, C. Neace, S. Keerthy, X. Liu, J. Dosescu and JA. Moshier. (1998) Human vaginal mucosal immune system : characterization and function. *Gen. Diagn. Pathol.* **143**, 271

Elliott, G.T., McLeod, R.A., Perez, J., and Von Eschen, K.B. (1993) Interim results of a phase II multicenter clinical trial evaluating the activity of a therapeutic allogeneic melanoma vaccine (Theraccine) in the treatment of disseminated malignant melanoma. *Semin Surg Oncol.* **9**, 264-272.

Elson CO. (1989) Cholera Toxin and its subunits as potential oral adjuvants. *Curr. Top. Microbiol. Immunol.* **146**, 29

Elson CO., and W. Ealding. (1984) Cholera toxin feeding did not induce oral tolerance in mice and abrogated oral tolerance to an unrelated protein antigen. *J. Immunol.* **133**, 2892.

Elson CO., and W. Ealding. (1987) Ir gene control of the murine secretory IgA response to cholera toxin. *Eur. J. Immunol.* **17**, 425.

Elson CO., SP. Holland, MT. Dertzbaugh, CF. Cuff and AO. Anderson. (1995) Morphologic and functional alterations of mucosal T cells by Cholera toxin and its B subunit. *J. Immunol.* **154**, 1032.

Elson CO., W. Ealding and J. Lefkowitz. (1984 b) A lavage technique allowing repeated measurement of IgA antibody in mouse intestinal secretions. *J. Immunol. Methods.* **67**, 101.

Erdile LF and B. Guy. (1997) OspA lipoprotein of Borrelia biurdogferi is a mucosal immunogen and adjuvant. *Vaccine*, **15**, 988.

Estrada A, Li B, Laarveld B. (1998) Adjuvant action of Chenopodium quinoa saponins on the induction of antibody responses to intragastric and intranasal administered antigens in mice. *Comp Immunol Microbiol Infect Dis.* **21**, 225.

Fries, L.F., Gordon, D.M., Richards, R.L., et al. (1992) Liposomal malaria vaccine in humans: A safe and potent adjuvant strategy. *Proc Natl Acad Sci* USA **89**, 358-362.

Giannasca PJ., KT. Giannasca, P. Falk, JI Gordon and MR. (1994) Neutra. Regional differences in glycoconjugates of intestinal M cells in mice : potential targets for mucosal vaccines. *Am. J. Physiol.* **267**, G1108.

Gizurarson S., V. Mjöll Jonsdottir and I. Heron. (1995) Intranasal administration of diphteria toxoid. Selecting antibody isotypes using formulations having various lipophilic characteristics. *Vaccine.* **13**, 617.

Glenn GM., T. Scharton-Kersten, R. Vassel, CP. Mallett, TL. Hale, and CR. Alving. (1998) Cutting edge : transcutaneous immunisation with cholera toxin protects mice against lethal mucosal toxin challenge. *J. Immunol.* **161**, 3211

Glenny A.T, Pope C.G., Waddington H., Wallace V. (1926) The antigenic value of toxoid precipitated by potassium alum. *J Path Bact.* **29**, 38-45.

Glück, R., Mischler, R., Finkel, B., Que. J.U., Scarpa, B. and Cryz, S.J.Jr (1994) Immunogenicity of new virosome influenza vaccine in elderly people. *Lancet* **344**, 160-163.

Goldenthal, K.L., Cavagnaro, J.A., Alving, C.R., and Vogel, F.R. (1993) NCVDG working groups: Safety evaluation of vaccine adjuvants: National cooperative vaccine development meeting working group. *AIDS Res Hum Retrovirus* **9**, S47-S51.

Gordon, D.M., McGovern, T.W., Krzych, U., *et al.* (1995) Safety, immunogenicity, and efficacy of a recombinantly produced Plasmodium falciparum circumsporozoite protein-hepatitis B surface antigen subunit vaccine. *J Infect Dis.* **171**, 1576-1585.

Gregoriadis, G. (1990) Immunological adjuvants: a role for liposomes. *Immunol. Today.* **11**, 89-97.

Gregoriadis, G., and Panagiotidi, C. (1989) Immunoadjuvant action of liposomes; comparison with other adjuvants. *Immun Lett.* **20**, 237-240.

Griffith, A.H. (1989) Permanent brain damage and pertussis vaccination: is the end of the saga in sight? *Vaccine* 7, 199-210.

Grob, P.J., Joller-Jemelka, H.I., Binswanger, U., *et al.* (1984) Interferon as an adjuvant for hepatitis B vaccination in non- and low-responder populations. *Eur. J. Clin. Microbiol.* **3**, 195-198.

Gupta, R.K., and Siber, G.R. (1994) Comparison of adjuvant activities of aluminum phosphate. calcium phosphate and stearyl tyrosine for tetanus toxoid. *Biologicals.* **22**, 53-63.

Gupta, R.K., and Siber, G.R. (1995a) Adjuvants for human vaccines-Current status, problems and future prospects. *Vaccine* **13**, 1263-1276.

Gupta, R.K., and Siber, G.R. (1995b) Adjuvant properties of aluminum and calcium compounds, in M.F. Powell and M.J. Newman (eds.), Vaccine Design: *The Subunit and Adjuvant Approach*. New York, Plenum Press, pp. 229-248.

Gupta, R.K., Relyveld, E.H., Lindblad, E.B., Bizzini, B., Ben-Efraim, S., and Gupta, C.K. (1993) Adjuvants-a balance between toxicity and adjuvanticity. *Vaccine* **11**, 294-306.

Guy B, C. Hessler, S. Fourage, P. Lecoindre, M. Chevalier, S. Peyrol, M. Boude J. Haensler, B. Rokbi and MJ. Quentin-Millet. (1998 c) Mucosal, systemic or combined therapeutic immunisations in cynomolgus monkeys naturally infected with Gastrospirillum hominis like organisms. *Vaccine Res.* **6**, 141.

Guy B., S Fourage, Ce Hessler, V Sanchez and MJ Quentin Millet. (1998 a) Effect of the nature of adjuvant and site of parenteral immunisation on the serum and mucosal immune responses induced by a nasal boost with a vaccine alone. *Clin. Diag. Lab. Immunol.* **5**, 732

Guy B., C Hessler, S Fourage, B Rokbi and MJ Quentin Millet. (1999 in press) Comparison between targeted and untargeted systemic immunisations with adjuvanted urease to cure Helicobacter pylori infection in mice. *Vaccine*

Guy B., C. Hessler, S. Fourage, J. Haensler, E. Vialon-Lafay, B. Rokbi and M.J. Quentin Millet. (1998 b) Systemic immunisation with urease protects mice against Helicobacter pylori infection. *Vaccine* **16**, 850.

Haensler, J., Trannoy, E., and Ronco, J. (1996) *Patent Application* WO 96/14831.

Haneberg B., D. Kendall, HM. Amerongen, FM. Apter, JP. Kraehenbuhl and MR. Neutra. (1994) Induction of specific IgA in the small intestine, colon-rectum, and vagina measured by a new method for collection of secretions from local mucosal surfaces. *Infect. Immun.* **62**, 15.

Hanke T., TJ. Blanchard, J. Schneider, CM. Hannan, M. Becker, SC. Gilbert, AVS. Hill, GL. Smith and A. McMichael. (1998) Enhancement of MHC class I restricted peptide specific T cell induction by a DNA prime/MVA boost vaccination regime. *Vaccine*, **16**, 439.

Hazama, M., Mayumi-Aono, A., Askawa, N., Kuroda, S., Hinuma, S. and Fujisawa, Y. (1993) Adjuvant-independent enhanced immune responses to recombinant herpes simplex virus type 1 glycoprotein D by fusion with biologically active interleukin-2. *Vaccine* **11**, 629-636.

Hoffman, S.L., Edelman, R., Bryan, I.P., et al. (1994) Safety, immunogenicity, and efficacy of a malaria sporozoite vaccine administered with monophosphoryl lipid A, cell wall skeleton of mycobacteria, and squalane as adjuvant, *Am J Trop Med Hyg.* **51**, 603-612.

Holmgren, J., Lycke, N., and Czerkinsky, C. (1993) Cholera toxin and cholera B subunit as oral-mucosal adjuvant and antigen vector systems, *Vaccine* **11**, 1179-1184.

Hopkins S., G. Fisher, JP. Kraehenbuhl and D. Velin. (1998) Nasal associated lymphoid tissue. A site for vaccination and pathogen entry.*STP Pharma Sc.* **8**, 47.

Hunter, R., Olsen, M., and Buynitzky, S. (1991) Adjuvant activity of non-ionic block copolymers. IV. Effect of molecular weight and formation on titre and isotype of antibody. *Vaccine* **9**, 250-255.

Imler JL. 1995 Adenovirus vactors as recombinant viral vaccines. *Vaccine*, **13**, 1143.

Isaka M., Y. Yasuda, S. Kosuka, Y. Miura, T. Taniguchi, K. Matano, N. Goto and K. Tochikubo. (1998) Systemic and mucosal immune responses of mice to aluminum adsorbed or aluminum-non-adsorbed tetanus toxoid administered intranasally with recombinant cholera toxin B subunit. *Vaccine*, **16**, 1620

Jabbal-Gill I., A. Neil Fisher, R. Rappuoli, S. Stewart Davis and L. Illum. (1998) Stimulation of mucosal and systemic antibody responses against Bordetella pertussis filamentous haemagglutinin and recombinant pertussis toxin after nasal administration with chitosan in mice. *Vaccine*, **16**, 2039.

Jacobson, M.A., Hardy, D., et al. (1996) Phase I trial of recombinant human interleukin 12 in HIV-infected subjects, 3rd *Conference on Retroviruses and Opportunistic Infections* 110.28 (Abstract).

Johnson, A.G. (1994) Molecular adjuvants and immunomodulators: New approaches to immunization, *Clin Microbiol Rev.* 7, 277-289.

Jones B., L. Pascopella and S. Falkow. (1995) Entry of microbes into the host : using M cells to break the mucosal barrier. *Current Opinion in Immunology*, 7, 474.

Jungers, P., Devillier, P., Salomon, H., et al. (1994) Randomised placebo-controlled trial of recombinant interleukin-2 in chronic uraemic patients who are non-responders to hepatitis B vaccine, *Lancet.* **344**, 856-857.

Kahn, J.O., Sinangil, F., Baenziger, J., Murcar, N., Wynne, D., Coleman, R.L., Steimer, K.S., Dekker, C.L., and Chernoff, D. (1994) Clinical and immunologic responses to human immunodeficiency virus (HIV) type 1 SF2 gpl20 subunit vaccine combined with MF59 adjuvant with or without muramyl tripeptide dipalmitoyl phosphatidylethanolamine in non-HIV-infected human volunteers, *J. Infect. Dis.* **170**, 1288-1291.

Kantele A., M. Häkkinen, Z. Moldoveanu, A. Lu, E. Savilahti, RD. Alvarez, S. Michalek and J. Mestecky. (1998) Differences in immune responses induced by oral and rectal immunisations with Salmonella typhi Ty21a : evidence for compartimentalization within the common mucosal immune system in humans. *Infect. Immun.* **66**, 5630.

Kasel, J.A., Couch, R.B., and Douglas, R.G. Jr. (1971) Antigenicity of alum and aqueous adenovirus hexon antigen vaccines in man *J. Immunol.* **107**, 916-919.

Keefer, M.C., Graham, B.S., McElrath, M.J., Matthews, T.J., Stablein, D.M., Corey, L. Wright, P.F., Lawrence, D., Fast, P.E., Weinhold, K., Hsieh, R.H., Chernoff, D., Dekker, C. and Dolin, R. (1996) Safety and immunogenicity of Env 2-3, a human immunodeficiency virus type 1 candidate vaccine, in combination with a novel adjuvant, MTP-PE/MF59. NIAID AIDS Vaccine Evaluation Group, *AIDS Res Hum Retroviruses* **12**, 683-693.

Keefer, M.C., Wolff, M., Gorse, G.J., Graham, B.S., Corey, L., Clements-Mann, M.L., Verani-Ketter, N., Erb, S., Smith, C.M., Belshe, R.B., Wagner, L.J., McElrath, M.J., Schwartz, D.H. and Fast, P. (1997) Safety profile of phase I and II preventive HIV type 1 envelope vaccination: experience of the NIAID AIDS Vaccine Evaluation Group, *AIDS Res Hum Retroviruses* **13**, 1163-1177

Kensil, C.R. (1996) Saponins as vaccine adjuvants. *Therapeutic Drug Carrier Systems* **13**, 1-55.

Keren DF., RA. McDonald and JL. Carey. (1988) Combined parenteral and oral immunisation results in an enhanced mucosal immunoglobulin A response to Shigella flexneri. *Infect. Immun.* **56**, 910.

Koutsoukos, M., Lerous, G., Vandepapeliere, P., *et al.*, (1994) Induction of cell mediated immune responses in man with vaccines against herpes simplex based on glycoprotein D, 34th *Interscience Conference on Antimicrobial Agents and Chemotherapy* 217 (Abstract).

Kozlowski PA., S. Cu-Uvin, MR. Neutra and TP. Flanigan. (1997) Comparison of the oral, rectal and vaginal immunisation routes for induction of antibodies in rectal and genital tract secretions of women. *Infect Immun.* **65**, 1387

Kremer L., L. Dupré, G. Riveau, A. Capron, and C. Locht. (1998) Systemic and mucosal immune responses after intranasal administration of recombinant Mycobacterium bovis BCG expressing GST from Schistosoma haematobium. *Infect. Immun.* **66**, 5669

Kuklin NA., M. Daheshia, PC. Marconi, DM. Krisky, RJ. Rouse, JC. Glorioso, E. Manican and BT. Rouse. (1998) Modulation of mucosal and systemic immunity by enteric administration of non replicating herpes simplex virus expressing cytokines. *Virology*, **240**, 245

Kuper CF., PJ Koornstra, DMH Hameleers, J. Biewenga, BJ. Spit, AM. Duijvestijn, PJC. Van Breda Vriesman and Taede Sminia. (1992) The role of nasopharyngeal lymphoid tissue .*Immunol.Today*, **13**:219

Lakew M., I. Nordstöm, C. Czerkinsky, and M. Quiding-Järbrink. (1997) Combined imunomagnetic cell sorting and ELISPOT assay for the phenotypic characterization of specific antibody-forming cells.*J.Immunol. Methods*, **203,** 193

Laufer DS., W. Hurni, B.: Watson, W. Miller, J. Ryan, D. Nalin and L. Brown. (1995) Saliva and serum as diagnostic media for antibody to Hepatitis A virus in adults and in individuals who have received an inactivated Hepatitis A vaccine. *Clin. Infect. Dis.* **20**, 868

Lawrence, G.W., Saul, A., Giddy, A.J., Kemp, R., and Pye, D. (1997) Phase I trial in humans of an oil-based adjuvant SEPPIC MONTANIDE ISA 720, *Vaccine* **15**, 176-178.

Leclerc, C., and Ronco, J. (1998) New approaches in vaccine development, *Immunol Today* **19**, 300-302.

Lehner T., Y. Wang, M. Cranage, LA. Bergmaier, E. Mitchell, L. Tao, G. Hall, M. Dennis, N. Cook, R. Brookes, L. Klavinskis, I. Jones, C. Doyle and R. Ward. (1996) Protective mucosal immunity elicited by targeted iliac lymph node immunisation with a subunit SIV envelope and core vaccine in macaques. Nature. *Medicine*, **2**, 767

Lemoine D, M. Francotte and V. Preat. (1998)Nasal vaccines. From fundamental concepts to vaccine development. *STP Pharma Sci.* **8**, 5.

Leroux-Roels, G., Moreau, E., Desombere, I., *et al.* (1994) Persistence of humoral and cellular immune response and booster effect following vaccination with herpes simplex (gD2t) candidate vaccine with MPL (abstr). 34th *Interscience Conference on Antimicrobial Agents and Chemotherapy* 250 (Abstract)

Leroux-Roels, G., Moreux E., Verhasselt, B., et al. (1993) Immunogenicity and reactogenicity of a recombinant HSV-2 glycoprotein D vaccine with or without monophosphoryl lipid A in HSV seronegative and seropositive subjects, 33rd *Interscience Conference on Antimicrobial Agents and Chemotherapy* 341 (Abstract).

Lin, R., Tarr, P.E., and Jones, T.C. (1995) Present status of the use of cytokines as adjuvants with vaccines to protect against infectious diseases, *Clin Infect Dis.* **21**, 1439-1449.

Livingston, P.O, Adluri, S., Helling, F., Yao, T.I., Kensil, C.R., Newman, M.J., and Marciani, D. (1994) Phase 1 trial of immunological adjuvant QS-21 with a GM2 ganglioside-keyhole limpet haemocyanin conjugate vaccine in patients with malignant melanoma, *Vaccine* **12**, 1275-1280.

Lowell GH., RW. Kaminski, TC. Vancott, B. Slike, K. Kersey, E Zawoznik, L. Loomis-Price, G. Smith, RR. Redfield, S. Amselem and DL. Birx. (1997) Proteosomes, emulsosomes, and CTB improve nasal immunogenicity of HIV gp 160 in mice : induction of serum, intestinal, vaginal, and lung IgA and IgG. *J. infect. Dis.* **175**, 292

Lycke N., and W. Strober. (1989 b) Cholera Toxin promotes B cell isotype differentiation. *J.Immunol.* **142,** 3781

Lycke N., T. Tsuji and J. Holmgren. (1992)The adjuvant effect of Vibrio cholerae and Escherichia coli heat labile enterotoxins is linked to their ADP ribosyltransferase activity. *Eur. J. Immunol.* **22,** 2277

Maassen CBM, JD Laman, MJ Heine den Bak-Glashouwer, FJ Tielen, JCPA van Holten Neelen, L. Hoogteijling, C. Antonissen, RJ. Leer, PH. Pouwels, WJA Boersma, and DM Shaw. (1999) Instruments for oral disease-intervention strategies : recombinant Lactobacillus casei expressing tetanus toxin fragment C for vaccination or myelin proteins for oral tolerance induction in multiple sclerosis. *Vaccine* **17**, 2117-2128

MacLean, G.D., Bowen-Yacyshyn, M.B., Samuel, J., *et al.* (1992) Active immunization of human ovarian cancer patients against a common carcinoma (Thomsen-

Friedereich) determinant using a synthetic carbohydrate antigen, *J Immunother.* **11**, 292-305.

MacLean, G.D., Reddish, M., Koganty, R.R., *et al.* (1993) Immunization of breast cancer patients using a synthetic sialyl-Tn glycoconjugate plus Detox adjuvant. *Cancer Immunol Immunother.* **36**, 215-222.

Malynn, B.A., Romeo, D.T., Wortis, H.H. (1985) Antigen-specific B cells efficiently present low doses of antigen for induction of T cell proliferation, *J. Immun.* **135**, 980-988.

Marinaro M, Boyaka PN, Finkelman FD, Kiyono H, Jackson RJ, Jirillo E, McGhee JR. (1997) Oral but not parenteral interleukin (IL)-12 redirects T helper 2 (Th2)-type responses to an oral vaccine without altering mucosal IgA responses. *J Exp Med.* **185**, 415

Martin, J.T. (1997) Development of an adjuvant to enhance the immune response to influenza vaccine in the elderly. *Biologicals* **25**, 209-213.

Mc Cluskie MJ., and HL. Davis. (1998) Cutting edge : CpG DNA is a potent enhancer of systemic and mucosal immune responses against Hepatitis B surface antigen with intranasal administration to mice. *J. Immunol.* **161**, 4463

McElrath, M;J. (1994) Adjuvant effects on human immune responses in recipients of candidate HIV vaccines. *IBC Conference: Novel Vaccine Strategies for Mucosal Immunization, Genetic Approaches and Adjuvants.* Rockville, MD, pp. 24-26.

McGee DW., Elson CO., and JR. McGhee. (1993) Enhancing effect of cholera toxin on interleukin 6 secretion by IEC-6 intestinal epithelial cells : mode of action and augmenting effect of inflammatory cytokines. *Infect. Immun.* **61**, 4637

McSorley S., C. Rask, R. Pichot, V. Julia, C. Czerkinsky and N. Gleichenhaus. (1998) Selective tolerization of Th1 like cells after nasal administration of a cholera toxoid-LACK antigen. *Eur. J. Immunol.* **28**, 424

Medaglini D, Oggioni MR, Pozzi G. (1998) Vaginal immunization with recombinant gram-positive bacteria. *Am J Reprod Immunol.* **39**, 199-208

Medaglini D, Pozzi G, King TP, Fischetti VA. (1995) Mucosal and systemic immune responses to a recombinant protein expressed on the surface of the oral commensal bacterium Streptococcus gordonii after oral colonization. *Proc Natl Acad Sci* U S A. **92**, 6868-72

Medaglini D, Rush CM, Sestini P, Pozzi G. (1997) Commensal bacteria as vectors for mucosal vaccines against sexually transmitted diseases: vaginal colonization with recombinant streptococci induces local and systemic antibodies in mice. *Vaccine* **15**, 1330-7

Mega J., JR. McGhee, and H. Kiyono. (1992) Cytokine and Ig- producing cells in mucosal effector tissues. Analysis of IL-5 and IFNγ producing T cells, T cell receptor expression, and IgA plasma cells from mouse salivary glands associated tissues. *J. Immunol.* **148**, 2030

Mengiardi B., R. Berger, M. Just and R. Glück. (1995) Virosomes as carriers for combined vaccines. *Vaccine*, **13**, 1306

Meuer, S., Dumann, H., Meyer zum Büschenfelde, K.H., and Köhler, H. (1989) Low-dose interleukin-2 induces systemic immune responses against HBsAg in immunodeficient non-responders to hepatitis B vaccination, *Lancet* **1**, 15-18.

Michel, M.L., Pontisso, P., Sobczak, E., Malpiece, Y., Streeck, R.E., and Tiollais, P. (1984) Synthesis in animal cells of hepatitis B surface antigen particles carrying a receptor for polymerised human serum albumin, *Proc. Natl. Acad. Sci.* USA **81**, 7708-7712.

Michetti P, Dorta G, Wiesel PH, Brassart D, Verdu E, Herranz M, Felley C, Porta N, Rouvet M, Blum AL, Corthesy-Theulaz I. (1999) Effect of Whey-Based Culture Supernatant of Lactobacillus acidophilus (johnsonii) La1 on Helicobacter pylori Infection in Humans. *Digestion* **60**, 203-209

Miettinen M., S. Matikainen, J. Vuopio-Varkila, J. Pirhonen, K. Varkila, M. Kurimoto, and I. Julkunen. (1998) Lactobacilli and streptococci induce IL12, IL18 and IFNg production in human peripheral blood mononuclear cells. *Infect Immun.* **66**, 6058

Mitchell, M.S., Harel, W., Kempf, R.A., *et al.* (1990) Active-specific immunotherapy for melanoma. *J Clin Oncol.* **8**, 856-869.

Mitchell, M.S., Kan-Mitchell, J., Kempf, R.A., *et al.* (1988) Active specific immunotherapy for melanoma: Phase I trial of allogeneic lysates and a novel adjuvant, *Cancer Res.* **48**, 5883-5893.

Moldoveanu Z, L. Love-Homan, W. Qiang Huang and AM. Krieg. (1998) CpG DNA, a novel immune enhancer for systemic and mucosal immunisation with influenza virus, *Vaccine* **16**, 1216

Monjour, L., Monjour, E., Vouldoukis, I., *et al.* (1986) Protective immunity against cutaneous leishmaniasis achieved by partly purified vaccine in a volunteer. *Lancet* **1**, 1490.

Mora AL., and JP. Tam. (1998) Controlled lipidation and encapsulation of peptides as a useful approach to mucosal immunisations. *J. Immunol.* **161**, 3616

Morein B., M. Villacres-Eriksson and K. Lovgren-Bengtsson. (1998) ISCOM, a delivery system for parenteral and mucosal vaccination. *Dev. Biol. Stand.* **92**, 33

Morris, W., Steinhoff, M.C., and Russell, P. (1994) Potential of polymer microencapsulation technology for vaccine innovation, *Vaccine* **12**, 5-11.

Munoz, J. (1964) Effect of bacteria and bacterial products on antibody response, *Adv.Immunol.* **4**, 397-440.

Nardelli B., PB. Haser and JP Tam. (1994) Oral administration of an antigenic synthetic lipopeptide (MAP-P3C) evokes salivary antibodies and systemic humoral and cellular responses. *Vaccine* **12**, 1335

Nardelli-Haefliger D., JP. Kraehenbuhl, R. Curtis III, F. Schödel, A. Potts, S. Kelly and P. de Grandi. (1996) Oral and rectal immunisation of adult female volunteers with a recombinant attenuated Salmonella typhi vaccine strain. *Infect. Immun.* **64**, 5219

Newman, M.J., Wu, Y.J., Gardner, B.H., Munroe ,K.J., Leombruno, D., Recchai, J., Kensi, C.R., and Coughlin, R.T. (1992) Saponin adjuvant induction of ovalbumin-specific CD8+ cytotoxic T lymphocyte responses. *J Immunol.* **148**, 2357-2362.

Nieminen T., H. Käythy, A. Virolainen and J. Eskola. (1998) Circulating antibody secreting cell response to parenteral pneumococal vaccines as an indicator of a salivary IgA antibody response. *Vaccine*, **16**, 313.

Okada E., S. Sasaki, N. Ishii, I. Aoki, T. Yasuda, K. Nishioka, J. Fukushima, JI. Miyazaki, B. Wahren and K. Okuda. (1997) Intranasal immunisation of a DNA Vaccine with IL-12 and GM-CSF expressing plasmids in liposomes induces strong mucosal and cell-mediated immune responses against HIV1 antigens. *J. Immunol.* **159**, 3638

Olberling, F., Morin, A., Duclos, B., *et al.* (1983) Enhancement of antibody response to a natural fragment of streptococcal M protein by Murabutide administered to healthy volunteers, *Int J Immunol* .398.

Ott, G., Barchfeld, G.L., Chernoff, et al. (1995a) MF59: Design and evaluation of a safe and potent adjuvant for human vaccines, in M.F. Powell and M.J.Newman (eds.), *Vaccine Design: The Subunit and Adjuvant Approach*, New York, Plenum Press, pp. 277-296.

Ott, G., Barehfeld, G.L., and Van Nest, G.(1995b) Enhancement of humoral response against human influenza vaccine with the simple submicron oil/water emulsion adjuvant MF59, *Vaccine* **13**, 1557-1562.

Paglia P., I Arioli, N. Frahm, T. Chakraborty, MP. Colombo and CA. Guzman. (1997) The defined attenuated Listeria monocytogenes Del.mpl2 mutant is an effective oral vaccine carrier to trigger a long lasting immune response against a mouse fibrosarcoma. *Eur. J. Immunol.* **27**, 1570

Patou, G., Scott, G.M., Kelsey, M.C., Playfair, J.H.L. (1989) Gamma interferon as an adjuvant to hepatitis B vaccine (abstr), *J Interferon Res.* **9**, S261.

Paul, W.E., and Seder, R.A. (1994) Lymphocyte responses and cytokines. *Cell* **76**, 241-251.

Payne, L.G., Jenkins, S.A., Andrianov, A., Roberts, B.E. (1995) Water-soluble phosphazene polymers for parenteral and mucosal vaccine delivery. *Pharm Biotechnol.* **6**, 473-493.

Payne, L.G., Van Nest, G., Barchfeld, G.L., Siber, G.R., Gupta, R.K., and Jenkins, S.A. (1998) PCPP as a parenteral adjuvant for diverse antigens. *Dev. Biol. Stand.* **92**, 79-87.

Peterson JW, SS. Saini, WD Dickey, GR Klimpel, JS. Bomalaski, MA. Clark, KJ Xu and AK. Chopra. (1996) Cholera toxin induces synthesis of phospholipase A2-activating protein. *Infect. Immun.* **64**, 2137

Powell, M.F., Eastman, D.J., Lim, A., Lucas, C., Peterson, M., Vennari., J., Weissburg, R.P., Wrin, T., Kensil, C.R., and Newman, M.J. (1995) Effect of adjuvants on immunogenicity of MN recombinant glycoprotein 120 in guinea pigs, *AIDS Res Hum Retroviruses* **11**, 203-209.

Powers, D.C., Hanscomes, P.J., and Pietrobon, P.J.F. (1995) In previously immunized elderly adults inactivated influenza A (H1N1) virus vaccines induce poor antibody responses that are not enhanced by liposome adjuvant, *Vaccine* **13**, 1330-1335.

Putkonen, P., Nilsson, C., Walther, L., Ghavamzadeh, L., Hild, K., Broliden, K., Biberfeld, G., and Thorstensson, R. (1994) Efficacy of inactivated whole HIV-2 vaccines with various adjuvants in cynomolgus monkeys, *J Med Primatol*.**23**, 89-94.

Quiroga, J.A., Castillo, I., Porres, J.C., *et al.* (1990) Recombinant gamma-interferon as adjuvant to hepatitis B vaccine in hemodialysis patients, *Hepatology* **12**, 661-663.

Ramon, G. (1925) Sur l'augmentation anormale de l'antitoxine chez les chevaux producteurs de serum antidiphterique. *Bull Soc Centr Med Vet* **101**, 227-234.

Ramon, G. (1926) Procedés pour accroitre la production des antitoxines. *Ann Inst. Pasteur* **40**, 1-10.

Relyveld, E.H. (1986) Preparation and use of calcium phosphate adsorbed vaccines. *Dev. Biol. Stand.* **65**, 131-136.

Rickman, L.S., Gordon, D.M., Wistar, R.Jr., Krzych, U., Gross, M., Hollingdale, M.R., Egan, J.E., Chulay, J.D., Hoffman, S.L. (1991) Use of adjuvant containing mycobacterial cell-wall skeleton, monophosphoryl lipid A and squalene in malaria circumsporozoite protein vaccine, *Lancet* **337**, 998-1001.

Robbins JB, R. Schneerson and SC Szu. (1995) Perspective : hypothesis : serum IgG antibody is sufficient to confer protection against infectious diseases by inactivating the inoculum. *J. Infect. Dis.* **171**, 1387

Roberts M., A. Bacon, R. Rappuoli, M. Pizza, I. Cropley, G. Douce, G. Dougan, M. Marinaro, J. McGhee and S. Chatfield. (1995) A mutant pertussis toxin molecule that lacks ADP-Ribosyltransferase activity, PT-9K/129G, is an effective mucosal adjuvant for intranasally delivered proteins. *Infect Immun.* **63**, 2100

Rollwagen FM., and S. Baqar. Oral cytokine administration. (1996*) Immunology Today*, **17**, 548

Ryan ET., JR Butterton, T. Zhang, MA. Baker, SL Stanley Jr., SB. Calderwood. (1997) Oral immunisation with attenuated vacine strains of Vibrio cholerae expressing a dodecapeptide repeat of the serine-rich Entamoeba histolytica protein fused to the Choler toxin B subunit induces systemic and mucosal antiamebic and anti V. cholerae antibody responses in mice. *Infect. Immun.* **65**, 3118

Salk, J. and Salk, D. (1977) Control of influenza and poliomyelitis with killed virus vaccines, *Science* **195**, 834-847.

Scalzo, A.A., Elliott, S.L., Cox, J., Gardner, J., Moss, D.J., and Suhrbier, A. (1995) Induction of protective cytotoxic T cells to murine cytomegalovirus by using a nonapeptide and a human-compatible adjuvant (Montanide ISA 720), *J Virol.* **69**, 1306-1309.

Schultz, N., Oratz, R., Chen, D., *et al.* (1995) Effect of DETOX as an adjuvant for melanoma vaccine, *Vaccine* **13**, 503-508.

Scolnick, E.M., McLean, A.A., Wesr, D.J., McAleer, W.J., Miller, W.J., Buynack, E.B. (1984) Clinical evaluation in healthy adults of a hepatitis B vaccine made by recombinant DNA, *JAMA* **251**, 2812-2815.

Shahum, E. and Therien, H.M. (1995) Liposomal adjuvanticity: effect of encapsulation and surface-linkage on antibody production and proliferative response, *Intl. Immunopharmacol.* **17**, 9-20.

Shinomyia N., M. Kumai, DG. Marsh, and SK. Huang. (1993) Detection of specific IgE secreting cells with an enzyme-linked immunospot assay. *J. Allergy Clin. Immunol.* **92**, 479

Sinha K, P. Mastroeni, J. Harrison, R. Demarco de Hormaeche and CE. Hormaeche. (1997) Salmonella typhimurium aroA, htrA, and aeoD htrA mutants cause progressive infection in athymic (nu/nu) BALB/c mice. *Infect. Immun.* **65**, 1566

Sizemore DR., AA Branstrom and JC Sadoff. (1995) Attenuated Shigella as a DNA delivery vehicle for DNA-mediated immunisation. *Science* **270**, 299

Smith, G.L., Mackett, M., and Moss, B. (1983) Infectious vaccinia virus recombinants that express hepatitis B virus surface antigen, *Nature* **302**, 490-495.

Soltysik, S., Wu, J.Y., Recchia, J., Wheele,r D.A., Newman, M.J., Coughlin, R.T., and Kensil, C.R. (1995) Structure/function studies of QS-21 adjuvant: assessment of triterpene aldehyde and glucuronic acid roles in adjuvant function, *Vaccine* **13**, 1403-1410.

Staats HF., RJ. Jackson, M. Marinaro, I. Takahashi, H. Kiyono and J. Mc Ghee. (1994) Mucosal immunity to infection with implications for vaccine development. *Current Opinion in Immunol. 6*, 572

Stewart, G.T. (1985) Whooping cough and pertussis vaccine: a comparison of risks and benefits in Britain during the period 1968-83. *Dev. Biol. Stand* **61**, 395-405.

Stewart-Tull, D.E.S. (1994) (Ed.) *The Theory and Practical Application of Adjuvants.* John Wiley and Sons Ltd, Chichester,.

Stoute, J.A., Moncef-Slaoui, D., Gray-Heppner, D., Momin, P., *et al.* (1997) A preliminary evaluation of a recombinant circumsporozoite protein vaccine against Plasmodium falciparum malaria, *The New England Journal of Medicine* **336**, 86-91.

Straus, S.E., Wald, A., Kost, R.G., McKenzie, R., Langenberg, A.G., Hohman, P., Lekstrom, J., Cox, E., Nakamura, M., Sekulovich, R., Izu, A., Dekker, C. and Corey, L. (1997) Immunotherapy of recurrent genital herpes with recombinant herpes simplex virus type 2 glycoproteins D and B: results of a placebo-controlled vaccine trial, *J. Infect. Dis.* **176**, 1129-1134

Stuart-Harris, C.H. (1969) Adjuvant influenza vaccines, *Bull Wld Hlth Org* **41**, 617-621.

Stürchler, D., Berger, R., Etlinge,r H., *et al.* (1989) Effects of interferons on immune response to a synthetic peptide malaria sporozoite vaccine in non-immune adults, *Vaccine* **7**, 457-46l.

Stürchler, D., Zimmer, G., Berger, R., *et al.* (1990) Interferon-alpha and synthetic peptide malaria sporozoite vaccine in non-immune adults: antibody response after 40 weeks, *Bull WHO* **68**, 38-41.

Sun JB., J. Holmgren and C. Czerkinsky. (1994) Cholera toxin B subunit : an efficient transmucosal delivery system for induction of peripheral immunological tolerance. *Proc. Natl. Acad. Sci.* USA . **91**,10795

Tacket CO., SM. Kelly, F. Schödel, G. Losonsky, JP. Nataro, R. Edelman, MM. Levine and R. Curtis III. (1997) Safety and immunogenicity of an attenuated Salmonella typhi vaccine vector strain expressing plasmid-encoded Hepatitis B antigens stabilized by the Asd-balanced lethal vector system. *Infect. Immun.* **65**, 3381

Taguchi T., JR. McGhee, RL Coffman, KW. Beagley, JH. Eldridge, K. Takatsu and H. Kiyono. (1990) Analysis of Th1 and Th2 cells in murine gut associated tissues; frequencies of CD4+ and CD8+ cells that secrete IFNg and IL5. *J. Immunol.* **145**, 68

Takahashi I., M. Marinaro, H. Kiyono, RJ. Jackson, I. Nakagawa, K. Fujihashi, S. Hamada, JD Clements, KL. Bost and J. McGhee. (1996) Mechanisms for mucosal immunogenicity and adjuvancy of Escherichia coli labile enterotoxin. *J. Infect. Dis.* **173**, 627

Tamura SI., A. Yamanaka, M. Shimohara, T. Tomita, K. Komase, Y. Tsuda, Y. Suzuki, T. Nagamine, K. Kawahara, H. Danbara, C. Aizawa, A. Oya and T. Kurata. (1994) Synergistic action of cholera toxin B subunit (and Escherichia coli heat labile toxin B subunit) and a trace amount of cholera whole toxin as an adjuavnt for nasal influenza vaccine. *Vaccine* **12**, 419

Telzak, E., Wolff, S.M., Dinarello, C.A., *et al.* (1986) Clinical evaluation of the immunoadjuvant murabutide, a derivative of MDP, administered with a tetanus toxoid vaccine, *J. Infect. Dis.* **153**, 628-633.

Thoelen, S., Van Damme, P., Mathei, C., Leroux-Roels, G., Desombere, I., Safary, A., Vandepapeliere, P., Slaoui, M. and Meheus, A. (1998) Safety and immunogenicity of a hepatitis B vaccine formulated with a novel adjuvant system. *Vaccine* **16**, 708-714

Todryck SM., CG. Kelly and T. Lehner. (1998) Effect of route of immunisation and adjuvant on T and B cell epitope recognition within a streptococcal antigen. *Vaccine* **16**, 174

Tough, D.F., Sun, S. and Sprent, J. (1997) T cell stimulation in vivo by lipopolysaccharide (LPS), *J. Exp. Med.* **185**, 2089-2094.

Trajman A., TT McDonald and CC. Elia. (1997) Intestinal immune cells in Strongyloides stercoralis infection. *J. Clin Pathol.* **50**, 991

Trauger, R.J., Ferre, F., Daigle, A.E., *et al.* (1994) Effect of immunization with inactivated gp120-depleted human immunodeficiency virus type 1 (HIV-l) immunogen on HIV-l immunity, viral DNA, and percentage of CD4 cells, *J Infect Dis* **169**, 1256-1264.

Triozzi, P.T., Martin, E.W., Gochnour, D., and Aldrich, W. (1993) Phase Ib trial of synthetic □ human chorionic gonadotropin vaccine patients with metastatic cancer, *Ann. NY. Acad. Sci.* **690**, 358-359.

Turner, J.L., Slade, H.B., Trauger, R.J., *et al.* (1992) Double-blind placebo-controlled dose ranging study of Salk immunogen in asymptomatic patients with early human immunodeficiency virus infection (PoB3043) (abstr). Program and abstracts, *VIII International Conference on AIDS/III STD World Congress (Amsterdam)* B94.

Unanue, E.R. (1985) Antigen-presenting function of the macrophage, *Ann. Rev. Immunol.* **2**, 395-428.

Valensi, J-P.M., Carlson, J.R. and Nest, G.A.V. (1994) Systemic cytokine profiles in BALB/c mice immunized with trivalent Influenza vaccine containing MF59 oil emulsion and other advanced adjuvants, *J. Immunol.* **143**, 4029-4039.

Valenzuela, P., Medina A., Rutter, W.J., Ammerer, G. and Hall, B.D. (1982) Synthesis and assembly of hepatitis B virus surface antigen particles in yeast, *Nature* **298**, 347-350.

van Besouw NM, van der Meide PH and Bakker NPM. (1994) The mitogen-induced generation of interferon gamma producing cells in cultures of rhesus monkey PBMC is age dependant. *J. Medical Primatology*, 23/ 42

Van Hoecke, C., Koutsoukos, M., Thiriat, C., *et al.* (1995) Humoral and cellular immune responses to three formulations of inactivated split influenza vaccine (ISIV) adjuvanted with QS-21, *35th Interscience Conference on Antimicrobial Agents and Chemotherapy*, Abstract 189.

VanCott JL., TA. Brim, RA. Simkins, and LJ. Saif. (1993) Isotype specific antibody secreting cells to transmissible gastroenteritis virus and porcine respiratory coronavirus in gut and bronchus associated lymphoid tisues of suckling pigs. *J. Immunol.* **150**, 3990

Vetvik H., HMS. Grewal, IL Haugen, C. Ahren and Bjorn Haneberg. (1998) Mucosal antibodies can be measured in air dried samples of saliva and feces. *J. Immunol. Methods.* **215**, 163

Villacres-Eriksson, M. (1995) Antigen presentation by naive macrophages, dendritic cells and B cells to primed T lymphocytes and their cytokine production following exposure to immunostimulating complexes, *Clin. Exp. Immunol.* **102**, 46-52.

Vogel, F.R. and Powell, M.F. (1995) A compendium of vaccine adjuvants and excipients. in M.F. Powell and M.J Newman (eds), *Vaccine Design: The Subunit and Adjuvant Approach.* New York, Plenum Press, pp.141-228.

Waldo FB., AWL. Van den Wall Bake, J. Mestecky and S. Husby. (1994)Suppression of the immune response by nasal immunisation. *Clin. Immunol. and Immunopathology.* **72**, 30

Walker RI. (1994)New strategies for using mucosal vaccination to achieve more effective immunisation. *Vaccine*, **12**, 87

Walker RI., and JD. Clements. (1993) Use of heat-labile toxin of enterotoxigenic Escherichia coli to facilitate mucosal immunisation. *Vaccine Research*, **2**, 1.

Wassef, N.M., Alving, C.R., and Richards, R.L. (1994) Liposomes as carriers for vaccines, *Immunomethods* **4**, 217-222.

Wiktor, T.J., Atanasiu, P., Bahmanyar, M., Boegel, K., Cox, J.H., Diaz, A.M., Fitzgerald, E.A., Kuwert, E., Netter, R., Selimov, M., Turner, G. and Van Steenis, G. (1978) Comparison studies on potency tests for rabies vaccines, *Dev. Biol. Stand.* **40**, 171-178.

Woolridge, R.L., Grayston, J.T., Chang, I.A., *et al.* (1967) Long-term follow-up of the initial (1959-1960) trachoma vaccine field on Taiwan, *Am J Ophthalmol.* **63**, 1650-1653.

Xu Amano J., RJ. Jackson, K. Fujihashi, H. Kiyono, HF. Staats and J. McGhee. (1994) Helper Th1 and Th2 cell responses following mucosal or systemic immunisation with cholera toxin. *Vaccine* **12**, 903.

Yamamoto M., DE Briles, S. Yamamoto, M. Ohmura., H. Kiyono and J. McGhee. (1998)A non toxic adjuvant for mucosal immunity to pneumococal surface protein A. *J. Immunol.* **161**, 4115

Zhou F., JP. Kraehenbuhl and M. Neutra. (1995)Mucosal IgA response to rectally administered antigen formulated in IgA-coated liposomes. *Vaccine*, **13**, 637

CHAPTER 3

Influence of Resident Intestinal Microflora on the Development and Functions of the Intestinal-associated Lymphoid Tissue

M C Moreau and V Gaboriau-Routhiau

3.1 Introduction

Gut-associated lymphoid tissue (GALT) is under constant exposure to environmental antigens. The digestive flora is the main antigenic stimulus. A huge population of live bacterial cells, estimated at 10^{14} in number, colonises the human gastrointestinal tract (Luckey and Floch, 1972). Bacterial numbers and composition vary considerably along the gastrointestinal tract, constituting complex ecosystems which depend on the physiology of the host and on interactions between bacteria. It has recently been shown that GALT has the ability to develop tolerance towards resident bacterial flora (Duchmann, 1995). Conversely, the digestive flora considerably influences the development and functioning of GALT. To understand the relationships between the digestive flora and GALT, it is important to consider the evolution of bacterial equilibrium during the main biological stages of life, from a digestive point of view, *i.e.* infancy (up to 2 years of age), adulthood and old age, as well as the bacterial colonisation of the different parts of the intestine.

In this chapter, we will begin by dealing with the role of the resident digestive flora on the development and functions of GALT. Then, we will focus on the neo-natal period which could be of particular importance for protection against some pathologies such as allergy and hypersensitivities.

3.2 Resident intestinal flora

3.2.1 Development of intestinal flora in newborns

Digestive flora in new-borns is developed sequentially according to the maturation of intestinal mucosa and dietary diversification.

In healthy conditions, the human baby's intestine is sterile at birth but, within less than 48 hours, 10^8 to 10^9 bacteria can be found in 1 g of faeces (reviewed in Raibaud, 1988; Hudault, 1996). The first bacteria

R. Fuller and G. Perdigon (eds.), Probiotics 3, 69–114.

colonising the baby's intestine come from the environment, with maternal faecal flora representing the most important and obviously best adapted source of bacterial contamination. However, there are large differences between the paucity of the bacterial species colonising the intestine of new-borns, and the very complex flora of the adult. Just after birth, only the facultative anaerobic bacteria *Escherichia coli* and *Streptococcus* can colonise the intestine of a baby. Two to 4 days later, an anaerobic flora can develop but only certain anaerobic bacteria, such as *Bifidobacterium, Bacteroides,* and *Clostridium,* are found. Although factors responsible for the growth of these first selected bacteria are not clearly identified, it is hypothesised that they may be endogenous factors, such as maturation of the intestinal mucosa, growth promoters or inhibitors present in the meconium, or exogenous factors. The main exogenous factor is the nature of the diet which plays a crucial role as shown by the differences between the intestinal flora of breast-fed babies and that of bottle-fed babies. In exclusively breast-fed babies, *Bifidobacterium, Escherichia coli* and *Streptococcus* compose the predominant faecal microflora, while in bottle-fed babies it consists of various bacteria, *i.e. Bifidobacterium, Bacteroides, Clostridia,* and other *Enterobacteria.* Thereafter, according to dietary diversification, the digestive flora is enriched by the development of other strictly anaerobic bacteria.

Weaning time is a crucial period during which deep changes in the digestive microflora equilibrium occur. Due to the instability of the baby's bacterial equilibrium and, consequently, the incapacity of the digestive flora to resist colonisation, the intestine can be colonised by opportunistic pathogens. The intestinal flora of human infants then reaches the stage of the adult flora at an age which has not yet been accurately defined, but which is presumably at about 2 years of age.

Bacterial colonisation in mice shows some differences with that of the human baby (Schaedler *et al.*, 1965; Moreau *et al.*, 1982). During the first week of life only facultative anaerobic bacteria, such as *Lactobacillus* and *Streptococcus,* colonise the new-born's intestine. Then, at the beginning of the second week of life, *Escherichia coli* reaches a high level. The first anaerobic bacteria develop at around day 15, when mice begin to take in solid food. The weaning time, at around 3 weeks of age, is correlated with the development of a lot of new bacterial strains, especially extremely oxygen-sensitive anaerobic bacteria which make up most of the flora at this time. During the weaning period the interactions between nutrients, digestive flora and GALT are closely dependent, making this period crucial to the development of the young. The digestive intestinal flora seems to be stabilised and representative of adult flora at around 6 weeks of age (Moreau *et al.*, 1986).

3.2.2 *Intestinal flora in adults*

More data is available on the location of bacterial flora in the different parts of the gut in human adults. The total bacterial count in gastric content is usually 10^3 to 10^4/g, with numbers being kept low due to pH acid. The situation is different in mice where facultative anaerobic bacteria, *Lactobacillus*, *Streptococcus*, are present at high levels throughout life. In humans, as in mice, the small intestine constitutes a transition zone with numbers of bacteria ranging from approximately 10^4 bacteria/ml of intestinal content in its proximal part to 10^7-10^8/ml at the ileocaecal region. In parallel, human microflora, essentially composed of Gram-positive facultative anaerobes, progressively enriches with Gram-negative species and a few strict anaerobes (Ducluzeau, 1989). The main factors limiting growth in the small intestine are rapid peristalsis (transit of content) and secretion of bile and pancreatic juice (King and Toskes, 1979).

The large intestine (*i.e.* caecum and colon) of humans and mice is the most intensely colonised region, essentially because of digestive stasis. It is generally accepted that faecal microflora adequately represents that of the colon. This large population (10^{10} to 10^{11} bacteria/g of intestinal content) is dominated by the strict anaerobes and also contains extremely oxygen-sensitive bacteria (Moore and Holdeman, 1974; Finegold *et al.*, 1983). The situation leads to a certain amount of difficulty in studying colonic microflora with classical microbiological methods which are based almost entirely on phenotypic approaches and the cultivation of bacteria on selective media. Although several hundred species of bacteria have been observed in the human colon only a few have been identified. The individual bacterial counts range over several orders of magnitude. Thus, bacterial species established at levels over 5.10^7-10^8 bacteria/g characterise the predominant microflora, whereas those below such a threshold compose the subdominant microflora. In fact, it is believed that only predominant bacteria are able to exert a measurable function. The complex human intestinal microflora is relatively stable in composition and the predominant species commonly isolated from the human colon belong to the genera *Bacteroides*, *Eubacterium*, *Bifidobacterium*, *Ruminococcus* and *Clostridium*. Subdominant species include enterobacteria, particularly *Escherichia coli*, and *Streptococci* (Savage, 1977; Finegold *et al.*, 1983; reviewed in Salminen *et al.*, 1998). Whereas *Lactobacilli* are predominant in mice, they are frequently subdominant in humans or cannot even be detected. Conversely, *Bifidobacterium*, which can be found at high levels in human flora, are absent from mice.

Table 3.1. Main physiologic functions of the indigenous intestinal microflora

Modification of intestinal content :	• pH, ↓ redox potential • production of metabolites (vitamins, digestive enzymes…) • reduction of metabolites (urea, cholesterol, triglycerides…)
Anatomic modification of the digestive tract :	• ↓ caecal volume • ↑ enterocytes renewal rate • ↓ villus morphometry
Modification of digestive physiology :	• ↑ transit of gastric and intestinal content • ↑ absorption of abiotic components
Improved resistance to gastrointestinal infection :	• barrier effect • modulation of toxin production in the intestine
Stimulation of immune functions	

Although the predominant human intestinal microflora is relatively stable from the perspective of bacterial genera, recent studies using 16S rRNA-based approaches have shown that each individual harbours a specific bacterial community which increases the complexity already described (MacCartney *et al.*, 1996; Zoetendal *et al.*, 1998). Nevertheless, the predominant microbial composition remains quite constant over a period of at least 6 months for healthy individuals (Zoetendal *et al.*, 1998). In addition to individual differences and the influence of age (infant *vs.* adult), some studies have shown that factors such as stress (Holdeman *et al.*, 1976) or antibiotic treatments (Borriello, 1995) also induce variations in human intestinal bacterial microflora, resulting in subdominant species or even pathogens becoming more dominant. Very little data exists on the evolution of intestinal microflora in the elderly. Nonetheless, bifidobacteria have been reported to decrease at old age, which may be related to a reduced adhesion to the intestinal mucus (Ouwehand *et al.*, 1999).

Indigenous intestinal microflora plays several roles, listed in Table 3.1. Two of them are especially important in human health: colonisation resistance to maintain microbial composition in an apathogenic and stable state (Van Der Waaij, 1993) and stimulation of the intestinal immune system, which will be developed below.

3.3 Influence of resident intestinal microflora on the development of GALT

The first year of life is a crucial period for human infants. At birth, the human GALT is poorly developed, while its functionality is essential for survival. The relationship between development and functionality of GALT is not clearly understood. GALT is quickly confronted with a large quantity of foreign antigens mainly represented by the digestive microflora. This period of time is also the moment when the risk of enteric infections and hypersensitivities to food proteins are the highest. Environmental and behavioural factors (stress, hormones, etc.) influence the development of GALT (Husband and Gleeson, 1996). Many observations support the notion that most mucosal immune cells are competent even before birth, but they need to undergo an activation process initiated by environmental signals. Experimental data reported here shows the enormous influence of the presence of digestive flora on GALT.

The digestive flora has a dual function. First of all, it is the main antigenic stimulus responsible for the activation and development of GALT. Secondly, through regulatory mechanisms, it modulates GALT functions. From these experimental studies, we can postulate that the digestive flora also plays an important role on the development and functions of GALT in humans.

To understand the effects of the digestive flora on the development of GALT, it is necessary to know what the structure of GALT is at birth and what changes appear after birth. As direct evidence from human subjects is scarce, we will report the possible roles of the digestive flora on these changes on the basis of experiments using germ-free (GF) animals.

3.3.1 Development of GALT in newborns

Peyer's patches

At birth, developed Peyer's patches (PP) are present in the human small intestine. They contain primary lymphoid follicles, T-cell dependent areas, a dome region and follicle-associated epithelium. However, as no antigenic stimulation exists in the foetus, secondary follicles with germinal centres are absent. The first activated lymphoid follicles with germinal centres appear several weeks after birth (reviewed in Brandtzaeg, 1998; MacDonald, 1994).

Lamina propria

The lamina propria (LP) of the small intestine is structurally well formed at birth but the cellularity is greatly reduced. There are no IgA-secreting cells (IgA-SC), while the machinery for production of secretory IgA (sIgA) response is in place before birth (J chain and secretory component). IgA-SC appear after 2-4 weeks of age and the number increases with time, reaching adult level by 1-2 years of age (Brandtzaeg, 1998; MacDonald, 1994). In contrast, saliva and serum levels of IgA take longer to reach adult concentration (around 6 years of age). In growing conventional (CV) mice, the first IgA immunocytes appear in the lamina propria at weaning time and a number equivalent to the adult stage is reached 3 weeks later, i.e. in 6-week-old mice (Crabbé *et al.*, 1970). The development is closely correlated to the increased level of IgA in serum. This difference between humans and mice could be due to the fact that there is only one class of IgA in mice and two subclasses, IgA1 and IgA2, in humans which seem to develop at different rates and respond to different antigenic stimuli. IgA1 is predominant in human serum and the adult level is reached at around 6 years of age. In intestinal mucosa, there is a heterogeneous distribution of the two IgA subclasses of immunocytes (reviewed in Brandtzaeg, 1995). IgA1 cells are in large number in the duodenum and jejunum (approximately 77%), whereas IgA2 cells predominate in the colon (64%). IgA2 are more resistant to microbial proteases than are IgA1. Moreover, an IgA1 antibody response is obtained after stimulation with a protein antigen (Underdown and Mestecky, 1994), while IgA2 antibodies are directed towards lipopolysaccharides (LPS) from Gram-negative bacteria which are abundant in the colon. A recent work (Kette *et al.*, 1995) has shown that an abnormal bacterial overgrowth in human jejunal segments alters the IgA subclass distribution with a preferential IgA2 production. Taken together, this data leads to the hypothesis that, among the unknown factors which influence a preferential IgA1 or IgA2 response, the presence of the digestive flora may be responsible for the induction of a preferential switch to a antibody response belonging to the IgA2 subclass.

There are few reports on LP T cells. At birth, the LP contains T cells which are capable of secreting cytokines such as IFN-γ and IL-2 when stimulated with superantigens (Lionetti *et al.*, 1993). They are predominantly of the helper phenotype (MacDonald, 1994). However, the majority of T cells colonise the LP only after antigenic activation (Halstensen *et al.*, 1990). It is conceivable that an expansion of T cells occurs in the LP after bacterial colonisation of the intestine and stimulation of the T cell precursors present in the PP.

Concerning endothelial adhesion molecules (ICAM-1, VCAM-1 and E-selectin), which play an important role in the recruitment of immune cells in the intestine, studies have shown that they are potentially present at birth and that antigenic stimulation leads to their expression on LP endothelium (Dohan *et al.*, 1993).

Epithelium

There are few intra-epithelial lymphocytes (IEL) in the intestinal epithelium of human new-borns. They are mainly $CD3^+CD8^+$ T cells. Their number increases slowly throughout pregnancy, but after birth it increases up to ten-fold by 1-2 years of age, suggesting the strong influence of antigenic stimulation on this post-natal expansion (Cerf-Bensussan and Guy-Grand, 1991). In mice, the homodimeric $\alpha\alpha$ $CD8^+$ subpopulation is present in suckling mice. The $\gamma\delta$-TCR appears during late foetal and perinatal development, while the $\alpha\beta$-TCR appear later, in adult life (Guy-Grand *et al.*, 1991)

In humans, the expression of the epithelial class II molecules at birth is the subject of controversy. According to several studies, their expression has been found to be present both before birth (MacDonald *et al.*, 1988) and after birth (Rognum *et al.*, 1992). In the latter case, the expression begins approximately one week after birth and reaches the adult level at around one month of age. In growing mice, MHC class II molecules are absent at birth but gradually increase on small intestinal epithelial cells after weaning (Hughes *et al.*, 1991).

Antigen-Presenting cells

Antigen-presenting cells (APC), represented by dendritic cells (DC) and macrophage populations, are located in the LP and PP. Lymph DC may arise from both sites. The major function of DC in immune response is thought to be the acquisition of antigen and its transport to draining lymph nodes where it is presented to T lymphocytes.

For human new-borns, no information is available regarding the distribution, numbers or function of APC in the intestine. Little data exists on mucosal DC from experimental animals. Measurement of the postnatal development of the airway intraepithelium DC network in rats showed that the number of DC expressing Ia molecules and the intensity of the Ia expression were low at birth and increased to adult levels around the time of weaning (MacWilliams and Holt, 1997). The same results were reported in neonatal mice where a small number of peritoneal macrophages and splenic adherent cells bear major histocompatibility complex (MHC) class II molecules. However, it was possible to increase the rate of postnatal development of the intestinal DC population in rats by i.p. administration of IFN-γ, suggesting that the maturation of DC could depend on inflammatory stimuli, and the establishment of the bacterial flora could afford such stimuli (MacWilliams and Holt, 1997).

The ability of DC to interact effectively with peripheral T cells did not occur until 3-4 weeks after birth in mice (Lu *et al.*, 1979). Because of the fundamental role of the APC in delivering adequate costimulatory signals to naive T cells, a deficiency in the APC function could be a chief explanation for the immunological immaturity of new-borns at the systemic level (Ridge *et al.*, 1996). This fact may explain why an antigenic stimulus in neonatal life is a tolerogenic rather than an immunogenic event.

3.4 Role of intestinal microflora on the development of GALT

According to substantial experimental data showing that extensive GALT modification occurs at weaning time in mice, it has often been postulated that such change could be due to the new antigenic proteins introduced in the diet. In fact, as previously mentioned, at weaning important changes in the digestive flora are directly correlated to dietary changes. To discriminate between the antigenic stimuli afforded by digestive microflora and dietary proteins on the development of GALT, GF rodents were used. The effect of the antigenic stimulation provoked by dietary proteins can be observed in GF animals fed on an antigen-free diet (Wostmann and Pleasants, 1991). On the basis of this data, it is obvious that the bacterial flora, instead of food antigens, is the major stimulus for the induction of the sudden increase in intestinal mucosal cellularity. It is now important to learn to what extent these effects are operative in humans.

In experimental studies, the role of the digestive flora is determined by comparison between GF and CV animals. As new-borns, GF animals exhibit an underdeveloped intestinal immune system which can be rapidly normalised by bacterial colonisation of the intestine with the faecal flora from a CV animal (i.e. oral inoculation with a fresh 1/100 dilution of CV faecal sample). It is, then, interesting to know the bacterial strains responsible for the immunomodulating effect observed. Gnotobiotic mice, ex-GF mice colonised with known bacteria which originate from human flora, are used for this purpose. After oral colonisation, the bacteria expand rapidly to colonise the intestine to a very high level within one day. A period of 3 weeks is estimated to be the time required for an optimal stimulatory effect on the digestive flora.

3.4.1 Peyer's patches

As in human new-borns, PP are poorly developed in GF mice. The germinal centres are absent, showing that their development is directly under the influence of the digestive flora (Parrot, 1976; Kramer and Cebra, 1995). $CD4^+$ T cells are found in Peyer's patches of GF mice but, in contrast to CV mice, they are CD45RBlow, indicative of naive or unprimed T cells. Colonisation of GF mice with intestinal flora shifts this population to a majority of CD45RBhigh, within 4-8 weeks, suggesting a non-specific role for resident bacterial flora in activating GALT $CD4^+$ T cells (Cebra *et al.*, 1999). Changes in bacterial intestinal colonisation lead to a modification in the number of M cells which are known to play a crucial role in the first step of the induction of mucosal immune responses (Smith *et al.*, 1987).

3.4.2 Lamina propria

PP are an important source of progenitor cells for intestinal IgA-SC (Craig and Cebra, 1971; Guy-Grand *et al.*, 1974). Another source of progenitor cells seems to be the $CD5^+$ B cells, also called B-1 cells, which are present in the peritoneal cavity in mice (Kroese *et al.*, 1989). It appears that up to 40% of LP IgA-SC are derived from B-1 cells in mice and humans (reviewed in Beagley *et al.*, 1998). Several authors have shown that the intestinal microbial flora plays a pivotal role on the development of the intestinal IgA-SC number. It is unknown if this effect is operative on the precursor cells present in the PP or/and on the $CD5^+$ B cells. However, according to Crabbé *et al.* (1968), who first reported that less than 10% of IgA-SC are present in GF mice as compared with CV mice, it is conceivable that the intestinal flora exerts its stimulating effect on both B cell lineages.

Three weeks after bacterial colonisation of the intestine, GF mice have an IgA-SC number equivalent to that found in CV mice. As in growing CV mice, the adult number is only reached at 6 weeks of age (Crabbé *et al.*, 1970), it has been suggested that the immaturity of the immune system of new-born and/or the suppressive effect of the mother's milk could be responsible for this delay. In fact, despite the beneficial effect of breast-feeding in new-borns, it is believed that maternal antibodies may have a suppressive effect on the development of mucosal immune responses in young, leading to a partially developed immune system at weaning (reviewed in Husband, 1996). Studies in mice nursing for a prolonged time have shown a reduced quantity of IgA in intestinal washings at 5 weeks of age compared to naturally weaned litters, suggesting an active role for maternal antibodies in delaying natural IgA responses (Kramer *et al.*, 1995). As previously described, studies in mice have shown that the sequential establishment of the digestive flora is strongly influenced by the diversification of the diet in infancy, and that weaning is a crucial period for the development of new bacteria in the intestine. Thus, the suppressive effect of the maternal antibody effect on the development of intestinal immune responses may be related to the paucity of the digestive flora which can only exert a partial stimulating effect on the intestinal IgA-SC number. To test this hypothesis, several models of gnotobiotic mice were created and then colonised by the entire digestive flora present in growing CV mice from 1 day after birth to 4 days after weaning (25 days of age) (Moreau *et al.*, 1982). IgA-SC numbers were evaluated by immunohistochemical observations 4 weeks after bacterial colonisation. In these experimental models, the effect of maternal milk and the immaturity of the neonate were discarded and only the stimulating effect of the digestive flora was tested. Digestive floras of mice 3 to 21 days old exerted only a partial stimulating effect on the intestinal IgA-SC number in gnotobiotic recipients (Table 3.2). However, gnotobiotic recipients colonised with the digestive flora of 25-day-old mice have a similar IgA-SC number to that found in adult CV mice.

Table 3.2. Effect of the sequential establishment of the digestive flora of growing conventional mice on the maturation of IgA plasma cells measured in gnotobiotic mice

Gnotobiotic mice harbouring the digestive flora of :	IgA plasma cell number /villus
Adult conventional mice	41± 1
Adult germ-free	4± 0.5
Growing conventional mice 1 to 4 days old	15 ± 2
Growing conventional mice 7 to 23 days old	23± 1
Growing conventional mice 25 days old	43 ± 1

Results are expressed in mean numbers ± SEM.

These results obviously show the important role played by the sequential establishment of the digestive flora in the sequential development of the intestinal IgA-SC and the pivotal role of the bacteria colonising the intestine after weaning in this process. Results have now been confirmed by other studies (Van Der Heijden *et al.*, 1989; Kramer *et al.*, 1995) showing that neither the age of weaning nor milk antibodies played a direct role in IgA-SC development, but rather that weaning itself has an impact through its effect on the digestive flora composition. Moreover, taking into account the 3-week delay between the bacterial stimulus and the intestinal IgA-SC response, these results showed that the neonate is capable of developing an IgA response at birth, the intensity of which depends on the stimulating capacity of the intestinal bacteria present in the intestine.

It is tempting to project such results into infants where the full development of the intestinal IgA-SC number observed at 2 years of age is correlated to the stabilisation of the digestive bacterial equilibrium.

Attempts have been made to elucidate the role played by individual bacterial strains present in the digestive flora of CV growing mice (Moreau *et al.*, 1978). From several gnotobiotic mice colonised with different single digestive bacteria, it was shown that Gram-positive bacteria had only a slightly stimulating effect (Table 3.3). The association of Gram positive bacteria led to a stimulatory effect which could be due to an additive effect. In contrast, a single Gram-negative bacterium, such as *E. coli* or *Bacteroides*, provoked a partial increase in the IgA-SC number.

Table 3.3. Effect of different bacterial strains isolated from the intestinal flora of growing conventional mice on the maturation of intestinal IgA plasma cells in gnotobiotic mice.

Bacterial strains	IgA plasma cell number/villus
Micrococcus	3± 1
Corynebacterium	3± 1
Eubacterium	5± 1
Lactobacillus	7± 1
Streptococcus	8 ± 2
Actinobacillus	10 ± 2
Escherichia coli	18 ± 3
Bacteroides	18 ± 3
E.coli + *Bacteroides*	17 ± 2
Conventional mice flora	41 ± 1
Germ-free mice	3 ± 1

Results are expressed in mean numbers ± SEM.

A similar stimulating effect was found with dead *E. coli* or *Bacteroides*, under the condition that the dead bacteria were given orally in the drinking water at a concentration of over 10^7 cells/ml (Moreau *et al.*, 1984). This effect was probably due to the lipopolysaccharides (LPS) present in the cell wall of Gram-negative bacteria, as demonstrated by MacGhee *et al.* (1984). Unfortunately, because of the difficulties in isolating and cultivating the EOS bacterial species which established after weaning, we failed to learn the bacteria, or the bacterial equilibrium which are responsible for the complete development of the IgA-SC numbers (Moreau *et al.*, 1978).

In contrast to extensive studies on LP plasma cells, there is considerably less information on the role of intestinal flora on development of LP T lymphocytes. In a study using pigs, Rothkotter *et al.*

(1991) showed that sub-populations of T cells differ substantially between GF and CV animals.

3.4.3 Epithelium

Intra-epithelial lymphocytes. IEL are found in both the small intestine and the colon in humans and mice. In mice there are marked differences in the distribution and percentages of IEL expressing αβ or γδ TCR between the large intestine, where the TCR-αβ T cells (αβ IEL) predominate, and the small intestine, where TCR-γδ T cells (γδ IEL) predominate. In human αβ IEL predominate both in the small intestine and the colon. (Beagley *et al.*, 1995).

The biological roles of IEL are still mysterious. To clarify the function of IEL, it would be interesting to know what their reactivity towards exogenous antigenic stimuli is. The numbers, phenotypes and cytolytic activities of IEL differ greatly between GF and CV mice, while αβ- and γδ-IEL seem to respond to different kinds of antigenic stimulation. There is a marked influence of the microbial intestinal colonisation on the number of single positive $CD4^+$ or $CD8^+$ αβ IEL, but little effect on the pool size of γδ-IEL (Bandeira *et al.*, 1990; Stepankova *et al.*, 1998). Moreover, Guy-Grand *et al.* (1991) have shown that the thymo-independent homodimeric αα $CD8^+$ subpopulation of IEL (all the γδ-IEL and part of the αβ IEL) is always present in GF mice. Thus, the subsets of IEL responding to the microbial stimulation are thymo-dependent precursor T cells present in PP. Conventionalisation of GF mice has shown that in 28 days the same percentage of αβ-IEL is reached as that found in CV mice (Umesaki *et al.*, 1993).

In a recent study, Kawaguchi *et al.* (1996) compare the effect of microbial and dietary antigens on the cytolytic activity of αβ-IEL and γδ-IEL in CV, GF and GF mice fed on an antigen-minimized diet (AgM-GF mice). Results show that the development of cytolytic activation of αβ-IEL is sharply attenuated in GF mice, but the number and cytotoxicity of γδ-IEL are comparable between CV and GF mice. In contrast, the cytolytic activities of γδ-IEL, as well as those of αβ-IEL, decrease remarkably in AgM-GF mice (Table 3.4).

Table 3.4. Effect of the deprivation of digestive microbial and food antigens on the number and cytolytic activity of IEL (from Kawaguchi-Miyashita *et al.*, 1996)

	Control mice (CV mice)	Microbial deprivation (GF mice)	Antigen deprivation (GF mice fed with an Ag-minimized diet)
IEL numbers			
• αβ-IEL	100%	50%	30%
• γδ-IEL	100%	100%	80% (NS)
Cytolytic activity			
• αβ-IEL	100%	50%	10%
• γδ-IEL	100%	100%	30%

Although the function of IEL is a subject of debate, these results showing that the cytolytic activity of γδ-IEL is only under the influence of the antigenic composition of the diet, suggest a role of the IEL subset in relationship with dietary antigens. Microbial antigens are quantitatively low in the small intestine, which is a relatively sterile environment, while food proteins are found in large quantities in the upper part of the small intestine. γδ-IEL respond to food proteins and proliferate more rapidly in the duodenum, where food antigens flow in large quantities, than in the ileum (Kawaguchi *et al.*, 1996). It has been suggested that γδ-IEL are involved in the induction and maintenance of oral tolerance to food-proteins (Ke *et al.*, 1997; Mengel *et al.*, 1995). Conversely, the observation that αβ-IEL, abundant in the colon, are deeply influenced in their number and cytolytic activity by the presence of the digestive microflora supports the idea that this population may act against enteric pathogens in the colon.

Human and murine αβ IEL have been shown to express an oligoclonal TCR repertoire. In mice, the same TCR repertoire appears to predominate in all the parts of the intestine, but it differs from mice with an identical genetic- and environmental background (Regnault *et al.*, 1994). Interestingly, the digestive flora is not responsible for oligoclonality of the repertoire since the TCRβ repertoire of the CD8αα or CD8αβ IEL populations in GF mice shows the same degree of oligoclonality as in CV mice (Regnault *et al.*, 1996). Recent studies in rats show that the microbial colonisation of GF rats influences the TCR Vβ repertoire of $CD8^+$ T cells. The proportions of Vβ8.2+ and Vβ10 increase, whereas Vβ8.5+ and Vβ16+ cells decrease somewhat (Helgeland *et al.*, 1996). These findings support the hypothesis that the

TCR α/β repertoire of IEL could be directed against bacterial antigens. In contrast, the TCR Vβ repertoire in mesenteric lymph nodes was not affected after microbial colonisation.

Class II molecules. The expression of MHC class II molecules on small intestinal epithelial cells is closely associated with bacterial colonisation of the intestine (Matsumoto *et al.*, 1992). The authors have shown that in GF mice, although class I molecules are expressed on the small intestinal epithelium, class II molecules are absent. In their study conventionalisation of GF mice provoked a gradual expression of class II molecules in the small intestine. However, there were differences in the delays and regions of expression of I-A and I-E molecules. The I-A molecule was induced on the villus tip and crypt epithelial cells 7 days after conventionalisation, whereas the I-E molecule was induced on the mid villus and crypt epithelial cells 14 days after conventionalisation. Both I-A and I-E molecules were fully expressed 21 days after conventionalisation. It has been shown that the expression of class II molecules is modulated by IFN-γ secretion (Vidal *et al.*, 1993) and bacterial colonisation might cause intestinal IEL to release IFN-γ.

In another study, using the kidney as representative of non-lymphoid tissue, class II molecules were expressed at the same level in GF and CV mice (Cokfield *et al.*, 1990). The discrepancy between the two studies may arise from different epithelium studied. Indeed, an equal presence of MHC class II-A was observed on spleen and lymph node cells from both CV and GF mice, suggesting the constitutive, antigen-independent expression of these molecules at the peripheral level.

3.4.4 Antigen-presenting cells

It appears that DC populations associated with airway and intestinal surfaces are cycling through these environments at a faster rate than those in other areas or tissues. This fact may be due to the stimulating effect of the mucosal bacterial flora and to a large antigenic load (Williams *et al.*, 1997). LPS, present in the cell wall of Gram-negative bacteria, has been described to increase levels of CMH II and B7 molecules (De Smedt *et al.*, 1996). In an another study, MacPherson *et al.*, (1995) have shown that i.v. administration of LPS in adult rats increases the release of intestinally derived DC into lymph and that TNF-α could play a role on the mechanisms underlying DC release. The source of intestinal TNF-α is still unclear. Mucosal mast cells present in the lamina propria are potential candidates for TNF-α release as it is stored in these cells (reviewed in Gordon *et al.*, 1990). However, it remains unknown exactly how mast cells respond to the resident bacterial flora. On the other hand, macrophages are also abundant in GALT and it has been shown that the colonisation of the intestine of gnotobiotic mice with *E. coli* stimulated the release of TNF-α by peritoneal, as well as bone-marrow derived macrophages (Nicaise *et al.*, 1995). Unfortunately, it remains unknown whether this stimulating effect is operative on intestinal macrophages. LP macrophages represent a specific subset of macrophages. They are derived from circulating blood monocytes, but their phenotype differs from that of the majority of blood monocytes. In humans, the most striking difference is the absence of CD14 on LP macrophages, a receptor for the LPS-binding protein, a serum protein that complexes with LPS (reviewed in Smith and Meng, 1997). This absence may play an important role in maintaining mucosal homeostasis by suppressing local macrophage activation and decreasing secretion of inflammatory cytokines. It is unknown whether the presence of bacterial intestinal flora is the environmental factor responsible for the down-regulation of $CD14^+$ expression on mucosal macrophages.

From an ecological point of view, we can speculate that, after birth, the colonisation of the intestine by *E.coli* may be a strong inflammatory stimulus responsible for the synthesis of inflammatory cytokines, IFN-γ and TNF-α, at the intestinal level, with consequences on the functionality of macrophages and DC. At the adult stage, when the level of *E. coli* decreased, another Gram-negative bacterium, *Bacteroides*, present in high levels, could be an important physiological source of LPS.

3.5 Influence of resident intestinal flora on the modulation of GALT functions

GALT generates two important immune functions. First is the immune exclusion performed by secretory IgA antibodies (SIgA Abs) to protect the mucosa by blocking microbial adhesion, microbial translocation and viral multiplication as well as by neutralising toxins. Second is a suppressive function, also called oral tolerance, characterised by regulatory mechanisms avoiding local and peripheral immune responses to harmless environmental antigens present in the intestine, such as bacterial antigens of the resident microflora or dietary proteins. Now, it is still unclear whether suppression of systemic immunity is accompanied by local SIgA production or not.

The early postnatal life is a period of high risk for intestinal disorders due to enteric pathogens and/or food hypersensitivities. During the neonatal period mammalian species exhibit some degree of reduced immunocompetence that could be attributed to functional immaturity in populations involved in immune intestinal responses. It could be also attributed to immunoregulatory mechanisms governing GALT functions. Apart from the role of intestinal flora on the development of GALT, the presence in great numbers of Gram-positive and Gram-negative bacteria containing immunomodulator components in their cell walls with adjuvant capacities (Johnson, 1994) may have modulating effects on GALT functions. Depending on the bacterial equilibrium, which can differ from one individual to another, immune responses elicited by GALT may be modulated differently. Gnotobiotic animal models are useful in analysing such modulating effects of digestive bacteria on GALT functions.

3.5.1 Secretory IgA antibody responses

The presence of the resident digestive flora exerts both direct and indirect effects on the SIgA responses. It induces secretion of natural SIgA Abs in response to bacterial antigens. In addition, it plays a modulating role on the specific SIgA response against some enteropathogens, as recently described with rotavirus (Moreau *et al.*, 1998a; 1998b). The regulatory mechanisms involved in producing such effects are unknown.

3.5.2 Intestinal microflora and natural SIgA antibodies

Sequential intestinal bacterial colonisation is responsible for the presence of natural SIgA Abs. They express polyreactivities and are, with other natural factors such as mucus and bile, the first line of defence at mucosal surfaces. Their efficiency is increased by binding an additional intestinal endogenous protein component, the fragment-binding protein (pFv), to form large complexes of high-agglutinating activity (Bouvet *et al.*, 1993; Bouvet and Fischetti, 1999). It has recently been shown that bacterial colonisation of GF rats with a human colonic flora favoured the release of pFv (Andrieux *et al.*, 1998). Both B-1 and B-2 cell lineages originating from the peritoneal cavity and Peyer's patches, respectively, seem to contribute to intestinal SIgA Abs responses. Recent studies have shown that B-1 and B-2 precursors of IgA intestinal B cells have different antigenic repertoires. B-1 cells mainly produce polyspecific natural Abs which bind to multiple unrelated antigens, predominantly microbial T-independent antigens, whereas B-2 cells respond predominantly to T-dependent antigens (reviewed in Beagley *et al.*, 1998). T-independent antigens are mainly found in micro-organisms and many of the LP IgA plasma cells secreting natural SIgA are postulated to originate from the B-1 cell lineage (Murakami and Honjo, 1995). The site where B-1 cells are stimulated, their path of migration to seed the LP and how they differentiate into IgA plasma cells are questions still awaiting answer.

The roles of natural SIgA Abs are not very well known. They have the potential to agglutinate multiple pathogens without delay or prior exposure. In healthy conditions, natural SIgA Abs could be important in inhibiting the microbial adherence and penetration of resident bacteria in the mucosa. SIgA are present at high levels in mucus, which is the first protective barrier against mucosal bacterial colonisation. Few bacterial species are closely associated with epithelium. Most of them are living in the mucus layer. It has been shown in rats that the adherence of bacteria to the intestinal mucosal surface is an important factor in bacterial translocation (Katamaya *et al.*, 1997). In neonatal rabbits, IgA supplementation abrogated bacterial translocation (Dickinson *et al.*, 1998). A majority of freshly isolated intestinal bacteria from a normal adult mouse are "coated" with SIgA (Kramer *et al.*, 1995). The relevance of this coating in the regulation of the intestinal microbial flora equilibrium is uncertain (Marcotte and Lavoie, 1996), but it could be important in protecting the systemic compartment from translocation of intestinal resident bacteria.

3.5.3 Intestinal microflora and modulation of SIgA anti-rotavirus response

Gastrointestinal infections and their consequences are a major clinical and economical problem. For example, *Salmonella typhi, Helicobacter pylori* in human adults and rotaviruses in infants cause mortality and morbidity worldwide. Little information is available regarding the role of resident intestinal bacteria on the modulation of the specific SIgA Ab response against enteropathogens. The first information has emerged from studies using lactic-acid producing bacteria as probiotics in mice (Perdigon *et al.*, 1995) and humans (Kaila *et al.*, 1992). Although it has not been demonstrated that probiotics can colonise the intestine as can resident bacteria, they can exert immunomodulating effects during their transit time.

Interestingly, in breast-fed babies a lactic-acid producing bacteria, *Bifidobacterium,* is one of the first anaerobic bacteria which colonise the baby's intestine. As it is commonly observed that breast-fed babies are more resistant to gastrointestinal infection, we hypothesised that the presence of *Bifidobacterium* in the resident digestive flora could have a stimulating effect on the SIgA Ab response against enteropathogens. To test this hypothesis an original model of adult mice infected with the heterologous simian rotavirus strain SA-11 was developed (Moreau *et al.*, 1998a; 1998b). Total and anti-rotavirus SIgA responses were evaluated both in faeces and in small intestine LP by enumerating IgA- (IgA-SC) and anti-rotavirus IgA secreting-cells (ARSC). To assess the respective immunomodulating role of two bacteria present in the baby's intestine, *Bifidobacterium* (Gram-positive bacteria) and *E. coli* (Gram-negative bacteria), two groups of gnotobiotic mice were created. Bacteria were allowed to colonise the intestine 3 weeks before viral infection to permit development of their immunological effect on GALT. Results on LP

ARSC and IgA-SC numbers are presented in Table 3.5. They were in good correlation with faecal measurements (Moreau *et al.*, 1998 a).

Table 3.5. Anti-rotavirus secreting cell (ARSC) and IgA-secreting cell (IgA-SC) numbers in small intestine lamina propria of CV, GF and gnotobiotic mice colonised with strains of *E. coli* or *Bifidobacterium.*

Groups of mice	ARSC/10^6 cells	IgA-SC/10^6 cells	Ratio of ARSC / IgA-SCx100
Conventional	100 ± 41**	206 000 ± 61 000**	0.26 ± 0.15**
Germ-free	447 ± 198	17 000 ± 8 000	3.80 ± 1.74
Bifidobacterium	5486 ± 2670**	33 000 ± 10 000	12.5± 5.65**
Escherichia coli	48 ± 11**	19 000 ± 6 000	0.63 ± 0.29 **

Results are expressed in mean numbers ± SEM of secreting-cells. ** P<0.01 with GF group.

Several conclusions have been drawn from the information found in this work. Firstly, whereas *Bifidobacterium* and *E.coli* were both established in high numbers in the intestine of gnotobiotic mice, they modulated the IgA anti-rotavirus response in a completely different way. The presence of *Bifidobacterium* had a strong adjuvant effect on the anti-rotavirus IgA response, whereas *E.coli* exerted an obvious suppressive effect. It is interesting to note that the low SIgA anti-rotavirus response obtained in CV mice may be explained by the presence of another Gram-negative bacterium, *Bacteroides*, which is present in very high levels in intestinal flora of adult CV mice. Secondly, in all groups of mice, the ARSC number did not depend on the total IgA-SC number, showing a lack of correlation between the modulating effect of bacteria on the SIgA anti-rotavirus response (virus-specific SIgA) and on the total SIgA response (natural SIgA). Finally, GF mice were able to mount a strong IgA anti-rotavirus response while GALT was poorly developed.

Other studies have shown an enhancement of serum or intestinal Ab response to orally administered antigens by Gram-positive bacteria (Herias *et al.*, 1998; Flo *et al.*, 1996), especially lactic-acid producing bacteria used as probiotics (see other chapters). The exact mechanisms underlying such effects at the intestinal level are poorly understood. Bacterial components are known to have immunomodulatory properties (Johnson, 1994). Cell walls of Gram-positive bacteria are rich in peptidoglycans, which have been specifically described as stimulating macrophage functions (reviewed in Hamann *et al.*, 1998). In contrast,

LPS is particularly abundant in Gram-negative bacteria and previous studies have shown its numerous effects on immunity, especially suppressive effects on immune responses (MacGhee *et al.*, 1984; Babb *et al.*, 1981; Kiyono *et al.*, 1980).

According to our results, the modulating effect of the digestive flora on natural and specific SIgA Ab responses were surprisingly uncorrelated. To our knowledge, this fact has never been discussed and we do not know the exact causes explaining such a lack of correlation. We can propose that it arises from a difference in B-1 and B-2 cell selection upon antigenic stimulation. Interesting results were obtained from previous studies measuring intestinal anti-*Salmonella* IgA plasma cell responses obtained after oral infection with *S. typhimurium* in non-responsive irradiated Xid mice reconstituted with responsive donor cells (Pecquet *et al.*, 1992). The authors showed that donor cells from the peritoneal cavity, enriched mainly with B-1 cells, were capable of giving a intestinal IgA Ab response, in contrast to B cells isolated from Peyer's patches, mainly of the B-2 type, which did not contribute to this response. Thus, we can postulate that thymo-independent bacterial antigens could act preferentially on B-1 cell lineage to secrete natural SIgA, whereas thymo-dependent antigens, such as viral proteins, might elicit B-2 cell lineage to secrete virus-specific SIgA. Moreover, the direct effect of bacterial components present in the cell walls and/or secreted by living bacteria, could also modulate the SIgA anti-rotavirus Ab response through non-specific cellular and molecular events. Stimulation of APC functions and cytokine synthesis may be involved as modulating events between the induction of the IgA response in Peyer's patches and secretion of SIgA in the intestinal lumen (reviewed in Krahenbuhl and Neutra, 1992). Mechanistic studies are required to clarify the molecular basis upon which resident bacteria modulate the SIgA Ab response to enteric pathogens.

The hypothesis of a possible dichotomy in virus-specific SIgA and natural SIgA responses may explain the results obtained by Cebra *et al.* (1995) in new-born mice. They described that 10-day-old suckling mice were as competent as 12-week-old mice at initiating a virus-specific SIgA response after enteric infection, whereas the complete development of the intestinal IgA plasma cell number was reached only 5-6 weeks later. Such results have also been described in humans. One-week-old babies were capable of developing protective immunity following oral vaccination with poliovirus or hepatitis B virus while the complete development of natural SIgA Abs takes several months in infants (reviewed in Bona and Bot, 1997). These observations address an important question about the immunological competence of new-borns to mount a SIgA Ab response. It is currently admitted that the ability of the immunologically naive new-born to generate a mucosal immune response depends on the functional capacity of GALT at birth but, taken together, all this data suggests that neonates are probably capable of mounting an active SIgA Ab response. Consequently, the ability to give a high specific sIgA anti-rotavirus Ab response could be correlated with the modulating effect of intestinal bacteria rather than with the development of GALT. This data could have important implications for oral vaccination of human new-borns. Numerous questions remain to be answered. They are discussed in Cebra *et al.* (1999).

In conclusion, experimental animal models of gnotobiotic mice brought to light the immunomodulating properties of two intestinal strains, *Bifidobacterium* and *E.coli,* on intestinal IgA anti-rotavirus response. Our results suggest the importance of the presence of *Bifidobacterium* in the baby's intestine in potentiating the synthesis of IgA Ab against viral enteropathogens. Foods promoting *Bifidobacterium* in the intestine could be instrumental in promoting a beneficial effect on health.

3.6 Oral tolerance

3.6.1 Definition

Oral tolerance (OT) is classically defined as the state of antigen-specific systemic immunological unresponsiveness induced by prior oral administration of the antigen and subsequent systemic exposure to the same antigen. it has been described in numerous animal models by using various antigens, especially particulate ones, such as sheep red blood cells (SRBC), or soluble ones, such as ovalbumin (OVA) (reviewed in Mowat, 1987). OT has also recently been described in humans (Husby *et al.*, 1994). its induction is believed to be of physiologic importance to avoid hypersensitivity reactions to dietary antigens. indeed, although small amounts of orally administered proteins escape enzymatic digestion in the intestine, they do not induce immune responses under healthy conditions (Husby *et al.*, 1985). recently, it has been hypothesised that a similar state of tolerance is established towards the indigenous gut microflora (Duchmann *et al.*, 1995). increasing interest in OT is also related to its potential role in the treatment of autoimmune diseases (reviewed in Weiner, 1997).

Orally fed antigens can suppress both specific humoral (IgG and IgE antibody responses) and cellular immune responses (reviewed in Strobel and Mowat, 1998). Cell-mediated immune responses, such as T-cell proliferation, delayed-type hypersensitivity (DTH) or contact sensitivity and $CD8^+$ cytotoxic T-cell responses, are generally easier to tolerate than humoral responses (Strobel and Ferguson, 1987), even in primed animals (Lamont *et al.*, 1988a; Peng *et al.*, 1989a). Nevertheless, IgE response seems to be remarkably sensitive to suppression when antigen is fed before or after parenteral immunisation with the same antigen (Saklayen *et al.*, 1984). Considering that IgE- and cell-mediated immune responses are frequently implicated in human food hypersensitivities (reviewed in Sampson and Burks, 1996), it seems logical that these immunological responses would be highly susceptible to regulatory mechanisms.

Systemic unresponsiveness is a long-lasting process which leads OT to be considered in terms of induction and maintenance. OT induction can be demonstrated very soon after feeding a protein, as it can be verified by parenteral immunisation with the same antigen within 7 days of feeding (Challacombe and Tomasi, 1980). However, its duration depends on the immune response studied. Studies on mice have shown that suppression of DTH lasts up to 17 months after one feeding of 20 mg OVA, whereas the suppression of the IgG antibody response does not last more than 3-6 months (Strobel and Ferguson, 1987).

3.6.2 Mechanisms of oral tolerance

It is now admitted that multiple mechanisms are involved in OT. Although debate about the relative role of each mechanism in OT still exists, it seems likely that they are not mutually exclusive. They have been extensively studied, especially in the last decade, and most of them have been described in detail in recent reviews (Weiner *et al.*, 1994; Weiner, 1997; Garside and Mowat, 1997; Strobel and Mowat, 1998). We will focus only on their major characteristics and on major questions still under debate.

Three principal immunological mechanisms have been implicated in OT: antigen-driven active cellular suppression, clonal anergy and clonal deletion of potentially reactive lymphocytes.

Active suppression was first described as a mechanism mediated by regulatory suppressive $CD8^{+}$T cells induced in GALT, which then migrate to the systemic immune system (reviewed in Mowat, 1987; Weiner *et al.*, 1994). More recently, it has been suggested that intestinal $CD8^{+}$ TcR-γδ+ IEL may be implicated in OT (Mengel *et al.*, 1995; Ke *et al.*, 1997). However, today, the requirement of $CD8^{+}$ T cells in induction and maintenance of OT does not seem so categorical, as OT can be induced in mice deficient or depleted of $CD8^{+}$ T cells (Lycke *et al.*, 1995; Garside *et al.*, 1995a; Barone *et al.*, 1995). In contrast, involvement of regulatory $CD4^{+}$ T cells in OT appears essential. It has been proposed that OT may reflect preferential activation of Th2 suppressive T cells and down-regulation of Th1 responses by Th2 cells *via* suppressive cytokines, such as IL-4, IL-10 and transforming growth factor (TGF)-β (Chen *et al.*, 1994). In relation to the cytokine-mediated active suppression, the phenomenon of "bystander suppression" has been described. Indeed, suppressive cytokines secreted after antigen-specific activation of regulatory T cells could suppress immune responses to an unrelated antigen anatomically colocalised with the fed antigen. Bystander suppression therefore represents an important potential in the treatment of autoimmune diseases where autoantigens are unidentified or available in extremely low quantities (reviewed in Weiner, 1997). However, OT to OVA can suppress both Th1 and Th2 responses and normal induction of OT is observed in both IL-4 and IL-10 deficient mice (Garside *et al.*, 1995b; Aroeira *et al.*, 1995). A recent study in a model of experimental autoimmune uveitis reported that IL-4 and IL-10 are both required for induction of OT (Rizzo *et al.*, 1999), underlining that the roles of IL-4 and IL-10 are still unclear. On the other hand, it has recently been proposed that a new subset of $CD4^+$ T cells, termed Th3 cells, primarily secreting TGF-β, may down-regulate properties for Th1 and other immune cells (reviewed in Thomas and Kemeny, 1998). The importance of TGF-β is further supported by prevention of bystander suppressive effects with anti-TGF-β antibodies (Powrie *et al.*, 1996).

The absence of both active suppression and reactive lymphocytes *in vivo*, in experimental models of OT, was thought to result from clonal deletion or anergy. Although clonal deletion of T cells has been demonstrated in several studies (reviewed in Garside and Mowat, 1997), experimental conditions, i.e. ingestion of very high doses of antigen, suggest that such deletion probably does not occur after induction of OT *in vivo*. In contrast, anergy is considered an important OT mechanism which may preferentially induce unresponsiveness of Th1 functions. It seems likely that anergy reflects aberrant presentation of a fed antigen by APC, leading to an absence of IL-2 secretion and T-cell activation.

Important questions about the way antigens are processed and presented remain, especially as to the location of antigen presentation and the APC involved. It is now proposed that APC may play a crucial role in the induction of OT, especially due to the presentation of the antigen to T cells associated with a failure of appropriate costimulation (reviewed in Strobel and Mowat, 1998; Brandtzaeg, 1998). Enterocytes expressing low levels of particular MHC class II molecules with no invariant chain and no costimulatory molecules, such as B7 or ICAM-1, had firstly been considered as potential tolerogenic APC (Vidal *et al*, 1993; reviewed in Mowat and Viney, 1997). Recent interesting studies tend to point towards a central role for dendritic cells (DC), thus opening new fields of investigation (reviewed in Strobel and Mowat, 1998). Expanding mature DC *in vivo* with the growth factor Flt3 ligand results in enhanced induction of OT in treated mice fed with low doses of soluble antigen which are inefficient in control mice (Viney *et al.*, 1998).

According to the concept that the mechanisms involved in OT may depend on different doses of fed antigen (reviewed in Weiner *et al.*,

1994), a new scheme of intestinal induction of OT proposes that patterns of tolerance may reflect the amounts of peptide/MHC complexes presented to T cells in the absence of costimulation. More recently, it has been suggested that CTLA-4, the high-affinity receptor for B7 molecules on T-cells, plays a crucial role in the induction of high-dose OT (Samoilova *et al.*, 1998).

In parallel, other experimental studies have suggested that the generation of a tolerogenic form of antigen that passes through the gut may also play an important role in the generation of OT. Bruce and Ferguson (1986a, 1986b) reported that serum from OVA-fed mice, transferred into naive recipients one hour after the feeding, induces suppression of systemic DTH responses, whereas serum from mice injected systemically with equivalent doses of OVA has no effect. However, the molecular nature of the tolerogen and how the intestine generates such material are still unclear. Moreover, the importance of intestinal enzymatic digestion of the antigen in induction of OT remains controversial, given that Louis *et al.* (1995) have paradoxically reported that specific systemic cellular hyporesponsiveness is also induced by one rectocolonic administration of 25 mg OVA. On the other hand, peripheral tolerance in the respiratory tract, especially suppression of the specific IgE response, has also been demonstrated in response to inhaled antigens (MacMenamin *et al.*, 1995).

3.6.3 Factors affecting oral tolerance

Although systemic suppression after antigen feeding is a general phenomenon, it is also possible to induce humoral and/or cellular systemic immune responses through the oral route and a number of factors have been reported to affect OT establishment. Moreover, several recent studies provide evidence that factors affecting OT and mechanisms governing OT are interrelated. These observations may have important implications for better understanding the development and treatment of hypersensitivities or autoimmune diseases. Only the major factors which influence OT are presented here and we particularly highlight the role of the indigenous gut flora.

Antigenic factors: Nature of antigen. Although OT can probably be induced to all thymus-dependent soluble antigens, it cannot be induced to thymus-independent ones (reviewed in Mowat, 1987). It also appears that particulate antigens, antigens associated with replicating bacteria or immune stimulating complexes (ISCOMs) tend to induce active immunity rather than tolerance (Dahlman *et al.*, 1992; Mowat *et al.*, 1993). It is hypothesised that such a difference may be related to their presentation in the gut and their preferential uptake by M cells overlying Peyer's patches.

On the other hand, OT cannot be induced to enzymatically-, chemically- or heat-denatured soluble antigens (Fritsché *et al.*, 1997; Peng *et al.*, 1995, 1998). It has been proposed that this may be related to the modification of the intestinal processing and absorption of the antigen and the resulting absence of any tolerogenic form of the antigen (Bruce and Ferguson, 1986a; Peng *et al.*, 1990).

Antigenic factors: Dose of antigen. The dose of antigen required for establishment of OT depends on the antigen used and on the systemic immune response studied. For example, studies on mice have shown that a single high dose (10-20 mg) of OVA induces suppression of both humoral and cell-mediated immune responses, whereas smaller doses can either induce suppression or enhance systemic responses (Lamont *et al.*, 1989). Moreover, suppression of the humoral response depends on the isotype considered. One oral dose of 1-5 mg OVA induces IgE unresponsiveness while the same doses leave IgG response unaffected. In contrast, repeated ingestion of a comparable dose (5 x 1 mg) suppress both IgE and IgG antibody responses (Saklayen *et al.*, 1984). However, we have reported that under the latter condition both IgE and IgG antibody suppression are of short duration (Moreau and Gaboriau-Routhiau, 1996), suggesting for the first time that factors which do not prevent the establishment of OT can disturb its maintenance.

Cell-mediated immune responses are easily tolerated as 100 µg of OVA is sufficient to suppress systemic DTH reactions in mice. Nevertheless, lower amounts of OVA (10-50 µg) induce priming for DTH response (Lamont *et al.*, 1989). This result suggests that small doses of dietary proteins, such as β–lactoglobulin or α–lactalbumin present in cow's-milk-based formula, and egg- or cow's-milk-proteins present in breast milk, may predispose susceptible neonates to food-hypersensitivity reactions.

Recent studies have shown that low versus high doses of antigen feeding influence the mechanisms involved in OT induction. Whereas low doses (5 x 1 mg) of the antigen hen egg lysozyme or autoantigen MBP induce cytokine-mediated active suppression, high doses (20 mg) of the antigen induce anergy. These two mechanisms are not mutually exclusive (Friedman and Weiner, 1994). This result confirms early studies by Gregerson *et al.* (1993) in the experimental model of autoimmune uveoretinitis. As previously reported in paragraph 3.6.2, the B7:CTLA-4 interaction at the intestinal level may be crucial in OT induction and the high dose of antigen may directly influence the costimulatory events, thus giving increasing importance to environmental parameters in the general process of OT.

Host factors: Genetic background of host. Early studies suggested the influence of the genetic background in the degree of suppression of both DTH and IgG responses after antigen feeding (Stokes *et al.*, 1983). It has been related to H-2 haplotype, H-2d mice being particularly sensitive to tolerance induction (Lamont *et al.*, 1988b). However, no direct proof has as yet been obtained.

Host factors: Influence of host age. The age at which antigens are first encountered by the host largely influences OT induction. Thus, mice do not become tolerant if fed OVA before 7 days of age and are even sensitised by early feeding or prenatal treatment (Strobel and Ferguson, 1984; Hanson, 1981). Similar observations have been reported in experimental models of autoimmune encephalomyelitis. Feeding myelin basic protein (MBP) to rats under 4 weeks of age results in priming instead of tolerisation (Miller *et al.*, 1994). In contrast, this is not observed in guinea pigs, which are more mature at birth (Heppell and Kilshaw, 1982; Telemo *et al.*, 1987). These results suggest that intestinal mucosal immaturity may prevent the induction of systemic unresponsiveness. The defect in oral tolerisation can be partially restored by transfer of mature adult splenocytes (Peng *et al.*, 1989b), suggesting that a more complex regulatory system may be involved. Interestingly, it has been thought that peripheral antigenic challenge during neonatal life represents a tolerogenic rather than an immunogenic event (Ridge *et al.*, 1996), highlighting differences between the peripheral and mucosal immune systems.

In humans, oral tolerisation has also been shown to be age-dependent, despite a more mature intestinal immune system at birth than that found in rodents. Neonates are more vulnerable to food hypersensitivities, especially to cow's milk proteins. In contrast to children receiving casein hydrolysate formula, it has been shown that both cellular and IgG antibody responses to cow's-milk-derived β-lactoglobulin are significantly increased in infants receiving cow's milk within the first months of life compared with infants receiving it only after the age of 9 months (Vaarala *et al.*, 1995). Nonetheless, it appears that these differences do not persist after 1 year of age. It is also noteworthy that systemic antibodies to food proteins are present in most normal individuals and do not correlate with any food hypersensitivity.

A deficiency in OT induction is also noticed at weaning (Strobel and Ferguson, 1984). However, it is still not known if it is related to the functioning of GALT or to gastrointestinal changes taking place during this period, especially modification of the gut microflora. Nevertheless, establishment of OT is crucial because of the numerous new dietary antigens encountered at weaning.

In parallel to host immaturity in the neonatal period, we have shown that ageing also influences OT, especially its long-term maintenance. Comparing 20-month-old and 2-month-old young adult CV mice fed with a single tolerogenic dose of 20 mg OVA, we observed that both IgG and IgE antibody suppression are induced but do not persist in old mice in contrast to young adult mice (Moreau and Gaboriau-Routhiau, 1996). Thus, as previously reported for repeated ingestion of small doses of antigen, these results confirm that factors which allow induction of OT can also prevent its maintenance, suggesting that different mechanisms may be involved in induction and maintenance of the OT process.

The age at which an antigen is introduced at the mucosal level has also been reported to influence OT mechanisms. Although both young (4 weeks of age) and adult (12 weeks of age) rats fed with OVA had reduced cell-mediated immune response, active suppression and bystander tolerance are shown in adult rats, whereas anergy is prevalent in young ones (Lundin *et al.*, 1996). No clear explanation has been proposed for this dichotomy, and it may be suspected that complex events occur at the mucosal level with the gut microflora acting as a crucial parameter.

Host factors: Intestinal permeability. Gut integrity and permeability of the intestinal epithelial layer seem to be determinant parameters in OT induction. Inflammatory reactions of the small intestinal mucosa and intestinal epithelial lesions are generally associated with increased intestinal permeability, which may result in abrogation of OT. Indeed, experimental studies in mice show that both graft-versus-host reaction (GvHR) and indomethacin-mediated increased intestinal permeability and induced inflammatory lesions of the intestine are associated with an abrogation of OT to OVA (Strobel and Fergusson, 1985; Louis *et al.*, 1996). Recently, by testing gut handling and processing of gliadin in mice with GvHR, Troncone *et al.* (1996) have reported that serum containing gut-absorbed gliadin fails to suppress systemic cellular immune responses when transferred intraperitoneally into naive recipients. However, comparable serum levels of gliadin between GvHR mice and normal ones have been detected (Troncone *et al.*, 1996). This data first suggested the importance of an intact gut epithelium in generating a tolerogenic serum factor. Secondly, one may wonder whether increased intestinal permeability might be the cause rather than the consequence of OT abrogation.

The hypothesis that the alteration of the intestinal mucosal epithelium and increased intestinal permeability to food proteins is probably not the primary cause of allergy but the secondary effect of an abnormal immunological response to food proteins is supported by several studies. Heyman *et al.* (1994) reported that the inflammatory cytokine tumour necrosis factor (TNF)-α is abnormally secreted by peripheral blood mononuclear cells (PBMC) taken from infants suffering cow's milk allergy. Interestingly, it was further established that this abnormal secretion results from a reduced threshold for PBMC immune reactivity to intact (i.e. non-intestinally processed) cow's milk proteins (Benlounes *et al.*, 1996). TNF-α directly alters the intestinal epithelial barrier permeability (Heyman *et al.*, 1994). In another clinical study, infants with cow's milk allergy displayed reduced permeability to β-lactoglobulin at normal values after cow's milk had been withdrawn from the diet (i.e. during the symptom-free period) (Saidi *et al.*, 1995). Taken together, this data would tend to show that increased permeability is not constitutive, and the increase in protein transport seems to be a consequence rather than a cause of food allergy due to inflammatory reactions at the gut level.

3.6.4 Role of resident intestinal microflora

Although indigenous gut microflora has been overlooked for a long time as an environmental parameter influencing GALT functions, increasing evidence now supports the idea that it could be an important environmental factor in modulating OT to dietary proteins. We will consider the role of gut microflora on both the induction and the maintenance of OT.

Influence on induction of OT. The influence of Gram-negative bacteria on OT induction was first suggested by Wannemuehler *et al.* (1982). Although OT, estimated by the antigen-specific IgM, IgG and IgA antibody suppression, cannot be induced in GF mice fed with SRBC, it can be restored in GF mice fed with 10 to 100 μg of lipopolysaccharides (LPS) the days before they are given SRBC. Moreover, in experiments using CV mice, it has been shown that LPS given orally with myelin basic protein may enhance tolerance development in experimental autoimmune encephalomyelitis (Khoury *et al.*, 1990). However, other studies demonstrated that the indigenous gut flora is not the basic requirement for OT induction in terms of humoral suppression, as it was possible to induce IgG and IgE antibody unresponsiveness in GF mice fed once with 20 mg of OVA (Moreau and Corthier, 1988; Moreau and Gaboriau-Routhiau, 1996). The differences observed in these two models may be related to the nature of the antigen, i.e. particulate vs. soluble. Nevertheless, Sudo *et al.* (1997) recently brought to light the role of a Gram-positive bacterium, *Bifidobacterium*, in the suppression of humoral antibody responses. *Bifidobacterium* can improve suppression of Th2-mediated immune response during the OT process. Comparing specific-pathogen free (SPF) mice, GF mice and gnotobiotic mice associated with *Bifidobacterium* and fed with tolerogenic doses of OVA, the authors show that OVA-specific IgE and IgG1 antibody levels, and IL-4 synthesis, are significantly reduced in SPF and *Bifidobacterium*–associated mice compared with GF counterparts. However, *Bifidobacterium* exerts its role only when associated in mice at the neonatal stage; it does not produce the same effect at an older age. The mechanisms involved are not clearly identified and further investigations are needed to elucidate the discrepancy between these results. It can, however, be conjectured that intestinal microflora, especially bacterial species present in the digestive tract as of the postnatal period, may exert a fundamental role on the development of normal GALT functions, such as OT induction.

Influence on maintenance of OT. Further observations support the idea that indigenous gut microflora also strongly influences the long-term duration of OT, humoral unresponsiveness being short-lived in GF mice. We have shown in CV mice that both IgG and IgE antibody unresponsiveness last up to 3 months after a tolerogenic 20 mg OVA-feeding, whereas in GF mice antibody unresponsiveness is short-lived, IgG antibody suppression lasting no more than 20 days (Moreau and Gaboriau-Routhiau, 1996). Long-term IgE antibody suppression is not altered in GF mice, confirming that IgE response may be more readily suppressed than other isotype responses (Moreau and Gaboriau-Routhiau, 1996).

More recently, experiments performed on gnotobiotic mice inoculated with known bacteria at the adult stage, have suggested that Gram-negative bacteria are involved in maintenance of OT to OVA. Gnotobiotic mice harbouring *E. coli* or *Bacteroides*, showed a long-term tolerance comparable to that observed in CV mice. In contrast, mice harbouring Gram-positive bacteria, such as *Bifidobacterium* or non-enterotoxigenic *Clostridium difficile,* showed tolerance similar to that observed in GF mice (Moreau *et al.*, 1998b).

Our preliminary results indicated that LPS could be involved in the effect of Gram-negative bacteria on OT maintenance. The influence of LPS on antigen presenting cells, such as dendritic cells (DC), may represent a new field of investigation. As previously reported (see paragraph 3.4.4.), recent studies suggest that LPS affects splenic DC populations and may regulate DC functions (De Smedt *et al.*, 1996; MacPherson *et al.*, 1995), which may have important consequences if confirmed with mucosal DC. It may thus be hypothesised that intestinal inflammation related to bacterial colonisation of the gut may stimulate TNF-α secretion and increase DC biological functions which may be involved in OT process.

On the other hand, it may be suggested that the influence of the indigenous gut microflora on intestinal permeability could be responsible for the effect on OT maintenance. Indeed, one study in suckling mice, assaying patterns of protein absorption in the neonatal period, has reported fourfold reduced intact horseradish peroxidase (HRP) transport in GF mice compared with the CV counterparts (Heyman *et al.*, 1986a). It can be hypothesised that the decline in permeability in GF mice may result from the absence of a basic physiological inflammation normally induced by the indigenous gut microflora, which could play a crucial role in the complete establishment of the OT process. Thus, whereas infancy is generally considered as a period during which the gastrointestinal barrier is immature, resulting in increased intestinal permeability to macromolecules, such a permeability may be necessary for normal OT induction. However, this possibility must be confirmed in adult mice.

Protective role of resident intestinal microflora. Clinical observations show that food hypersensitivities are most common in human infants, particularly at the time of weaning. At weaning, the switch of diet generally alters colonisation resistance and predisposes the child to enteric infections and diarrhoeas. Studies on mice have shown that both cholera toxin (CT) and *E. coli* heat-labile enterotoxin (LT), secreted by *Vibrio cholerae* and enterotoxigenic *E. coli*, respectively, abrogate OT induction, in terms of systemic humoral immunity, to an antigen given simultaneously by the oral route (Elson and Ealding, 1984; Clements *et al.*, 1988; Snider *et al.*, 1994; Pierre *et al.*, 1992). The gut microflora is not directly involved in the toxin-mediated abrogative process, as shown by the fact that it exists in both CV and GF mice (Gaboriau-Routhiau and Moreau, 1996). Therefore, the transient presence of enterotoxins in young children, especially at weaning, may interfere with the OT process, resulting in food hypersensitivities. It is interesting to note that not all enterotoxins affect OT. Neither *Staphylococcus aureus* enterotoxin B nor *Clostridium perfringens* type A enterotoxin prevent induction and maintenance of OT to OVA in mice (Gaboriau-Routhiau and Moreau, 1997).

The relationships between gut microflora, the influence of enterotoxins and mechanisms governing OT are still not understood. The influence of enteropathogens, responsible for acute diarrhoea, on changes in intestinal permeability to intact macromolecules has been studied. However, the correlation between diarrhoea and changes in intestinal permeability is still controversial. LT has been reported to increase intestinal permeability to macromolecules in CV mice (Verma *et al.*, 1994). In contrast, *in vitro* studies have shown that CT does not alter permeability to HRP (Heyman *et al.*, 1986b). Therefore, it is not known whether altered permeability can be implicated in the toxin-mediated abrogation of OT.

We recently demonstrated another fundamental role of the indigenous gut microflora on the OT process by showing that its presence allows the recovery of suppressive mechanisms after the transient CT- or

LT-mediated breakdown of OT (Gaboriau-Routhiau and Moreau, 1996). Kinetics of the anti-OVA IgG antibody responses show that a hyporesponsive state occurs in CV mice fed with CT- or LT-plus OVA as compared with control mice, but that it does not occur in GF mice. Thus, in children, it may be important to preserve the normal gut microflora, as it could, in time, play a crucial role, such as improving recovery of tolerance.

Investigating the protective effect of the indigenous gut microflora further *in vivo*, we observed that it also decreases susceptibility of the individual to the LT-mediated effect on OT induction (Gaboriau-Routhiau and Moreau, 1996). However, this was only effective when the microflora was associated in neonates, highlighting the importance of its natural establishment during the neonatal period (Gaboriau-Routhiau, manuscript in preparation). As previously suggested by Sudo *et al.* (1997), it may be supposed that the gut microflora is important in contributing to the functioning of intestinal immunity as well as to protecting it and that the neonatal period is crucial for the normal establishment and development of GALT immune functions. Hence, we believe that in the neonatal and weaning periods it is important to preserve the intestinal microflora. Its alteration, e.g. during antibiotic treatment, may impair the intestinal barrier to intact proteins which may be related to increased food hypersensitivities in children.

In conclusion, although the influence of the indigenous gut microflora on induction and maintenance of OT and mechanisms involved in this complex phenomenon are not yet fully understood, indications exist that the gut microflora plays a critical role. We have reported that environmental parameters, such as the dose of antigen, the age of the host and the composition of the gut microflora, can influence induction and/or maintenance of OT, suggesting that OT may be divided into two stages characterised by their sensitivity to environmental parameters. We would therefore hypothesise that OT is a dynamic process during which sequentially suppressive mechanisms, leading to the induction and the long-term persistence of suppression, might be involved. It would now be interesting to identify the mechanisms which correlate with short- and long-term persistence of tolerance induced by protein feeding.

3.7 Neonatal period: a critical stage in the prevention of short and/or long-term pathologies?

There is increasing evidence that the neonatal period could be important in the aetiology of some pathologies, such as allergies, coeliac disease, diabetes and inflammatory bowel diseases (IBD) developing in infancy and/or later. According to the importance of the neonatal period for the interactions between GALT, the digestive flora and nutrition, questions can be asked about environmental factors which can affect these interactions, especially early dietary diversification and antibiotherapies. Through the examples given here we would like to show that the resident digestive flora has a fundamental role in maintaining health and preventing disease and that it must be considered as a true part of the body.

3.7.1 Neonatal period and immaturity of GALT

The high prevalence of dietary hypersensitivities and enteric infections in the neonate is believed to be due to the immaturity of GALT functions. Hypersensitivities to cow's milk proteins and egg albumin occur in approximately 3-10% of infants during the first two years of life in contrast to 0.001-0.5% of adults (reviewed in: Sampson and Burks, 1996; Monneret-Vautrin, 1996; Koning *et al.*, 1996; Björkstén, 1998). Food hypersensitivities are mainly characterised by an elevated IgE response (allergy) with respiratory and/or skin symptoms (atopic dermatitis) or by an intestinal cellular immune response with digestive symptoms (diarrhoeas, abdominal pain). After 2 years of age most infants no longer develop food allergies. Those who continue to develop allergies do so mainly towards fish and egg proteins. However, development of food allergies during early life seems to be correlated with a high risk of developing allergies to inhalant allergens in adulthood (Holt and Macaubas, 1997).

The paradigm of Th1/Th2 subclasses of $CD4^+$ T cells, well established in murine models, has lent insight into one of the mechanisms involved in allergies. The balance between Th1/Th2 cytokines is considered to be critical for IgE production, even if regulatory mechanisms of allergies are much more complex than the sole Th1/Th2 balance since high IgE levels can be found in healthy children. $CD4^+$ T cells expressing the Th2 cytokine profile release IL-4 and IL-5 which are potent inducers for IgE and recruitment of eosinophils, respectively. It is known that there is a mutual opposition between Th1 and Th2 cells, Th1 cytokines, especially IFN-γ, down-regulating the Th2 function. Neonates generally display polarised expression of Th2-like cytokines as foetal development occurs in a Th2 cytokine profile to avoid foetal rejection (Warner *et al.*, 1996). Thus, mechanisms acting on the switch of Th2 to Th1 after birth must be induced. IL-12, produced by various types of APC, strongly activates Th1 cells thus producing IFN-γ (Trinchieri, 1993). Arulanaudam *et al.* (1999) have shown that neonates have a reduced expression of IL-12 in the spleen and that administration of recombinant IL-12 redirects the new-born immune system towards a Th1-

type cytokine profile with IFN-γ production. An important question is whether the digestive flora is capable of polarising the Th1/Th2 balance. This fact could be of importance in allergic diseases. Recent exciting experiments have shown that conventionalisation of GF mice by the resident intestinal flora of CV mice enhanced IL-12 production in the spleen (Nicaise *et al.*, 1999). These findings suggest that bacterial colonisation after birth could be effective in polarising the Th2 profile towards a Th1 profile. It could be of particular interest during the neonatal period since, as recently described, IL-12 cannot reverse Th2 response into Th1 in adult human atopic patients in contrast to non-atopic patients (Hilkens *et al.*, 1996). In fact, this data addresses the question of the importance of the roles of IL-12 and IFN-γ during the neonatal period to the reversibility of Th2 to Th1 cells later in life and, consequently the importance of the first bacteria colonising the intestine in this process.

3.7.2 Neonatal period and nutrition

GALT is the primary target of all types of dietary constituents. A majority of human studies conclude that exclusive breast-feeding for at least one month prevents the development of allergies to cow's milk proteins and other allergic manifestations up to 3 years of age (reviewed in Vanderplas, 1998). However, the long-term beneficial effect of breast feeding and preventive nutrition of new-borns in avoiding dietary hypersensitivities remains controversial. Human milk contains components enhancing maturation of the intestinal mucosa of new-born infants (reviewed in Björkstén, 1998; Husband and Gleeson, 1996). It also promotes the *Bifidobacterium* establishment in the intestine. As described above from experimental animal models, *Bifidobacterium* could enhance the anti-rotavirus SIgA response in babies. On the other hand, from the results of Sudo *et al.* (1997), the very early presence of *Bifidobacterium* in the intestine may down-regulate development of IgE antibody responses and the resulting susceptibility to food allergic diseases. These data may underline the importance of *Bifidobacterium* establishment in the gut during the post-natal period, highlighting breast-milk feeding or use of *Bifidobacterium* as probiotic, in atopic neonates.

The moment new food proteins can be introduced in the baby's diet is often questioned and exclusively breast-feeding during the first 5-6 months of life is now recommended for infants predisposed to allergy. Exclusively breast-feeding for too long can delay the development of natural SIgA production by preventing changes in intestinal flora. In contrast, too early an introduction of new dietary antigens can lead to short and/or long term detriment including allergies or coeliac disease. Coeliac disease or gluten-sensitive enteropathy affects susceptible infants and adults who develop inflammatory intestinal symptoms after gluten ingestion. From interesting experimental studies, it has been demonstrated in rats that the early introduction of gliadin is responsible for the coeliac disease aetiology but, in this case, the presence of the intestinal flora has no influence (Stepankova *et al.*, 1996).

In autoimmune diabetes, it has been suggested that cross-reactions between caseins and unknown pancreatic self-antigens in early life could be the cause of the disease (reviewed in Kolb and Pozilli, 1999). Cross-reactions between intestinal bacteria and self-epitopes (mimicry epitopes) have also been suspected in the development and prevention of the disease (Singh and Rabinovitch, 1993).

3.7.3 Neonatal period and intestinal flora

Over the last forty years, there has been an increase in the prevalence of allergic diseases in western industrialised countries (reviewed in Björkstén, 1998). Environmental changes must play a role since genetic factors have not changed. Among a long list of factors, disturbances of the intestinal microflora due to early dietary diversification and/or antibiotherapies may have important short- and long-term consequences on infants.

In 1989, Strachman stated the hypothesis that, in western countries, the decrease of natural infections in infants could be a cause of the increase in the prevalence of allergic diseases. This fact could be due to a disruption in driving the profile of Th2 to Th1. However, Ruuska (1992) reported that infants who had a significantly greater number of episodes of acute diarrhoea than those who did not, developed food allergy. These contradictory results could arise from the different types of food hypersensitivity studied, i.e. allergy *vs.* DTH, where Th2 or Th1 unbalanced polarisation is involved, respectively. In an interesting critical review, Wold (1998) discusses the Strachman's "hygiene hypothesis". More than infections, Wold argues that the hygienic lifestyle can lead to an alteration of the normal intestinal colonisation pattern in infancy, thus disturbing the OT process. Indeed, reduced intestinal colonisation of *E. coli* in Swedish neonates is reported. As described above, the presence of intestinal flora in early life plays important inductive and protective roles on the OT process, especially with the importance of *E. coli.* We suggest that the use of antibiotics as current treatment during infancy is more responsible for strong modifications or destruction of the intestinal flora than are postnatal hygiene habits developed in western countries and that such antibiotic use could have harmful consequences on GALT. Establishment of intestinal flora in the sterile intestine of a baby at birth and profound changes taking place at weaning time can be considered as physiological stresses leading to inflammatory cytokine secretions (Sarandakou *et al.*, 1998) which might be important in inducing development and functioning of GALT. Thus, frequent antibiotherapies with the result of successive destruction, colonisation and modification of the intestinal flora equilibrium can lead to disturbances in the regulatory mechanisms with harmful consequences to GALT functions in preventing immunopathological reactions.

From the list of questions arising from the aetiology of IBD, the role of the neonatal period in the establishment of tolerance to its own intestinal flora has been mentioned. Recently, Duchmann *et al.* (1995) provided evidence that, under healthy conditions, GALT does not develop immune responses towards resident bacteria and a breakdown of tolerance could be the cause of immune reactions to the resident intestinal flora leading to IBD. In experimental studies, Karlsson *et al.* (1999) have shown that induction of OT to a transgenic *E. coli* producing OVA was possible if the strain colonised the intestine just after birth, whereas colonisation at adult stage primed mice to the bacterial antigens. In other studies using spontaneously colitic C3H/HeBr adult mice, a surprising humoral immune reactivity in serum has been found directed predominantly towards antigens of facultative anaerobes, which were in low number in faeces (Brandwein *et al.*, 1997). Facultative anaerobes are present in high levels during the neonatal period, and then their numbers decrease in adult faecal flora. This antibody response may result from a disordered immune response starting very early in life and leading to pathology later on.

3.8 Conclusions

The intestinal flora exerts a strong effect both on GALT activation and development and on the regulatory mechanisms involved in the maintenance of the steady-state at the intestinal level. This effect is probably different according to the bacterial equilibrium which is present in the different parts of the intestine. A delicate balance exists in the intestine between the bacterial flora and the immune status of the host. Aberrations in the dynamic balance, either at the microbial level (e.g. antibiotic therapies) or at the control level of GALT functions (breakdown of OT) may have harmful consequences. Thus, a lot of questions have to be answered to maintain human health. For instance, the reversibility of the effects of the intestinal flora on GALT is poorly understood. This knowledge is important as regards the consequences existing after long-term antibiotherapies, elemental enteral diet, or total parenteral nutrition in humans. Experimental studies have brought to light changes that occur in GALT after such diets and their relationship to intestinal bacterial modifications (Guihot *et al.*, 1997). In neonates, many observations support the notion that most mucosal immune cells are competent even before birth, but they need to undergo an activation process initiated by environmental signals. According to Ridge *et al.* (1996), orientation to tolerance or activation to an antigen is not determined by the self or non-self origin of the antigen but rather by the conditions under which it is introduced. Mature virgin T cells can be activated, tolerated or switched to Th1 or Th2 responses according to the dose of antigen, the type of adjuvant and the type of APC. From this point it follows that the role of the intestinal bacterial colonisation could be important in controlling the type of immune response. Consequently, particular attention has to be focused on the intestinal flora development during the neonatal period when the induction of lifelong regulatory immune mechanisms could be established.

Few attempts have been made to elucidate the mechanisms of intestinal bacteria in modulating the immune system, especially at the intestinal level. Small amounts of LPS and PG derived from the intestinal flora may be indispensable to the development, maintenance and good functioning of the immune system. However, there is as yet no information regarding the exact role of these bacterial components when they issue from digestive flora. Moreover, living bacteria secrete metabolites resulting from intestinal fermentation which can have immunomodulating effects (Siavoshian *et al.*, 1996; reviewed in Salminen *et al.*, 1998). Particular interest must be paid to the role of the intestinal flora on the APC due to the fundamental role they play in innate and adaptive immunity (Medzhitov and Janeway, 1997).

In addition to its effects on GALT, the intestinal flora influences peripheral immunity in a protective manner. Intestinal microbial colonisation is responsible for the enhancement of natural IgG1, IgG2a and IgG2b Abs in serum (Bos *et al.*, 1988), which have been shown to strongly influence the B-cell repertoire (Freitas *et al.*, 1991). The consequences on human health are important as a vast majority of natural IgG display reactivity towards self antigens and could play a role in the regulation of peripheral tolerance (reviewed in Kaveri *et al.*, 1998). Other experimental studies have demonstrated that the presence of intestinal flora protects experimental animals from pathologies such as arthritis (Van der Broek *et al.*, 1992) and anaemia (Milon *et al.*, 1992). As well as causing detrimental effects at the intestinal level, antibiotherapies may have an impact at the peripheral level. Recent study has shown that B-cell activity measured *in vitro* is depressed in infants receiving antibiotic treatments (Cukrowska *et al.*, 1999).

It is widely recognised that the features of mucosal immunity described here have mainly been discovered and investigated in rodents. We need to know to what extent these phenomena and their regulation are operative in man, with the aim of applications for human health (Fergusson, 1996). It is necessary to develop appropriate biomarkers for direct studies in humans, and gnotobiological experiments, as described here, are convenient for such investigations.

Acknowledgement

We wish to thank Donald White for the English correction of the chapter.

Dedication

We would like to dedicate this chapter to Anne Fergusson who died some months ago at the age of 57 years. An important clinical researcher in the field of intestinal immunity, she was above all else a very nice woman.

References

Andrieux, C., Pirès, R., Moreau, M.C. and Bouvet, J.P. (1998) Release of soluble co-receptor (Protein Fv) of secretory immunoglobulins after colonization of axenic rats by the human gut flora, *Scand. J. Immunol.*, **48**, 192-195.

Aroeira, L.S., Cardillo, F., De Albuquerque, D.A., Vaz, N.M. and Mengel, J. (1995) Anti-Il-10 treatment does not block either the induction or the maintenance of orally induced tolerance to ovalbumin, *Scand. J. Immunol.*, **41**, 319-323.

Arulanandam, B.P., VanCleave, V.H. and Metzger, D.W. (1999) IL-12 is a potent neonatal vaccine adjuvant; *Eur. J. Immunol.*, **29**, 256-264.

Babb, J.L., Kiyono, H., Michalek, S.M. and McGhee, J.R., (1981) LPS regulation of the immune response: suppression of immune response to orally administered T-independent antigen, *J. Immunol.*, **127**, 1052-1057.

Bandeira, A., Mota-Santos, T., Itohara, S., Degermann, S., Heusser, C., Tonegawa, S. and Coutinho, A. (1990) Localization of γ/δ T cells to the intestinal epithelium is dependant of normal microbial colonization, *J. Exp. Med.*, **172**, 239-244.

Barone, K.S., Jain, S.L. and Michael, J.G. (1995) Effect of *in vivo* depletion of $CD4^+$ and $CD8^+$ cells on the induction and maintenance of oral tolerance, *Cell. Immunol.*, **163**, 19-29.

Beagley, K.W., Fujihashi, K., Lagoo, A. S., Lagoo-Deenadaylan, S., Black, C. A., Sharmanov, A.T., Yamamoto, M., McGhee, J.R., Elson, C. O. and Kyiono, H. (1995) Differences in intraepithelial lymphocyte T cells subsets isolated from murine small versus large intestine, *J. Immunol.*, **154,** 5611-5619.

Beagley, K. W., Bao, S. and Husband, A.J. (1998) Mucosal IgA responses in cytokine knockout mice: Differential cytokine requirement for IgA secretion by B-1 and B-2 cells, *Mucosal Immunol. Update*, **6**, No 4, 15-19.

Benlounes, N., Dupont, C., Candalh, C., Blaton, M.A., Darmon, N., Desjeux, J.F. and Heyman, M. (1996) The threshold for immune cell reactivity to milk antigens decreases in cow's milk allergy with intestinal symptoms, *J. Allergy Clin. Immunol.*, **98**, 781-789.

Björkstén, B. (1998) Environmental influence on the development of childhood immunity, *Nutr. Rev.*, **56**, S106-S112.

Bona, C. and Bot, A. (1997) Neonatal immunoresponsiveness, *The Immunologist*, **5**, 5-9.

Borriello, S.P. (1995) Clostridial disease of the gut, *Clin. Infect. Dis.*, **20** (Suppl 2), S242-S250.

Bos, N.A., Meeuwsen, G., Wostman B.S., Pleasants, J.R. and Benner, R. (1988) The influence of exogenous antigenic stimulation on the specificity repertoire of background immunoglobulin-secreting cells of different isotypes, *Cell. Immunol.*, **112**, 371-380.

Bouvet, J.P., Pirès, R., Iscaki, S. and Pillot, J. (1993) Nonimmune macromolecular complexes of Ig in human gut lumen: probable enhancement of antibody functions, *J. Immunol.*, **151**, 2562-2571.

Bouvet, J.P. and Fischetti, V.A. (1999) Diversity of antibody-mediated immunity at the mucosal barrier, *Infect. Immun.*, **67**, 3687-3691.

Brandtzaeg, P. (1995) Molecular and cellular aspects of the secretory immunolobulin system, *APMIS*, **103**, 1-19.

Brandtzaeg, P. (1998) Development and basic mechanisms of human gut immunity, *Nutr. Rev.*, **56**, S5-S18.

Brandwein, S.L., MacCabe, R.P., Cong, Y., Wiates, K.B., Ridwan, B.U., Dean, P.A., Ohkusa, T., Birkenmeier, E.H., Sundberg, J.P. and Elson, C.O. (1997) Spontaneously colitic C3H/HeJBir mice demonstrate selective antibody reactivity to antigens of the enteric bacterial flora, *J. Immunol.*, **159**, 44-52.

Bruce, M.G. and Ferguson, A. (1986a) Oral tolerance to ovalbumin in mice : studies of chemically modified and "biologically filtered" antigen, *Immunology*, **57**, 627-630.

Bruce, M.G. and Ferguson, A. (1986b) The influence of intestinal processing on the immunogenicity and molecular size of absorbed, circulating ovalbumin in mice, *Immunology*, **59**, 295-300.

Cebra, J. J., Bos, N. A., Cebra, E. R., Kramer, D. R., Kroese, F. G. M. and Schrader, C. E. (1995) Cellular and molecular biologic approaches for analyzing the *in vivo* development and maintenance of gut mucosal IgA responses, in Mestecky *et al.*, (eds), *Advances in Mucosal Immunology*, Plenum press, New-York, pp 429-434.

Cebra, J.J., Jlang, H.Q., Sterzl, J. and Tlaskalova-Hogenova, H. (1999) The role of mucosal microbiota in the development and maintenance of the mucosal immune system, in Ogra *et al.*, (eds), *Mucosal Immunology*, Academic Press, pp 267-280.

Cerf-Bensussan, N. and Guy-Grand, D. (1991) Intestinal intraepithelial lymphocytes, *Gastroenterol. Clin. North Am.*, **20**, 549-576.

Challacombe, S.J. and Tomasi, T.B. (1980) Systemic tolerance and secretory immunity after oral immunization, *J. Exp. Med.*, **152**, 1459-1472.

Chen, Y., Kuchroo, V.K., Inobe, J.I., Hafler, D.A. and Weiner, H.L. (1994) Regulatory T cell clones induced by oral tolerance: Suppression of autoimmune encephalomyelitis, *Science*, **265**, 1237-1240.

Clements, J.D., Hartzog, N.M. and Lyon, F.L. (1988) Adjuvant activity of *Escherichia coli* heat-labile enterotoxin and effect on the induction of oral tolerance in mice to unrelated protein antigens, *Vaccine*, **6**, 269-277.

Cockfield, S.M., Urmson, J., Pleasants, J.R. and Halloran, P.F. (1990) The regulation of expression of MHC products in mice, *J. Immunol.*, **144**, 2967-2974.

Crabbe, P., Bazin, H., Eyssen, H. and Heremans, J.F. (1968) The normal microbial flora as a major stimulus for proliferation of plasma cells synthetizing IgA in the gut, *Int. Arch. Allergy*, **34**, 362-375.

Crabbe, P., Nash, D., Bazin, H., Eyssen, H. and Heremans, J.F. (1970) Immunohistochemical observations on lymphoid tissues from conventional and germ-free mice, *Lab. Invest.*, **22**, 448-457.

Craig, S.W. and Cebra, J.J. (1971) Peyer's patches an enriched source of precursors for IgA-producing immunocytes in the rabbit, *J. Exp. Med*, **134**, 188-200.

Cukrowska, B., Lodinovà-Zadnikovà, R., Sokol, D. and Tlaskalova-Hogenovà, H. (1999) In vitro immunoglobulin response of fetal B-cells is influenced by perinatal infections and antibiotic treatment: a study in preterm infants, *Eur. J. Pediatr.*, **158**, *in press*.

Dahlman, A., Ahlstedt, S., Hanson, L.A., Telemo, E., Wold, A.E. and Dahlgren, U.I. (1992) Induction of IgE antibodies and T-cell reactivity to ovalbumin in rats colonized with *Escherichia coli* genetically manipulated to produce ovalbumin, *Immunology*, **76**, 225-228.

De Smedt, T., Pajak, B., Muraille, E., Lespagnard, L., Heinen, E., De Baetselier, P., Urbain, J., Leo, O. and Moser, M. (1996) Regulation of dendritic cell numbers and maturation by lipopolysaccharide *in vivo*, *J. Exp. Med.*, **184**, 1413-1424.

Dickinson, E. C., Gorga, J. C., Garett, M., Tuncer, R., Boyle, P., Walkins, S.C., Alber, S.M., Parizhskaya, M., Trucco, M., Rowe, M. I. and Ford, H. R. (1998) Immunoglobulin A supplementation abrogates bacterial translocation and preserves the architecture of the intestinal epithelium, *Surgery*, **124**, 284-290.

Dohan, A., MacDonald, T.T. and Spencer, J. (1993) The ontogeny of adhesion molecule expression in the human intestine, *Clin. Exp. Immunol.*, **91**, 532-537.

Duchmann, R., Kaiser, I., Hermann, E., Mayet, W., Ewe, K., Meyer zum Buschenfelde, K.H. (1995) Tolerance exists towards resident intestinal flora but is broken in active inflammatory bowel disease, *Clin. Exp. Immunol.*, **102**, 448-455.

Ducluzeau, R. (1989) Role of experimental microbial ecology in gastroenterology, in E. Bergogne-Berezin (ed.), *Microbial Ecology and Intestinal Secretions*, Springer-Verlag, Paris, pp 7-26.

Elson, C.O. and Ealding, W. (1984) Cholera toxin feeding did not induce oral tolerance in mice and abrogated oral tolerance to an unrelated protein antigen, *J. Immunol.*, **133**, 2892-2897.

Fergusson, A. (1996) Mucosal immunology: from bench to the bedside and beyond, *Immunology*, **89**, 475-782.

Finegold, S.M., Sutter, V.L. and Mathisen, G.E. (1983) Normal indigenous intestinal flora, in D.J. Hentges (ed.), *Human Intestinal Microflora in Health and Disease*, Academic Press, New York, pp 3-31.

Flo, J., Goldma, H., Roux, M.E. and Massoud, E. (1996) Oral administration of a bacterial immunomodulator enhances the immune response to cholera toxin, *Vaccine*, **14**, 1167-1173.

Freitas, A.A., Viale, A.C., Sunblad, A., Heusser, C. and Coutinho, A. (1991) Normal serum immunoglobulins participate in the selection of peripheral B-cell repertoires, *PNAS*, **88**, 5640-5644.

Friedman, A. and Weiner, H.L. (1994) Induction of anergy or active suppression following oral tolerance is determined by antigen dosage, *PNAS*, **91**, 6688-6692.

Fritsché, R., Pahud, J.J., Pecquet, S. and Pfeifer, A. (1997) Induction of systemic immunologic tolerance to β–lactoglobulin by oral administration of a whey protein hydrolysate, *J. Allergy Clin. Immunol.*, **100**, 266-273.

Gaboriau-Routhiau, V. and Moreau, M.C. (1996) Gut flora allows recovery of oral tolerance to ovalbumin in mice after transient breakdown mediated by cholera toxin or *Escherichia coli* heat-labile enterotoxin, *Pediatr. Res.*, **39**, 625-629.

Gaboriau-Routhiau, V. and Moreau, M.C. (1997) Oral tolerance to ovalbumin in mice: Induction and long-term persistence unaffected by *Staphylococcus aureus* enterotoxin B and *Clostridium perfringens* type A enterotoxin, *Pediatr. Res.*, **42**, 503-508.

Garside, P., Steel, M., Liew, F.Y. and Mowat, A.M. (1995a) $CD4^+$ but not $CD8^+$ T cells are required for the induction of oral tolerance, *Int. Immunol.*, **7**, 501-504.

Garside, P., Steel, M., Worthey, E.A., Satoskar, A., Alexander, J., Bluethmann, H., Liew, F.Y. and Mowat, A.M. (1995b) T helper 2 cells are subject to high dose oral tolerance and are not essential for its induction, *J. Immunol.*, **154**, 5649-5655.

Garside, P. and Mowat, A.M. (1997) Mechanisms of oral tolerance, *Critical Reviews in Immunology*, **17**, 119-137.

Gordon, J., R., Burd, P.R. and Galli, S. (1990) Mast cells as a source of multifunctional cytokines, *Immunol. Today*, **11**, 458-464.

Gregerson, D.S., Obritsch, W.F. and Donoso, L.A. (1993) Oral tolerance in experimental autoimmune uveoretinitis. Distinct mechanisms of resistance are induced by low vs high dose feeding protocols, *J. Immunol.*, **151**, 5751-5761.

Guihot, G., Merle, V., Leborgne, M., Pivert, G., Corriol, O., Brousse, N., Ricour, C. and Colomb V. (1997) Enteral nutrition modifies Gut-Associated Lymphoid Tissue in rat regardless of the molecular form of nitrogen supply, *J. Pediatr. Gastroenter. Nutr.*, **24,** 153-161.

Guy-Grand, D., Griscelli, C. and Vassali, P. (1974) The gut-associated lymphoid system: nature and properties of large dividing cells, *Eur. J. Immunol.*, **4**, 435-443.

Guy-Grand, D., Cerf-Bensussan, N., Malissen, B., Malassis-Seris, M., Briottet, C. and Vassali, P. (1991) Two gut intraepithelial CD8+ lymphocyte populations with different T cell receptors: a role for the gut epithelium in T cell differentiation, *J. Exp. Med.*, **173**, 471-481.

Halstensen, T. S., Scott, H. and Brandzeag, P. (1990) Human CD8+ intraepithelial T lymphocytes are mainly CD45RA-RB+ and show increased co-expression of CD45R0 in celiac disease, *Eur. J. Immunol.*, **20**, 1825-1829.

Hamann, L., El-Samalouti, V., Ulmer A.J., Flad, H.D. and Rietschel, E. T (1998) Components of gut bacteria as immunomodulators, *Int. J. Food Microbiol.*, **41**, 141-154.

Hanson, D.G. (1981) Ontogeny of orally induced tolerance to soluble proteins in mice. I. Priming and tolerance in newborns, *J. Immunol.*, **127**, 1518-1524.

Helgeland, L., Vaage, J.T., Rolstad, B., Midtvedt, T. and Brandzaeg, P. (1996) Microbial colonization influences composition and T-cell receptor Vβ repertoire of intraepithelial lymphocytes in rat intestine, *Immunology*, **89**, 494-501.

Heppell, L.M. and Kilshaw, P. (1982) Immune responses in guinea pigs to dietary protein. I. Induction of tolerance by feeding ovalbumin, *Int. Arch. Allergy Appl. Immunol.*, **68**, 54-59.

Herias, M.V., Midved, T., Hanson, L.A. and Wold, A.E. (1998) Increased antibody production against gut-colonizing *E.coli* in the presence of the anaerobic bacterium *Peptostreptococcus*, *Scand. J. Immunol.*, **48**, 277-282.

Heyman, M., Crain-Denoyelle, A.M., Corthier, G., Morgat, J.L. and Desjeux, J.F. (1986a) Postnatal development of protein absorption in conventional and germ-free mice, *Am. J. Physiol.*, **14**, G326-G331.

Heyman, M., Dumontier, A.M. and Desjeux, J.F. (1986b) Intestinal barrier to intact horseradish peroxidase in experimental secretory diarrhea, *J. Pediatr. Gastroenterol. Nutr.*, **5**, 463-466.

Heyman, M., Darmon, N., Dupont, C., Dugas, B., Hirribaren, A., Blaton, A.M. and Desjeux, J.F. (1994) Mononuclear cells from infants allergic to cow's milk secrete tumor necrosis factor alpha, altering intestinal function, *Gastroenterology*, **106**, 1514-1523.

Hilkens, C.M.U., Messer, G., Tesselaar, K., Van Rietschoten, A.G.I., Kapsenberg, M. and Wierenga, E.A. (1996) Lack of IL-12 signaling in human allergen-specific Th2 cells, *J. Immunol.*, **157**, 4316-4321.

Holdeman, L.V., Good, I.J. and Moore, W.E.C. (1976) Human fecal flora: Variation in bacterial composition within individuals and a possible effect of emotional stress, *Appl. Environ. Microbiol.*, **31**, 359-375.

Holt, P.G. and Macaubas, C. (1997) Development of long term tolerance versus sensitisation to environmental allergens during the perinatal period, *Curr. Opin. Immunol.*, **9**, 782-787.

Hudault, S. (1996) Microbial colonisation of the intestine of newborn, in J.G. Bindels, A.C. Goedhart and H.K.A. Visser (eds), *Recent developments in infant nutrition*, Kluwer Academic Publishers, Dordrecht, pp 307-317.

Hughes, A., Bloch, K.J., Bhan, A.K., Gillen, D., Giovino, V.C. and Harmatz, P.R. (1991) Expression of MHC class II (Ia) antigen by the neonatal enterocytes: the effect of treatment with interferon-gamma, *Immunology*, **72**, 491-496.

Husband, A.J. and Gleeson, M. (1996) Ontogeny of mucosal immunity. Environmental and behavioral influences, *Brain Behavior Immun.*, **10**, 188-204.

Husby, S., Jensenius, J.C. and Svehag, S.E. (1985) Passage of undegraded dietary antigen into the blood of healthy adults. Quantification, estimation of size distribution and relation of uptake to levels of specific antibodies, *Scand. J. Immunol.*, **22**, 83-92.

Husby, S., Mestecky, J., Moldoveanu, Z., Holland, S. and Elson, C.O. (1994) Oral tolerance in humans – T cell but not B cell tolerance after antigen feeding, *J. Immunol.*, **152**, 4663-4670.

Johnson, A.G. (1994) Molecular adjuvants and immunomodulators: new approaches to immunization, *Clin. Microbiol. Rev.*, **7**, 277-289.

Kaila, M., Isolauri, E., Soppi, E., Virtanen, E., Laine, S., and Arvilommi, H. (1992) Enhancement of the circulating antibody secreting cell response in human diarrhea by a human *Lactobacillus* strain, *Pediatr. Res.*, **32,** 141-144.

Karlsson, M.R., Kabu, H., Hanson, L.A., Telemo, E. and Dahlgren, U.I.H. (1999) Neonatal colonization of rats induces immunological tolerance to bacterial antigens; *Eur. J. Immunol.*, **29**, 109-118.

Katamaya, M., Xu, D.Z., Specian, R.D. and Deitch, E.A. (1997) Role of bacterial adherence and the mucus barrier on bacterial translocation: effects of protein malnutrition and endotoxin in rats, *Ann. Surg.*, **225**, 317-326.

Kaveri, S.V., Lacroix-Desmazes, S., Mouthon, L. and Kazatchkine, M.D. (1998) Human natural autoantibodies: Lessons from physiology and prospects for therapy, *The Immunologist*, **6**, 227-233.

Kawaguchi-Miyashita, M., Shimizu, K., Nanno, M., Shimada, S., Watanabe, T., Koga, Y., Matsuoka, Y., Ishikawa, H., Hashimoto, K. and Ohwaki, M. (1996) Development and cytolytic function of intestinal intraepithelial T lymphocytes in antigen-minimized mice, *Immunology*, **89**, 268-273.

Ke, Y., Pearce, K., Lake, J.P., Ziegler, H.K. and Kapp, J.A. (1997) $\gamma\delta$ T lymphocytes regulate the induction and maintenance of oral tolerance, *J. Immunol.*, **158**, 3610-3618.

Kette, K., Baklien, K., Bakken, A., Kral, J.G., Fausa, O. and Brandzaeg, P. (1995) Intestinal B-cell isotype response in relation to local bacterial load: Evidence for immunoglobulin A subclass adaptation. *Gastroenterology*, **109**, 819-825.

Khoury, S.J., Lider, O., Al-Sabbagh, A. and Weiner, H.L. (1990) Suppression of experimental autoimmune encephalomyelitis by oral administration of myelin basic protein. III. Synergistic effect of lipopolysaccharide, *Cell. Immunol.*, **131**, 302-310.

King,C.E. and Toskes, P.P. (1979) Small intestine bacterial overgrowth, *Gastroenterology*, **76**, 1035-1055.

Kiyono, H., Babb, J.L., Michalek, S. and McGhee, J.R. (1980) Cellular basis for elevated IgA responses in C3H/HeJ mice, *J. Immunol.*, **125**, 732-737.

Kolb, H. and Pozilli, P. (1999) Cow's milk and type I diabetes: the gut immune system deserves attention, *Immunol. Today*, **20**, 108-110.

Koning, H, Baert, M.R.M., Oranje, A.P., Savelkoul, H.F.J. and Neijens, H.J. (1996) Development of immune functions related to allergic mechanisms in young children, *Pediatr. Res.*, **40**, 363-375.

Krahenbuhl, J.P and Neutra, M. (1992) Molecular and cellular basis of immune protection of mucosal surfaces, *Physiol. Rev.*, **72**, 853-879.

Kramer, D.R. and Cebra, J.J. (1995) Early appearance of "natural" mucosal IgA responses and germinal centers in suckling mice developing in the absence of maternal antibodies, *J. Immunol.*, **154**, 2051-2062.

Kroese, F.G.M., Butcher, E.C., Stall, A.M., Lalor, P.A., Adams, S. and Herzenberg, L. A. (1989) Many of the IgA producing cells in murine gut are derived from self-replenishing precursors in the peritoneal cavity, *Int. Immunol.*, **1**, 75-80.

Lamont, A.G., Bruce, M.G., Watret, K.C. and Ferguson, A. (1988a) Suppression of an established DTH response to ovalbumin in mice by feeding antigen after immunization, *Immunology*, **64**, 135-140.

Lamont, A.G., Mowat, A., Browning, M.J. and Parrott, D.M.V. (1988b) Genetic control of oral tolerance to ovalbumin in mice, *Immunology*, **63**, 737-739.

Lamont, A.G., Mowat, A. and Parrott, D. (1989) Priming of systemic and local delayed-type hypersensitivity responses by feeding low doses of ovalbumin to mice, *Immunology*, **66**, 595-599.

Lionetti, P., Breese, E. and Spencer, J. (1993) Activation of V-β3+ T cells and tissue damage in human small intestine induced by the bacterial superantigen, *Staphylococcus aureus* enterotoxin B, *Eur. J. Immunol.*, **23**, 664-668.

Louis, E., Franchimont, D., Lamproye, A., Van Kemseke, C., Schaaf, N., Mahieu, P. and Belaiche, J. (1995) Systemic immune response after rectocolonic administration of ovalbumin in mice, *Int. Arch. Allergy Immunol.*, **108**, 19-23.

Louis, E., Franchimont, D., Deprez, M., Lamproye, A., Schaaf, N., Mahieu, P. and Belaiche, J. (1996) Decrease in systemic tolerance to fed ovalbumin in indomethacin-treated mice, *Int. Arch. Allergy Immunol.*, **109**, 21-26.

Lu, C.Y., Calamai, E.G. and Unanue, E.R. (1979) A defect in the antigen-presenting function of macrophages from neonatal mice, *Nature*, **282**, 327-329.

Luckey, T.D. and Fioch, M.H. (1972) Introduction to intestinal microecology, *Am. J. Clin. Nutr.*, **25**, 1291-1295.

Lundin, B.S., Dahlgren, U.I.H., Hanson, L.A. and Telemo, E. (1996) Oral tolerization leads to active suppression and bystander tolerance in adult rats while anergy dominates in young rats, *Scand. J. Immunol.*, **43**, 56-63.

Lycke, N., Bromander, A., Ekman, L., Grdic, D., Hornquist, E., Kjerrulf, E., Kopf, M., Kosco-Vilbois, M., Schon, K. and Vajdy, M. (1995) The use of knock-out mice in studies of induction and regulation of gut mucosal immunity, *Mucosal Immunol. Update*, **3**, 1-8.

MacCartney, A.L., Wenzhi, W. and Tannock, G.W. (1996) Molecular analysis of the composition of the bifidobacterial and lactobacillus microflora of humans, *Appl. Environ. Microbiol.*, **62**, 4608-4613.

MacDonald, T.T., Weinel, A. and Spencer, J. (1988) HLA-DR expression in human fetal intestinal epithelium, *Gut*, **29**, 1342-1348.

MacDonald, T.T. (1994) Development of mucosal immune function in man: potential for GI disease states, *Acta Pediatr. Japonica*, **36**, 532-536.

MacMenamin, C., McKersey, M., Kühnlein, P., Hünig, T. and Holt, P.G. (1995) γδ T cells down-regulate primary IgE responses in rats to inhaled soluble protein antigens, *J. Immunol.*, **154**, 4390-4394.

MacPherson, G.G., Jenkins, C.D., Stein, M.J. and Edwards, C. (1995) Endotoxin-mediated dendritic cell release from the intestine. Characterization of released dendritic cells and TNF dependence, *J. Immunol.*, **154**, 1317-1322.

MacWilliam, AS. and Holt, P.G. (1997) Mucosal dendritic cells in the respiratory tract, *Mucosal Immunol. Update*, **5**, 21-25.

Mc Ghee, J.R., Michalek, S.M., Kiyono, H., Eldrigde, J.H., Colwell, D.E., Williamson, S.I., Wannemuehler, M.J., Jirillo, E., Mosteller, L.M., Spalding, D.M., Hamada, S., Gollahon, K.A., Morisaki, I., Gregory, R.L. and Koopman, W.J. (1984) Mucosal immunoregulation: environmental lipopolysaccharide and GALT T lymphocytes regulate the IgA response, *Microbial. Immunol.*, **28**, 261-280.

Marcotte, H. and Lavoie, M.C. (1996) No apparent influence of immunoglobulins on indigenous oral and intestinal microbiota in mice, *Infect. Immun.*, **64**, 4694-4699.

Matsumoto, S., Setoyama, H. and Umesaki, Y. (1992) Differential induction of major histocompatibility complex molecules on mouse intestine by bacterial colonization, *Gastroenterology*, **103**, 1777-1782.

Medzitov, R. and Janeway, C.A. (1997) Innate immunity: impact on the adaptative immune response, *Curr.Opin. Immunol.*, **9**, 4-7.

Mengel, J., Cardillo, F., Aroeira, L.S., Williams, O. and Russo, M. (1995) Anti-γδ T cell antibody blocks the induction and maintenance of oral tolerance to ovalbumin in mice, *Immunology Letters*, **48**, 97-102.

Miller, A., Lider, O., Abramsky, O. and Weiner, H.L. (1994) Orally administered myelin basic protein in neonates primes for immune responses and enhances experimental autoimmune encephalomyelitis in adult animals, *Eur. J. Immunol.*, **24**, 1026-1032.

Milon, G, Moreau, M.C., Lebastard, M. and Marshall, G. (1992) Hematopoiesis during infection in mice: an inducible, genetically controlled response mediated by CD4+ T cells homing in their bone marrow, in R. van Furth (ed), *Mononuclear phagocytes*, Kluwer Academic Publishers, The Netherlands, pp 50-54.

Monneret-Vautrin, D.A. and Kanny, G. (1996) Allergies alimentaires, *Rev. Prat. (Paris)*, **46**, 961-967.

Moore, W.E.C. and Holdeman, L.V. (1974) Human fecal flora: the normal flora of 20 Japanese-Hawaiians, *Applied Microbiol.*, **27**, 961-979.

Moreau, M.C., Ducluzeau, R., Guy-Grand, D. and Muller M.C. (1978) Increase in the population of duodenal IgA plasmocytes in axenic mice monoassociated with different living or dead bacterial strains of intestinal origin, *Infect. Immun.*, **21**, 532-539.

Moreau, M.C., Raibaud, P. and Muller, M.C. (1982) Relation entre le développement du système immunitaire intestinal à IgA et l'établissement de la flore microbienne dans le tube digestif du souriceau holoxénique, *Ann. Immunol. (Inst. Pasteur)*, **133D**, 29-39.

Moreau, M.C., Ducluzeau, R., Muller, M.C., and Raibaud, P. (1984) Effect of *Escherichia coli* strain on intestinal IgA plasmocyte stimulation and serum antibody response in gnotobiotic mice, *Progress Clin. Biol. Res.*, **181**, 391-395.

Moreau, M.C., Corthier, G., Muller, M.C., Dubos, F. and Raibaud, P. (1986) Relationships between rotavirus diarrhea and intestinal microflora establishment in conventional and gnotobiotic mice, *J. Clin. Microbiol.*, **23**, 863-868.

Moreau, M.C., and Corthier, G. (1988) Effect of the gastrointestinal microflora on induction and maintenance of oral tolerance to ovalbumin in C3H/HeJ mice, *Infect. Immun.*, **56**, 2766-2768.

Moreau, M.C. and Gaboriau-Routhiau, V. (1996) The absence of gut flora, the doses of antigen ingested and aging affect the long-term peripheral tolerance induced by ovalbumin feeding in mice, *Res. Immunol.*, **147,** 49-59.

Moreau, M.C., Bisetti, N. and Dubuquoy, C. (1998a) Immunomodulating properties of a strain of *Bifidobacterium* used as probiotic on the fecal and cellular intestinal IgA antirotavirus responses in mice, in M Sadler and M Saltmarsh (ed), *Functional Foods,* The Royal Society of Chemistry, pp 47-54.

Moreau, M.C., Gaboriau-Routhiau, V., Dubuquoy, C., Bisetti, N., Bouley, C. and Prevoteau, H. (1998b) Modulating properties of intestinal bacterial strains, *Escherichia coli* and *Bifidobacterium*, on two specific immune responses generated by the gut, *i.e.* oral tolerance to ovalbumin and intestinal IgA anti-rotavirus response, in gnotobiotic mice, in Talwar G.P., Nath I., Ganguly N.K. and Rao K.V.S. (eds), *The 10th International Congress of Immunology*, Monduzzi Editore, Bologna, pp 407-411.

Mowat, A..M. (1987) The regulation of immune responses to dietary protein antigens, *Immunol. Today*, **8**, 93-98.

Mowat, A.M., Maloy, K.J. and Donachie, A.M. (1993) Immune-stimulating complexes as adjuvants for inducing local and systemic immunity after oral immunization with protein antigens, *Immunology*, **80**, 527-534.

Mowat, A.M. and Viney, J.L. (1997) The anatomical basis of intestinal immunity, *Immunological Reviews*, **156**, 145-166.

Murakami, M and Honjo, T. (1995) Involvement of B-1 cells in mucosal immunity and autoimmunity, *Immunol. Today*, **16**, 534-538.

Nicaise, P., Gleizes, A., Forestier, F., Sandre, C., Quero, A.M. and Labarre, C. (1995) The influence of *E.coli* implantation in axenic mice on cytokine production by peritoneal and bone marrow-derived macrophages, *Cytokine*, **7**, 713-719.

Nicaise, P., Gleizes, A., Sandre, C., Kergot, R., Lebrec, H., Forestier, F., and Labarre, C. (1999) The intestinal microflora regulates cytokine production positively in spleen-derived macrophages but negatively in bone marrow-derived macrophages, *Eur. Cytokine. Net.*, **10**, *in press*.

Ouwehand, A.C., Isolauri, E., Kirjavainen, P.V. and Salminen, S.J. (1999) Adhesion of four Bifidobacterium strains to human intestinal mucus from subjects in different age groups, *FEMS Microbiol. Letters*, **172**, 61-64.

Parrott, D.M.W. (1976) The gut-associated lymphoid tissue and gastrointestinal immunity, in Fergusson A, MacSween NRM (eds), Immunological aspects of the liver and gastrointestinal tract, Lancaster: MTP Press, pp 1-32.

Pecquet, S., Ehrat, C. and Ernst, P. (1992) Enhancement of mucosal antibody responses to *Salmonella typhimurium* and the microbial hapten phosphorylcholine in mice with X-linked immunodeficiency by B-cell precursors from the peritoneal cavity, *Infect. Immun.*, **60**, 503-509.

Peng, H.J., Turner, M.W. and Strobel, S. (1989a) The kinetics of oral hyposensitization to a protein antigen are determined by immune status and the timing, dose and frequency of antigen administration, *Immunology*, **67**, 425-430.

Peng, H.J., Turner, M.W. and Strobel, S. (1989b) Failure to induce oral tolerance to protein antigen in neonatal mice can be corrected by transfer of adult spleen cells, *Pediatr. Res.*, **24**, 486-490.

Peng, H.J., Turner, M.W. and Strobel, S. (1990) The generation of a "tolerogen" after ingestion of ovalbumin is time-dependant and unrelated to serum levels of immunoreactive antigen, *Clin. Exp. Immunol.*, **81**, 510-515.

Peng, H.J., Chang, Z.N., Han, S.H., Won, M.H. and Huang, B.T. (1995) Chemical denaturation of ovalbumin abrogates the induction of oral tolerance of specific IgG antibody and DTH responses in mice, *Scand. J. Immunol.*, **42**, 297-304.

Peng, H.J., Chang, Z.N., Lin, S.Y., Han, S.H. and Chang, C.H. (1998) Chemical denaturation of ovalbumin abrogates the induction of oral tolerance of mouse reaginic antibody responses, *Scand. J. Immunol.*, **47**, 475-480.

Perdigon, G., Alvarez, S., Gobbato, N., De Budeguer, M.V., and De Ruiz Holgado, A.A.P. (1995) Comparative effect of the adjuvant capacity of *Lactobacillus casei* and lipopolysaccharide on the intestinal secretory antibody response and resistance to *Salmonella* infection in mice, *Food Agricultural Immunol.*, **7**, 283-294.

Pierre, P., Denis, O., Bazin, H., Mbella, E.M. and Vaerman, J.P. (1992) Modulation of oral tolerance to ovalbumin by cholera toxin and its B subunit, *Eur. J. Immunol.*, **22**, 3179-3182.

Powrie, F., Carlino, J., Leach, M.W., Mauze, S. and Coffman, R.L. (1996) A critical role for transforming growth factor-β but not interleukin 4 in the suppression of T helper type 1-mediated colitis by CD45RB^{low} CD4^{+} T cells, *J. Exp. Med.*, **183**, 2669-2674.

Raibaud, P. (1988) Factors controlling the bacterial colonization of the neonatal intestine, in Hanson L.A.(ED), *Biology of Human Milk*, Raven press, New York, pp 205-219.

Regnault, A., Cumano, A., Vassali, P., Guy-Grand, D. and Kourilsky, P. (1994) Oligoclonal receptor of the CD8αα and the CD8αβ TCR-αβ murine intestinal intraepithelial T lymphocytes: evidence for the random emergence of T cells, *J. Exp. Med.*, **180**, 1345-1349.

Regnault, A., Levraud, J.P., Lim, A., Six, A., Moreau, M.C., Cumano, A. and Kourilsky, P. (1996) The expansion and selection of T cell receptor α/β intestinal intraepithelial T cell clones, *Eur. J. Immunol.*, **26**, 914-921.

Ridge, J.P., Fuchs, E.J. and Matzinger, P. (1996) Neonatal tolerance revisited: turning on newborn T cells with dendritic cells, *Science*, **271**, 1723-1726.

Rizzo, L.V., Morawetz, R.A., Miller-Rivero, N.E., Choi, R., Wiggert, B., Chan, C.C., Morse III, H.C., Nussenblatt, R.B. and Caspi, R.R. (1999) Il-4 and Il-10 are both required for the induction of oral tolerance, *J. Immunol.*, **162**, 2613-2622.

Rognum, T.O., Stoltenberg; L., Vege, A. and Brandzaeg, P. (1992) development of intestinal mucosal immunity in fetal life and in first postnatal months, *Pediatr. Res.*, **32**, 145-149.

Rothkotter, H.J., Ulbrich, H and Pabst, R. (1991) The postnatal development of gut lamina propria lymphocytes: number, proliferation and T and B cell subsets in conventional and germ-free pigs, *Pediatr. Res.*, **29**, 237-242.

Ruuska, T. (1992) Occurrence of acute diarrhea in atopic and nonatopic infants: the role of prolonged breast-feeding, *J. Pediatr. Gastroenterol. Nutr.*, **14**, 27-33.

Saidi, D., Heyman, M., Kheroua, O., Boudraa, G., Bylsma, P., Kerroucha, R., Chekroun, A., Maragi, J.A., Touhami, M. and Desjeux, J.F. (1995) Jejunal response to β-lactoglobulin in infants with cow's milk allergy, *C. R. Acad. Sci.* Paris, **318**, 683-689.

Saklayen, M.G., Pesce, A.J., Pollak, V.E. and Michael, J.G. (1984) Kinetics of oral tolerance: Study of variables affecting tolerance induced by oral administration of antigen, *Int. Archs. Allergy Appl. Immunol.*, **73**, 5-9.

Salminen, S., Bouley, C., Boutron-Ruault, M.C., Cummings, J.H., Franck, A., Gibson, G.R., Isolauri, E., Moreau, M.C., Roberfroid, M. and Rowland, I. (1998) Functional food science and gastrointestinal physiology and function, *British J. Nutr.*, **80** (suppl. 1), S147-S171.

Samoilova, E.B., Horton, J.L., Zhang, H., Khoury, S.J., Weiner, H.L. and Chen, Y. (1998) CTLA-4 is required for the induction of high dose oral tolerance, *Int. Immunol.*, **10**, 491-498.

Sampson, H.A. and Burks, A.W. (1996) Mechanisms of food allergy, *Annu. Rev. Nutr.*, **16**, 161-177.

Sarandakou, A., Giannaki, G., Malamitsi-Putchner, A., Rizos, D., Hourdaki; E., Protonotariou, E. and Phocas, I. (1998) Inflammatory cytokines in newborn infants, *Mediators Inflamm.*, 7, 309-312.

Savage, D.C. (1977) Microbial ecology of the gastrointestinal tract, *Annu. Rev. Microbiol.*, **31**, 107-133.

Schaedler, R.W., Dubos, R. and Costello, R. (1965) The development of the bacterial flora in the gastrointestinal tract of mice, *J. Exp. Med.*, **122**, 59-66.

Siavoshian, S., Blottiere, H.M., Bentouimou, N., Cherbut, C., and Galmiche, J.P. (1996) Butyrate enhances major histocompatibility complex class I, HLA-DR and ICAM-1 antigen expression on differentiated human intestinal epithelial cells, *Eur. J. Clin. Invest.*, **26**, 803-810.

Singh, B. and Rabinovitch, A. (1993) Influence of microbial agents on the development and prevention of autoimmune diabetes, *Autoimmunity*, **15**, 209-213.

Smith, M.W., James, P.S. and Tivey, D.R. (1987) M cell numbers increase after transfer of SPF mice to a normal animal house. *Am. J. Path.*, **128,** 385-389.

Smith, P.D. and Meng, G. (1997) Mucosal macrophages in infection and immunity, *Mucosal Immunol. Update*, **5**, 32-34.

Snider, D.P., Marshall, J.S., Perdue, M.H. and Liang, H. (1994) Production of IgE antibody and allergic sensitization of intestinal and peripheral tissues after oral immunization with protein Ag and cholera toxin, *J. Immunol.*, **153**, 647-657.

Stepankova, R., Sinkora, J., Hudcovic, T., Kozakova, H. and Tlaskalova-hogenova, H. (1998) Differences in development of lymphocyte subpopulations from GALT of germ-free and conventional rats: effect of aging, *Folia Microbiol.*, **43**, 531-534.

Stokes, C.R., Swarbrick, E.T. and Soothill, J.F. (1983) Genetic differences in immune exclusion and partial tolerance to ingested antigens, *Clin. Exp. Immunol.*, **52**, 678-684.

Strachan, D. (1898) Hay, fever, hygiene and household size, *Brit. J. Med.*, **289**, 1259-1260.

Strobel, S. and Ferguson, A. (1984) Immune responses to fed protein antigen in mice. III. Systemic tolerance or priming is related to age at which antigen is first encountered, *Pediatr. Res.*, **18**, 588-594.

Strobel, S., Mowat, A.M. and Ferguson, A. (1985) Prevention of oral tolerance induction to ovalbumin and enhanced antigen presentation during graft-versus-host reaction in mice, *Immunology*, **56**, 57-64.

Strobel, S. and Ferguson, A. (1987) Persistence of oral tolerance in mice fed ovalbumin is different for humoral and cell-mediated immune responses, *Immunology*, **60**, 317-318.

Strobel, S. and Mowat, A.M. (1998) Immune responses to dietary antigens: oral tolerance, *Immunol. Today*, **19**, 173-181.

Sudo, N., Sawamura, S.A., Tanaka, K., Aiba, Y., Kubo, C. and Koga, Y. (1997) The requirement of intestinal bacterial flora for the development of an IgE production system fully susceptible to oral tolerance induction, *J. Immunol.*, **159**, 1739-1745.

Telemo, E., Jacobsson, I., Weström, B. and Folkesson, H. (1987) Maternal dietary antigens and the immune response of the offspring in the guinea pig, *Immunology*, **62**, 35-38.

Thomas, M.J. and Kemeny, D.M. (1998) Novel CD4 and CD8 T-cell subsets, *Allergy*, **53**, 1122-1132.

Trinchieri, G. (1993) Interleukin-12 and its role in the generation of Th1 cells, *Immunol. Today*, **14**, 335-338.

Troncone, R., Caputo, N., Zibella, A., Russo, R., Rossi, M., Gianfrani, C., Stern, M., Wieser, H. and Auricchio, S. (1996) Defective "gut processing" of gliadin in mice with graft-versus-host enteropathy, *Int. Arch. Allergy Immunol.*, **109**, 44-49.

Umesaki, Y., Setoyama, H., Matsumoto, S. and Okada, Y. (1993) Expansion of α/β T-cell receptor-bearing intestinal intraepithelial lymphocytes after microbial colnization in germ-free mice and its independence from thymus, *Immunology*, **79**, 32-37.

Underdown, B. and Mestecky, J. (1994) Mucosal immunoglobulins, in Ogra *et al.*, (eds), Handbook of Mucosal Immunology, Academic Press, Orlando, Florida, pp 79-97.

Vaarala, O., Saukkonen, T., Savilahti, E., Klemola, T. and Akerblom, H.K. (1995) Development of immune response to cow's milk proteins in infants receiving cow's milk or hydrolyzed formula, *J. Allergy Clin. Immunol.*, **96**, 917-923.

Vanderplas, Y. (1998) Myths and facts about breastfeeding: Does it prevent later atopic allergy? *Nut. Res.*, **18**, 1373-1387.

Van Den Broek, M.F, Van Bruggen, M.C.J., Koopman, J.P., Hazenberg, M.P. and Van Der Berg, W.B. (1992) Gut flora induces and maintains resistance against streptococcal cell wall-induced arthritis in F344 rats, *Clin. Exp. Immunol.*, **88**, 313-317.

Van Der Heijden, P.J., Bianchi, A.T.J., Heidt, P.J., Stok; W. and Bokhout, B.A. (1989) Background (spontaneous) immunoglobulin production in the murine small intestine before and after weaning. *J Reprod. Immunol.*, **15**, 217-227.

Van Der Waaij, D. (1993) Mechanisms involved in the development of the intestinal microflora in relation to the host organism: Consequences for colonization resistance, in C.E. Hormaeche, C.W. Penn and C.J. Smyth (eds.), *Molecular biology of bacterial infection: Current status and future perspectives*, University Press, Cambridge, pp 1-12.

Verma, M., Majumdar, S., Ganguly, N.K. and Walia, B.N.S. (1994) Effect of *Escherichia coli* enterotoxins on macromolecular absorption, *Gut*, **35**, 1613-1616.

Vidal, K., Samarut, C., Magnaud, J.P., Revillard, J.P. and Kaiserlian, D. (1993) Unexpected lack of reactivity of allogeneic anti-Ia monoclonal antibodies with MHC class II molecules expressed by mouse intestinal epithelial cells, *J. Immunol.*, **151**, 4642-4650.

Viney, J.L., Mowat, A.M., O'Malley, J., Williamson, E. and Fanger, N.A. (1998) Expanding dendritic cells *in vivo* enhances the induction of oral tolerance, *J. Immunol.*, **160**, 5815-5825.

Wannemuehler, M.J., Kiyono, H., Babb, J.L., Michalek, S.M. and McGhee, J.R. (1982) Lipopolysaccharide (LPS) regulation of the immune response: LPS converts germfree mice to sensitivity to oral tolerance induction, *J. Immunol.*, **129**, 959-965.

Warner, J.A., Jones, A.C., Miles, E.A., Colwell, B.M. and Warner, J.O. (1996) Maternofetal interaction and allergy, *Allergy*, **51**, 447-451.

Weiner, H.L., Friedman, A., Miller, A., Khoury, S.J., Al-Sabbagh, A., Santos, L., Sayegh, M., Nussenblatt, R.B., Trentham, D.E. and Hafler, D.A. (1994) Oral tolerance: Immunologic mechanisms and treatment of animal and human organ-specific autoimmune diseases by oral administration of autoantigens, *Annu. Rev. Immunol.*, **12**, 809-837.

Weiner, H.L. (1997) Oral tolerance: Immune mechanisms and treatment of autoimmune diseases, *Immunol. Today*, **18**, 335-343.

Weinstein, P. D. and Cebra, J.J. (1991) The preference for switching to IgA expression by Peyer's patch germinal center B cells is likely due to the intrinsic influence of their environment, *J. Immunol.*, **147**, 4126-4135.

Williams, N. A., Harper, H.H. and Cochrane, L. (1997) Antigen presenting cells of the small intestinal lamina propria, *Mucosal Immunol. Update*, **5**, 29-32.

Wold, A.E. (1998) The hygiene hypothesis revised: is the rising frequency of allergy due to changes in the intestinal flora?, *Allergy*, **53**, 20-25.

Wostmann, B.S. and Pleasants, J.R. (1991) The germ-free animal fed chemically defined diet: a unique tool, *Proc. Soc. Exp. Biol. Med.*, **198**, 539-546.

Zoetendal, E.G., Akkermans, A.D.L. and De Vos, W.M. (1998) Temperature gradient gel electrophoresis analysis of 16S rRNA from human fecal samples reveals stable and host-specific communities of active bacteria, *Appl. Environ. Microbiol.*, **64**, 3854-3859.

CHAPTER 4

Antitumour Activity of Lactic Acid Bacteria

I Kato

4.1 Introduction

Since ancient times, lactic acid bacteria have influenced human dietary habitats. The products fermented by the bacteria are consumed in many different forms. Metchnikoff proposed beneficial effects from the consumption of fermented milk products such as yoghurt on human health at the beginning of the 20th century. Since this time, studies have demonstrated that lactic acid bacteria inhabit the human gastrointestinal tract, together and with various other microorganisms form on intestinal microflora, which affects physiological functions in the host. It has gradually become clear that the intestinal microflora have both negative and positive effects on human health, however, lactic acid bacteria are beneficial to human health.

Certain microorganisms such as *Mycobacterium bovis* BCG, *Propionibacterium acnes*, and *Streptococcus pyogenes* are known to exhibit remarkable antitumour activity and to act as immunopotentiators. A preparation of *S. pyogenes* has been clinically used as an immunopotential antitumour agent for over 20 years in Japan. BCG has also been administered by intravesical injection for superficial bladder cancer. These microorganisms can stimulate nonspecific (macrophage functions and natural killer cell activity) and specific (T and B cell functions) resistance, and are referred to as Biological Response Modifiers (BRMs).

Consumption of fermented milk or lactic acid bacteria enhances the immune response and increases resistance to neoplasms and various infections. It also improves digestion and assimilation, aids in normalization of the microflora, prevents diarrhoea and constipation, and decreases the serum cholesterol level. Roles for lactic acid bacteria and their fermented products in antitumour activity and the modification of various biological responses have been reported. Reddy *et al.* (1973) demonstrated that the feeding of yoghurt inhibited growth of Ehrlich ascites tumour in the peritoneal cavity. Goldin and Gorbach (1980) reported on the effect of a dietary supplement of *Lactobacillus acidophilus* on intestinal cancer induced by 1,2-dimethylhydrazine

R. Fuller and G. Perdigon (eds.), Probiotics 3, 115–138.

dihydrochloride in F344 rats. It was found that *L. acidophilus* delayed the onset of experimental colon cancer. Perdigon *et al.* (1986; 1987; 1988; 1994; 1995) indicated that feeding of lactic acid bacteria and yoghurt augmented systemic immune responses (macrophage function and number of immunoglobulin secreting cells) as well as local immune responses (IgA secretion into intestine). Furthermore, they (1990; 1991) demonstrated that feeding of milk fermented with *L. casei* and *L. acidophilus* prevented gastrointestinal infection by *Salmonella typhimurium* and *Escherichia coli*. They suggested that these biological activities were a result of the immunomodulating abilities of lactic acid bacteria and fermented products.

4.2 Effects of carcinogenesis in an epidemiological study

Consumption of fermented dairy products has been proposed to provide protection against carcinogenesis. Several epidemiological studies have examined the relationship between consumption of various foods including fermented dairy products and carcinogenesis in various organs such as the colorectum (Boutron, *et al.*, 1996; Kearney, *et al.*, 1996; Kampman, *et al.*, 1994a; 1994b; 1994c), pancreas (Bueno de Mesquita, *et al.*, 1991), breast (Van't Veer, *et al.*, 1989; 1991), ovary (Cramer, *et al.*, 1989; Simard, *et al.*, 1991), and oesophagus (Cook Mozaffari, *et al.*, 1979).

A case-control study for cancer of the exocrine pancreas was carried out in the Netherlands during 1984-88 (Bueno de Mesquita, *et al.*, 1991). From the results for 164 patients and 480 controls, it was concluded that consumption of fermented milk products influenced the development of pancreatic carcinoma.

It is proposed that colorectal cancer risk is associated with intake of vegetable fiber, calcium, and dairy products. In a case-control study, which was set up in France between 1985 and 1990 by Boutron *et al.* (1996), the relationship between dairy products and the risk of small adenoma (154 patients), large adenoma (208 patients), and colorectal cancer (171 patients) was investigated. It was found that consumption of yoghurt inversely correlated with the risk of developing large adenomas but other dairy foods (milk and cheese) showed no relationship with adenoma and cancer. In contrast, Kampman *et al.* (1994) reported that intake of milk and fermented dairy products did not relate to adenoma in the US or colon cancer in the Netherlands.

For breast-cancer occurrence in the Netherlands, van't Veer, *et al.* (1989; 1991) reported an association of consumption of fermented milk products among 133 breast cancer patients and 289 control subjects. They suggested that consumption of a large amount of fermented milk products and Gouda cheese reduces the risk of developing breast cancer. They observed no relationship between consumption of milk and breast cancer, and concluded that the lactic acid bacteria contained in fermented milk and cheese might provide protection against carcinogenesis of breast cancer by modifying the enterohepatic circulation or stimulating an immunological response.

4.3 Antitumour activity of lactic acid bacteria administered *via* the parenteral route

From the collection of lactic acid bacteria in our institute, we selected strains that possessed strong antitumour activity. Against solid tumour and ascites tumour forms, the antitumour activities of 26 strains of lactobacilli were examined (Fig. 4.1). For the solid form, lactic acid bacteria were injected 5 times intravenously after a subcutaneous inoculation of Sarcoma 180, and tumour weight was determined on the 21st day. To examine the activity against the ascites tumour form, bacteria were injected 5 times intraperitoneally after intraperitoneal inoculation of Sarcoma 180, and the mortality of mice was monitored for 40 days. All 5 strains of *L. casei* tested and one strain of *L. plantarum* markedly suppressed the growth of Sarcoma 180 in solid and ascites form. We selected one of these bacteria, *Lactobacillus casei* YIT 9018 (LC), which showed 82.7% inhibition for solid form and enhanced the survival rate (216%) for ascites form.

4.3.1 In animal models

LC showed antitumour activities against various transplantable tumours of rodents (Table 4.1). Besides that of allogeneic tumor (Sarcoma 180), the growth of syngeneic tumours (Meth A, MCA K-1, L1210, C57AT1, 3LL, B16 and K234) was suppressed by the administration of LC *via* various routes in mice. In Donryu rats, LC also inhibited the growth of ascites hepatomas (AH 130, AH 55, AH 7974 and AH 41C) and prolonged the lifespan of the animals.

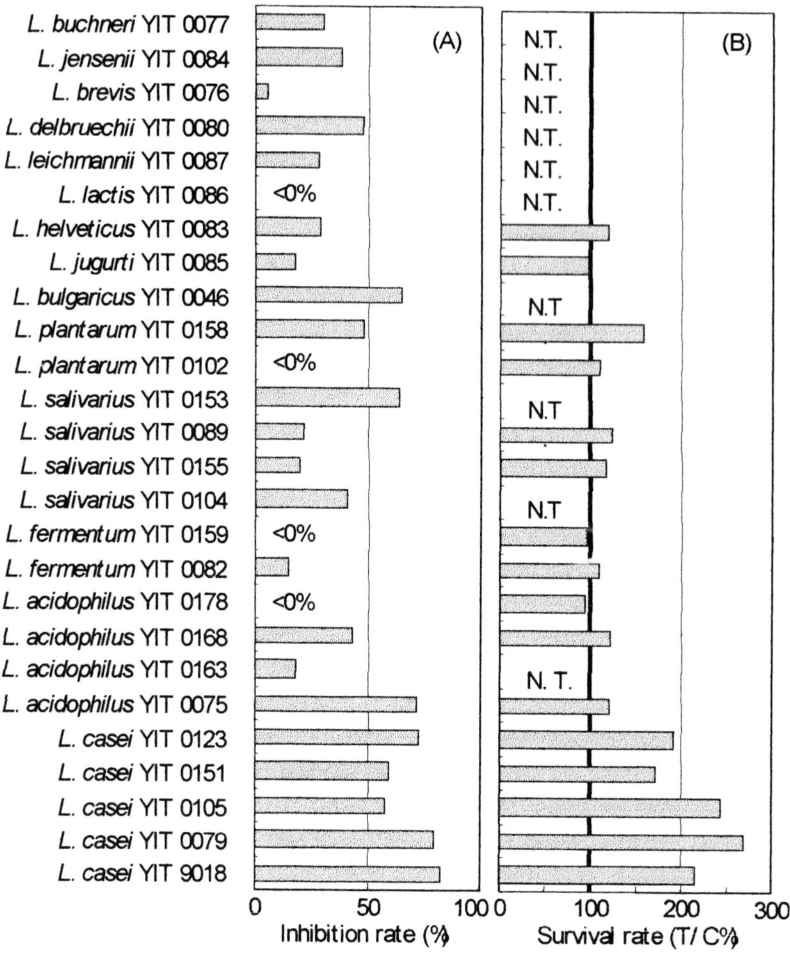

Figure 4.1. Antimour activities of lactobacilli against (A) the solid form and (B) the ascites form of Sarcoma 180 in ICR mice.

In clinical trials, a preparation of heat-killed LC significantly prolonged survival in patients with malignant pleural effusions of lung cancer. In an experimental model of malignant pleurisy with Meth A in BALB/c mouse, it was clearly shown that intrapleural injection of LC prolonged the survival of BALB/c mice inoculated intrapleurally with Meth A tumour cells. In this model, intrapleural injection of Meth A cells resulted in subsequent growth of the tumour cells and the mice died from the tumour with increased pleural effusion. LC was as effective as other preparations of antitumoural microorganisms such as *S. pyogenes*, *P. acnes* and BCG in preventing intrapleural tumour growth (Matsuzaki *et al.*, 1988a).

Table 4.1. Antitumour activity of LC

Tumours	Transplanted sites	Animals	Injection routes	Dose (mg/kg)	Antitumour effect	
Meth A	i.pl.	BALB/c mouse	i.pl.	4 x 5	T/C	250
Meth A	i.p.	BALB/c mouse	i.p.	5 x 5	T/C	>157
L1210	i.p.	DBA/2 mouse	i.p.	10 x 3	T/C	138
C57AT1	i.p.	C57BL/6 mouse	i.p.	2 x 5	T/C	134
Sarcoma 180	i.p.	ICR mouse	i.p.	2 x 5	T/C	>209
Meth A	s.c.	BALB/c mouse	i.p.	10 x 5	I.R.	87.6
MCA K-1	s.c.	BALB/c mouse	i.p.	10 x 5	I.R.	61.3
Meth A	s.c.	BALB/c mouse	i.v.	10 x 5	I.R.	88.2
MCA K-1	s.c.	BALB/c mouse	i.v.	2 x 5	I.R.	60.4
Sarcoma 180	s.c.	ICR mouse	i.v.	10 x 5	I.R.	75.9
3LL	s.c.	C57BL/6 mouse	i.v.	10 x 4	T/C	>132
B16	s.c.	C57BL/6 mouse	i.v.	10 x 5	T/C	>150
B16-F10	i.v.	C57BL/6 mouse	i.v.	10 x 5	T/C	134
AH 130	i.v.	Donryu rat	i.v.	10 x10	T/C	181
AH 55	i.v.	Donryu rat	i.v.	10 x10	T/C	159
AH 7974	i.v.	Donryu rat	i.v.	10 x10	T/C	139
AH 41C	i.v.	Donryu rat	i.v.	10 x10	T/C	>178
Meth A	s.c.	BALB/c mouse	s.c.	30 x 7	I.R.	72.9
Meth A	s.c.	BALB/c mouse	i.t.	4 x 5	I.R.	88.4
Meth A	s.c.	BALB/c mouse	i.t.	4 x 5	T/C	>152
K234	s.c.	BALB/c mouse	i.t.	4 x 5	T/C	>162
B16-BL6	s.c.	C57BL/6 mouse	i.t.	10x 4	I.R.	81.9
B16-BL6	s.c.	C57BL/6 mouse	i.t.	10x 4	T/C	156
B16-F10	s.c.	C57BL/6 mouse	i.t.	10x 5	T/C	142

i.pl.: intrapleural, i.p.: intraperitoneal, i.v.: intravenous, s.c.: subcutaneous,
i.t.: intratumoural, i.d.: intradermal,
T/C (%) = (mean survival day of tested mice / mean survival day of control mice) x 100.
I.R. (%) = (1-mean tumour weight of tested mice / mean tumor weight of control mice) x 100.

LC suppressed not only the growth of but also metastasis from the primary tumour. Pulmonary metastasis developed following subcutaneous inoculation of Lewis lung carcinoma cells in C57BL/6 mice. Intralesional and intravenous injection of LC to primary tumour caused a decrease in the number of metastatic nodules in lung and prolongation of the survival period. In strain-2 guinea pigs inoculated with line-10 hepatoma, lymph node metastasis was suppressed by LC-injection and 50% of mice were free of metastasis in contrast to 0% of mice in the control group at 73 days after inoculation of primary tumour (Matsuzaki *et al.*, 1985). Furthermore, LC showed remarkable anti-metastatic activity against a highly metastatic variant of B16 melanoma (B16-BL6) in C57BL/6 mice (Matsuzaki *et al.*, 1987; 1988b). The surgical excision of tumour, resulting from B16-BL6 inoculation into the front footpad of mice, induced both lymph node and lung metastasis. The intralesional and intravenous injection of LC significantly inhibited the metastasis in axillary lymph node and lung. And the injection of LC augmented *in vitro* cytolytic activity against B16-BL6 cells and natural killer activity of axillary lymph node cells. Watanabe (1996) demonstrated that intraperitoneal injection of LC caused a decrease in the incidence of spontaneous thymic lymphoma and prolongation of survival in AKR mice.

4.3.2 Immunomodulation

As part of the mechanism of the antitumour effect of LC, a close relationship between the antitumour activity and augmentation of the host-mediated response of LC was suggested. Macrophages were directly activated by LC and became cytotoxic against tumour cells. Peptone-induced peritoneal macrophages of BALB/c mouse were cultured for 24 hrs with LC *in vitro*. After removing bacterial cells, the macrophages were cultured with tumour cells, and subsequently the extent to which tritium-thymidine was incorporated into tumour cells was evaluated. It was found that LC could directly induce the expression of cytotoxic macrophages (Table 4.2).

Table 4.2. Induction of cytostatic activity of macrophages against various tumour cells *in vitro*

Target tumour cells	Cytostatic activity (% growth inhibition)
Meth A	100
RL♂1	71
P815	62
YAC 1	87

Peritoneal exudate macrophages, which had been induced by i.p. injection of proteose-peptone, were cultured with or without LC (50 μg/ml) for 24 hrs, and then the cytostatic activity of the macrophages against each tumour cell was determined.

In vivo, the phagocytic activity toward sheep red blood cells and cytostatic activity to EL4 tumour cells of peritoneal macrophages was augmented by the intraperitoneal injection of LC. And the phagocytic

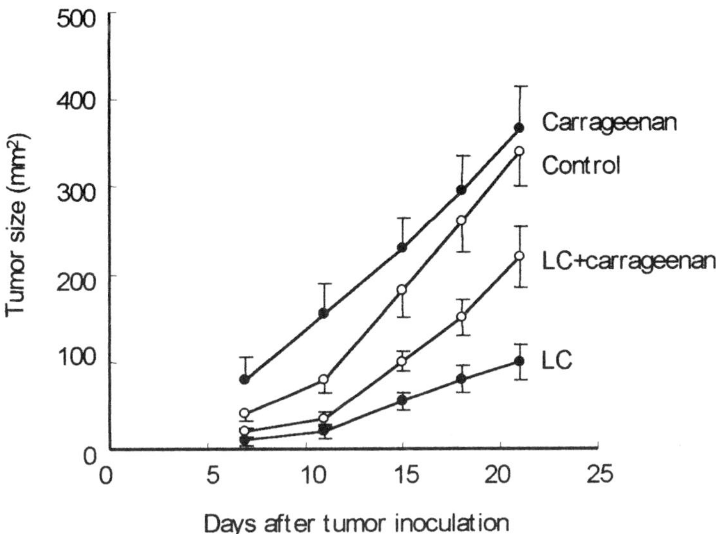

Figure 4. 2. Effect of carrageenan on the antitumor activity of LC. Sarcoma 180 tumour cells were subcutaneously inoculated into ICR mice.
Carrageenan (20 mg/kg) was intraperitoneally injected on day -2, and LC was intravenously injected on day +1, +2, +3, +4, and +5.

activity of the reticuloendothelial system as determined by the carbon clearance test was also augmented (Kato *et al.*, 1983). The production of oxygen radicals and a cytotoxic factor for tumour cells by macrophages or Kupffer cells was up-regulated by LC-injection (Hashimoto *et al.*, 1984; 1985). Intraperitoneal injection of LC induced tumouricidal macrophages in a neutralization test (Kato *et al.*, 1985). Furthermore, the antitumour activity of LC against Sarcoma 180 was partially suppressed by injection of carrageenan or silica particles acting as macrophage inhibitors (Fig. 4.2). These results showed that the macrophages activated by LC played important roles in LC-induced antitumour activities.

Natural killer cells are essential to the prevention of tumour growth in the host. LC augmented natural killer cell activity in spleen of BALB/c mice (Kato *et al.*, 1984). Intravenous injection of LC induced splenic natural killer cell activity 5-fold compared with the value in non-treated control mice. Another lactic acid bacterium (*L. fermentum* YIT 0159), which possessed no antitumour activity, did not augment natural killer cell activity. The augmentation of natural killer activity by LC was observed in tumour-bearing mice (Table 4.3). These observations indicated a close relationship between the antitumour effect of LC and augmentation of natural killer cell activity by LC.

Table 4.3. Augmentation of natural killer activity of Meth A bearing BALB/c mice

Mice	Treatment	Natural killer activity (%)	Tumour weight (g)
Normal	Saline	4.3 ± 0.7	
	LC	34.3 ± 1.5	
10-days Meth A bearing	Saline	9.7 ± 1.3	0.19 ± 0.03
	LC	19.4 ± 2.6	0.11 ± 0.02
20-days Meth A bearing	Saline	9.4 ± 0.8	1.05 ± 0.17
	LC	19.6 ± 1.4	0.64 ± 0.20

Meth A cells (5 x 10^5/mouse) were inoculated subcutaneously into BALB/c mice. Lc (250 μg/mouse) was injected intravenously 3 days before natural killer assay. Values represent the mean ± S.E. (n =5).

Table 4.4. Effect of $CD4^+$ or $CD8^+$ T cell depletion on the antitumour activity of LC in Meth A bearing mice

Treatment	Tumour weight, g (inhibition ratio, %)		
	Exp. 1	Exp. 2	Exp. 3
Mouse IgG2b	2.56 ± 0.33	2.06 ± 0.50	1.61 ± 0.76
Mouse IgG2b + LC	0.59 ± 0.27 (77.0)	0.56 ± 0.24 (72.8)	0.46 ± 0.16 (71.4)
Anti-CD4	2.76 ± 0.50	Not done	1.31 ± 0.58
Anti-CD4 + LC	1.24 ± 0.49 (55.1)	Not done	0.62 ± 0.29 (54.0)
Anti-CD8	Not done	3.06 ± 0.71	3.06 ± 0.39
Anti-CD8 + LC	Not done	0.84 ± 0.29 (72.5)	0.89 ± 0.27 (70.9)

Meth A cells 5 x 10^5/mouse were inoculated into BALB/c mice after the injection of anti-CD4 or anti-CD8 antibody. LC (250 μg/mouse) was injected at 3, 6, 9, 12, and 15 days after tumour inoculation. Tumours were weighed on the 21st day.

T cells play an important role in antitumour immunity as effector cell. LC induced tumour-specific and T cell-dependent antitumour immunity. When a mixture of LC and tumour cells was injected into mice, systemic antitumour immunity developed. This antitumour response is cellular not humoral or tumour specific. The effector cells expressed Thy1 antigen on their surface (Yasutake *et al.*, 1984 a). To clarify the T cell dependency in LC-induced antitumour activity, *in vivo* depletion of the T cell subpopulation using anti-CD4 and anti-CD8 antibody was performed (Hayashi and Okwaki, 1989). Splenic T cells were depleted by the intravenous injection of antibody, then the antitumour activity of LC against Meth A tumour in the T cell-depleted mice was determined. The antitumour activity of LC was decreased by the depletion of $CD4^+$ but not $CD8^+$ cells (Table 4.4). $CD4^+$ T cells have a function as helpers/inducers in host-immune responses. Perhaps, LC displayed antitumor activity through the modification of $CD4^+$ T cell functions such as production of cytokines and induction of killer cells.

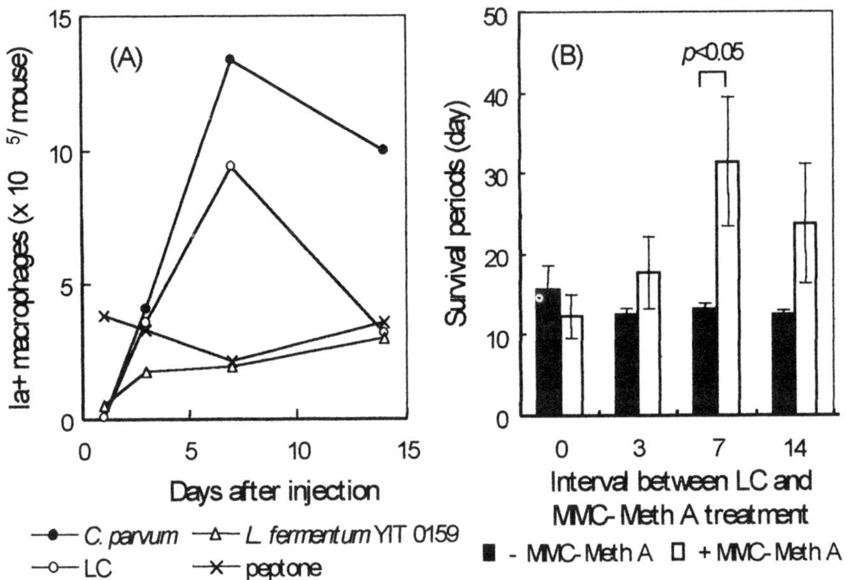

Figure 4.3. Coincidence of induction of Ia^+ macrophage by LC and acquisition of tumour specific immune response by MMC-Meth A and LC.

(A) Microorganism (500μg/mouse) was intraperitoneally injected into BALB/c mouse. Peritoneal exudate cells were stained with anti-I-A^d antibody and FITC-anti-mouse IgG, and Ia^+ macrophages were determined. (B) LC (500 μg/mouse) was intraperitoneally injected into BALB/c mice, then MMC-Meth A cells (5 x 10^6) were injected at various intervals. Viable Meth A cells (10^6) were implanted in the peritoneal cavity 14 days after MMC-Meth A. Survivors were monitored for 40 days.

We demonstrated a correlation between the induction of a T cell-mediated antitumour response and macrophage activation by LC (Kato *et al.*, 1988). In animal systems, T cell-dependent antitumour responses are induced by the immunization of inactivated tumour cells. When mitomycin-treated Meth A cells (MMC-Meth A) were instilled intraperitoneally, Thy 1-positive T cells possessing antitumour activity appeared in the peritoneal cavity. On the other hand, MHC class II antigen (Ia antigen in mouse) is essential to the interaction of antigen presenting cells and T cells. Ia-antigen positive cells act as accessory cells in the induction of antigen-specific T cells. Following injection of LC, the expression of Ia-positive macrophages was induced in the peritoneal cavity. The induction showed a maximum both quantitatively and qualitatively at 7 days after injection. The timing of the maximum induction coincided with the most effective period for induction of the T cell-mediated antitumor response (Fig. 4.3) and the antitumour activity was abolished by treatment of anti-Ia antigen *in vivo*. The results showed that macrophage activation by LC was an important step in the acquisition of T cell mediated antitumour immunity. As to the mechanism of antitumour activity of LC, we suggested that T cells contribute to the development of tumour-specific antitumour activity, and macrophages activated by LC contribute directly to the killing of tumour cells and to the generation of T cell-mediated antitumour activity.

While presenting antigen particles to T cells and B cells, macrophages simultaneously release a cytokine known as interleukin-1 (IL-1), which stimulates T and B cells. IL-1 secreted by macrophages promotes the maturation of B cells and induces stem cells in the bone marrow to differentiate into T and B cells and to multiply. Helper T cells stimulated by IL-1 secreted other cytokines, such as IL-2. IL-2 launches attacks on antigens by increasing the number of killer T cells, promotes production of antibodies by increasing the number of B cells and steps up the phagocytic activity of macrophages. Mouse resident macrophages and human peripheral blood cells, co-cultured with LC secreted IL-1 *in vitro*, and augmented secretion of colony-stimulating factors (CSFs) from fibroblasts and endothelial cells. The injection of LC by various routes (intraperitoneally, intravenously and subcutaneously) stimulated myelopoietic capacity *via* CSF-production and augmented protective ability against X-ray-irradiation in mice (Nanno *et al.*, 1986; Nomoto *et al.*, 1991). IL-1 stimulates production of IL-2 from T cells and the expression of IL-2 receptors on the surface of T cells. IL-2 stimulates the proliferation of T cells, and induces lymphokine-activated killer cell activity. Production of IL-2 was augmented by LC-injection (Matsuzaki *et al.*, 1990b).

Interferon-gamma (IFN-γ) is produced by helper T cells and is an essential cytokine in the development of cellular immunity and in induction of tumour-specific immunity. IFN-γ can activate cytocidal macrophages, natural killer cells, and cytotoxic T cells. IL-12 is an IFN-γ-inducible cytokine. IL-12 is secreted by B cells, dendritic cells, and macrophages. When ovalbumin (OVA)-priming splenocytes were cultured with OVA in the absence or presence of LC, LC induced IFN-γ production in a dose dependent manner (Shida *et al.*, 1998). But another strain of lactic acid bacteria, *L. johnsonii* did not enhance IFN-γ production. In our recent study (Kato *et al.*, 1999), a similar enhancement of IFN-γ production by LC was observed. LC enhanced IFN-γ production from splenocytes stimulated with concanavalin A. The IFN-γ production was decreased by addition of anti-IL-12 antibody. And macrophages activated by LC were essential in the production of IFN-γ by splenic T cells. LC had no direct effect on T cell functions (proliferation and cytokine production). Based on the above findings, we concluded that LC directly activated macrophages, to produce IL-12 and accessory cells, which subsequently led to a dominant state of cellular immunity.

4.3.3 In clinical trials

A therapeutic trial involving human neoplasms using a preparation of heat-killed LC was performed from 1983 in Japan. For patients with carcinoma of the uterine cervix, subcutaneous injection of the LC preparation combined with radiation therapy prolonged survival and the relapse-free interval compared to radiation alone (Okawa *et al.*, 1989; 1993). In patients with malignant pleural effusions secondary to lung cancer, the intrapleural instillation of doxorubicin plus the LC preparation produced a significant prolongation of survival, and improvement in performance status and symptoms (chest pain, chest discomfort, and anorexia) compared to the administration of doxorubicin alone (Masuno *et al.*, 1991). Both trials indicated LC is an effective adjuvant immunotherapeutic agent.

4.4 Antitumour activity of lactic acid bacteria administered *via* a non-parenteral route

4.4.1 Against transplantable tumours in animal models

The antitumour activity of LC given *via* a non-parenteral route, against various transplantable tumours in rats and mice has been reported.

Asano *et al.* (1986) gave oral gavage of live LC to C3H/He mice for 10 consecutive days from 7 days after subcutaneous inoculation of mouse bladder tumour, MBT-2. At 21 days after the inoculation, treated mice showed a significant decrease of tumour weight compared with untreated controls. In Donryu rats, ascitic hepatoma cells (AH130 or AH41C) were injected intravenously and LC was administered for 10 days from 3 days after the injection. Compared with rats not given LC, rats treated with LC had a longer survival period (Yokokura *et al.*, 1984).

Patients with colon and gastric cancer frequently suffer from hepatic metastasis and this is a significant factor in the choice of postoperative adjuvant therapy. The prophylactic effects of various immunomodulative substances on hepatic metastasis have been studied in animals. The therapeutic effect of LC has been assessed in an experimental model of hepatic metastasis from gastrointestinal cancer (Tazawa *et al.*, personal communication). When 2.5 x 10^6 ascites hepatoma (AH60C) cells were inoculated into the portal vein of Donryu rats, haematogenous hepatic metastasis occurred in 84.6% (11/13) of control rats at 11 days after the tumour-inoculation. The metastatic incidence was 45.5% (5/11) of tested rats dosed orally with LC for 10 consecutive days. LC-treated rats showed fewer metastases (47.3 ± 27.3) in the liver than control rats (80.8 ± 23.1).

Table 4. 5. Antitumour response to secondary tumours induced by resection of the primary tumours and oral administration of LC

Sample	Dose	N	Footpad thickness (mm, mean ± S.E.)		
			Day 7	Day 14	Day 21
Control	DW (x 7)	11	2.93 ± 0.07	5.08 ± 0.19	7.52 ± 0.29
LC	0.25 x 10^9	10	2.87 ± 0.07	5.09 ± 0.18	7.21 ± 0.47
LC	0.5 x 10^9	10	2.84 ± 0.09	4.26 ± 0.35	5.59 ± 0.68*
LC	1.0 x 10^9	11	2.62 ± 0.05*	3.70 ± 0.37*	5.27 ± 0.60*

After resection of primary Colon 26 tumours for sensitization, Colon 26 tumour cells were inoculated into the footpad of BALB/c mice to form the secondary tumours. LC was administered orally for 7 days and the footpad thickness was measured. * $p<0.05$

We showed that tumour-specific responses were augmented by oral administration of LC (Kato *et al.,* 1994). Colon 26 tumour cells (5x10^5 cells) were intradermally inoculated in the abdomen of C57BL/6 mice and the tumour mass was completely resected 5 days later. At 3 days after tumour resection, 1 x 10^5 Colon 26 cells were subcutaneously injected into a footpad of each mouse. LC was orally administered for 7 days and the effect on the secondary tumour was assessed by measurement of footpad thickness. The growth of secondary tumour was significantly suppressed by LC compared with the control group (Table 4.5). The antitumour effect of LC was only exerted when Colon 26 was the secondary tumour and not when the secondary tumour was Meth A. So we suggest that LC induced a tumour-specific host immune response to the primary tumour, indicating that LC has systemic immunopotentiating activity.

4.4.2 Suppression of carcinogenesis in animal models

Many chemicals have been shown to have a carcinogenic potential in animals, and have been used in the study of organ-specific carcinogenesis and its suppression. N-butyl-N(4-hydrobutyl)nitrosamine (BBN) is known to induce bladder tumours at high frequency when administered orally to rats and mice. Since most BBN-induced tumours in rodents are superficial, well-differentiated, transitional cell carcinomas, BBN has been used in experiments on bladder carcinogenesis to create a model of human superficial bladder cancer. The effect of administration of LC on BBN-induced bladder carcinogenesis in male Wistar rats has been studied (Tomita *et al.*, 1994). To induce bladder tumours, 0.05% BBN in drinking water was provided to the rats *ad libitum* for 7 weeks. LC was administered by oral gavage twice a week according to various schedules relative to exposure to BBN. At 22 weeks after the start of exposure to BBN, bladder weight, tumour volume, and histological findings were determined. The mean bladder weight and the mean tumour volume per bladder were significantly lower in the LC treated groups than in the control group. The grade of malignancy of the induced bladder tumours was significantly lower in the concomitant treatment group than in the control group (Table 4.6). Using C3H/He mice, a suppressive effect of LC on BBN-induced bladder carcinogenesis was also demonstrated (Ohtani *et al.,* 1993). Mice were given 0.05% BBN in drinking water for 10 weeks and simultaneously administered LC by oral gavage twice a week for 10 weeks. Twenty-five weeks after the start of the experiment, the mice were sacrificed. The incidence of bladder carcinogenesis was 66.7 % (20/30) in mice treated with LC compared with 90.0% (27/30) in mice treated with placebo. There was a significant reduction in the LC group ($p<0.05$ analyzed by the chi-squared test).

Table 4. 6. Prevention of BBN-induced bladder carcinogenesis by LC

Treatment period of LC	N	Bladder weight (g)			Tumour volume per bladder (mm^3)		
		Mean	±	SD	Mean	±	SD
Control (Non-treatment)	16	1.63	±	1.45	1875.7	±	1839.5
22 weeks (throughout the study)	20	0.66	±	0.48**	567.0	±	591.9*
7 weeks (simultaneous with exposure to BBN)	20	0.80	±	0.87*	975.9	±	1203.5
15 weeks (after exposure to BBN)	18	1.08	±	0.90	907.6	±	775.3*

Wister rats were given BBN-containing drinking water for 7 weeks and treated orally with LC. At 22 weeks after the start of exposure to BBN, the urinary bladder was harvested and the tumor volume was determined.
$^{*}p<0.05$, $^{**}p<0.01$

Subcutaneous injection of 3-methylcholanthrene, a known potent carcinogen, also induces tumours in mice. The effect of LC on subcutaneous tumours induced by 3-methylcholanthrene was examined (Fig. 4.4). Mice received a single subcutaneous injection of 0.5 mg of 3-methylcholanthrene, and were given LC by oral gavage for 5 days before injection and twice weekly thereafter for 150 days. The final tumour incidence was 59.0% in mice treated with LC compared with 91.8% in control mice, indicating marked suppression of methylcholanthrene-induced carcinogenesis by oral administration of LC.

Oral administration of LC suppressed chemically induced carcinogenesis. We suggest that this suppression may result from the eradication of cancer cells *via* augmentation of immune surveillance by LC. And suppression of carcinogenesis by LC may involve another mechanism, i.e., modification of the metabolism and excretion of chemical carcinogens as a result of alteration of the intestinal flora. When protein-rich foods such as meat are heated, large amounts of heterocyclic amines are produced. Most of these heterocyclic amines are reported to have mutagenic and carcinogenic potential. In humans, it has been reported that intake of cooked meat containing carcinogenic heterocyclic amines increases the urinary excretion of mutagens. Hayatsu and Hayatsu (1993) assessed the effect of live LC on the increase of urinary mutagenicity after ingestion of cooked meat in 6 healthy volunteers. The urinary mutagenicity observed in the LC-treated period was only 6-66% (average 47.5%) of that observed in the LC-untreated period. This finding confirmed the administration of LC decreased the passage of dietary mutagens from the intestine into the urine. Since a decrease of urinary mutagenicity may mean decreased systemic exposure to mutagens, oral administration of LC may be effective in reducing the risk of carcinogenesis from intestinal sources.

There may be various ways in which exogenous lactobacilli reduce the risk of carcinogenesis from intestinal sources. Exogenous lactobacilli may enable the intestinal flora to metabolize dietary mutagens into non-mutagenic substances in the intestinal tract. Alternatively, bacterial cells may be directly bound to mutagens in the intestinal tract, thereby inhibiting their intestinal absorption. Morotomi and Mutai (1986) showed absorption of mutagens by intestinal microorganisms. Among the mutagens tested, Trp-P-1 and Trp-P-2 were absorbed by various species of intestinal bacteria, including *Bifidobacterium*, *Lactobacillus* and *Bacteroides*. LC exhibited a high binding affinity for the above mutagens as well as other mutagens, including IQ, MeIQ, and MeIQx.

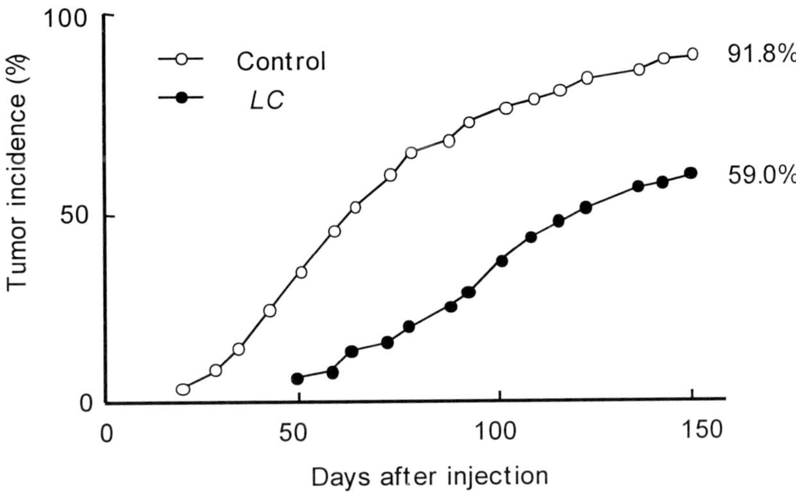

Figure 4.4. Effect of administration of LC on methylcholanthrene-induced carcinogenesis in BALB/c mice.
3-methylcholanthrene (0.5 mg) was injected subcutaneously to each mouse on day 0. The mice were given water containing LC or tap water from 5 days to 1 day before injection of the carcinogen and two days per week thereafter for 150 days.

4.4.3 Immunomodulation

It is well known that in tumour-bearing animals and humans, immunity is impaired due to the presence of the tumour. In particular, suppression of T cell activity may be of great concern from the aspect of preventing cancer recurrence. We examined the effect of LC on the activity of T cells obtained from BALB/c mice with Colon 26 tumour (Kato *et al.*, 1994). When splenocytes were stimulated with T cell mitogen (concanavalin A and phytohemagglutinin) and cytokines (IL-1 and IL-2), the proliferative activity of splenocytes from tumour bearer was suppressed compared with normal mice. Oral treatment of LC facilitated the restoration of T cell proliferative activity in tumour-bearing mice (Fig. 4.5).

In another experiment, oral treatment with LC augmented IFN-γ production by splenocytes obtained from normal and tumour-bearing mice (Kato *et al.*, 1999).

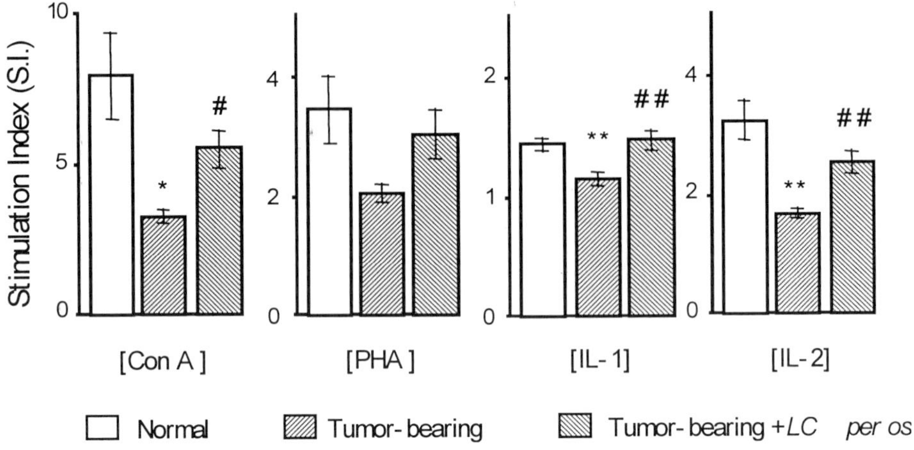

Figure 4.5. Effect of oral administration of LC on the proliferative activity of splenocytes.
Colon 26 tumour cells were inoculated into the hind footpad of BALB/c mice. And LC was given orally for 7 consecutive days. The next day, splenocytes were obtained and cultured with mitogens or cytokines. The results are presented as the mean S.I. values and S.E. of 4 mice. Significant differences: * $p<0.05$, ** $p<0.01$ versus Normal group, and # $p<0.05$, ## $p<0.01$ versus Tumour-bearing group.

4.4.4 In clinical trials

Although surgical resection transurethrally is usually performed to treat superficial bladder cancer and the therapy prolongs the survival of the patients, the rate of recurrence of this cancer is high. Intravesical instillation of various chemotherapeutic agents or *Mycobacterium bovis* BCG has proved to have great efficacy though it occasionally produces adverse reactions. Aso *et al.* (1992; 1995) reported on the prophylactic efficacy of oral administration of a viable LC preparation on the recurrence of superficial bladder cancer after transurethral resection in a double blind trial. The recurrence-free rate at one year after transurethral resection was 79.0% in the LC group (10^{10} cells, 3 times/day) and 54.9% in the placebo group. By Cox multivariate analysis, the risk of recurrence in the placebo group was 2.58-fold higher than that in the LC group. Adverse reactions (diarrhoea, constipation and elevation of the hepatic transaminase) were transient and mild in the LC group. These results show that LC preparations may be useful in prophylactic therapy against bladder cancer without serious adverse effects and will effectively improve the quality of life (QOL) of the patients.

In patients with Dukes A colon cancer, immunomodulatory effects of oral administration of a LC preparation were determined. Flow cytometric analysis revealed an increase of helper T cells $CD4^{+}CD45RA^{-}$

and natural killer cells ($CD57^{+}CD16^{+}$) and suppressor T cells ($CD8^{+}CD11b^{+}$) in the peritoneal blood of patients treated with the LC preparation (Sawamura *et al.*, 1994).

4.5 Antitumour activity of cell fragment from lactic acid bacteria

As described above, some lactic acid bacteria have potential antitumour activity against experimental and transplantable tumours in animals. It is known that the adjuvant active principle of antitumoural bacteria, such as *Mycobacterium bovis* BCG and *Propionibacterium acnes*, is the cell wall fraction, and that the minimum adjuvant-active structure of bacterial cell wall is muramyl-L-alanyl-D-isoglutamine (MDP).

The product from the cell wall of *L. bulgaricus* has shown antitumour activity and activation of macrophage function (spreading, phagocytosis, and production of IL-1 and TNF-alpha) (Davidkova, 1992; Popova, 1993). Sekine *et al.* (1985; 1994; 1995) reported that a cell wall preparation isolated from *Bifidobacterium infantis* has potential antitumour activity against syngeneic Meth A fibrosarcoma in BALB/c mice. The preparation activates nonspecific immunity, as well as T cell mediated immunity (delayed type hypersensitivity and antitumour neutralizing activity). The antitumour activity of LC was abrogated by the treatment of *N*-acetylmuramidase, a lytic enzyme for cell wall of Gram-positive bacteria, and the protoplasts of LC did not show antitumour activity (Yasutake *et al.*, 1984b). So, the cell wall fraction from lactic acid bacteria possessing antitumour and immunopotentiating activities is the active component.

The cell surface structure of lactobacilli is composed of a cell wall (peptidoglycan layer), polysaccharides as accessory polymers of the cell wall, and lipoteichoic acid elongated from the cell membrane (Fig. 4.6). The basal composition and structure of the peptidoglycan layer is similar throughout the genus. On the other hand, the polysaccharides of the cell wall have various structures, and the differences of antigenicity and physiological activity between strains originate from this diversity of polysaccharide structure. De Ambrosini *et al.* (1996) examined the effect of oral administration of peptidoglycans from five bacterial strains on phagocytosis of peritoneal macrophages. Even though the chemical composition of the peptidoglycans was the same, only those from *L. casei* stimulated phagocytic activity of macrophages: the peptidoglycans from the other four strains were not effective. They concluded the biological activity is unlikely to be due to the peptidoglycan structure.

Matsuzaki *et al.* (1990a) reported antitumoural components of LC. Intact cell wall from LC was prepared by treatment with detergents, solvents and enzymes. Surface polysaccharide fraction and cell wall

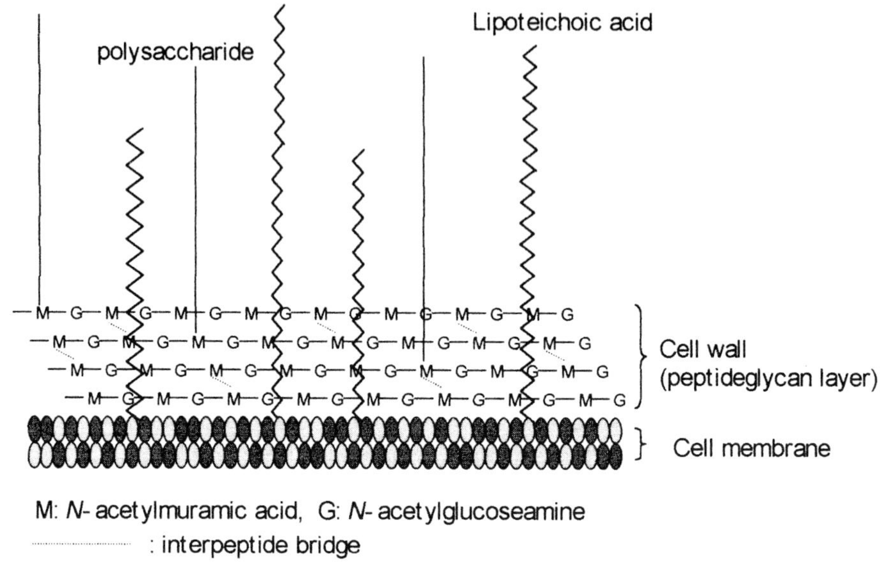

Figure 4.6. Structure of cell surface of Gram-positive bacteria

fraction lacking polysaccharides were also prepared. The intact cell wall showed the same level of antitumour activity as whole LC against Meth A fibrosarcoma. Solubilized polysaccharides and polysaccharide-removed-cell wall fractions did not have any antitumour activity. The chemical characteristics of the polysaccharide-peptidoglycan complex from LC have been reported (Nagaoka *et al.*, 1990). The peptidoglycan layer from LC consists of *N*-acetylmuramic acid, *N*-acetylglucosamine and four amino acids, i.e. lysine, aspartic acid, glutamic acid and alanine. The polysaccharide-peptidoglycan complex from LC had a high concentration of rhamnose. The growth of Meth A inoculated subcutaneously was markedly suppressed by the intratumoural injection of the polysaccharide-peptidoglycan complex (inhibition ratio: 70.4%). The combined structure of polysaccharides and peptidoglycan is indispensable for the antitumour activity of LC. Although it was supposed that the variation in antitumour efficiency among lactobacilli results from the diversity of the composition and the structure of the polysaccharide-peptidoglycan complex, further examination is required to clarify the relationship between the antitumour activity and the structure of *L. casei*.

4.6 LAB and the formation of aberrant crypt foci

The consumption of lactic acid bacteria and its fermented milk as probiotics were expected to prevent the incidence of colon cancer. An aberrant crypt focus (ACF) is a precursor lesion of colon indicating the initiation of the carcinogenic process following oral administration of chemical carcinogens, such as azoxymethane and 1,2-dimethylhydrazine. Some reports indicated that the feeding of *Bifidobacterium* or *Lactobacillus* decreased the ACF formation by azoxymethane or 1,2-dimethylhydrazine in colon of F344 rats. Kulkarni and Reddy (1994) demonstrated that the feeding of lyophilized cultures of *B. longum* significantly inhibited the ACF formation (53%) induced by azoxymethane and the crypt multiplicity in the colon. Similar observations using *B. longum* have been reported (Sekine *et al.*, 1997; Rowland *et al.*, 1998; Challa *et al.*, 1997). Arimochi *et al.* (1997) reported the effect of intestinal bacteria on the formation of azoxymethane-induced ACF in the SD rat colon. They used five intestinal bacteria, *Lactobacillus acidophilus, Bifidobacterium adolescentis, Bacteroides fragilis, Escherichia coli and Clostridium perfringens*. The culture supernatant of *L. acidophilus* had an inhibitory effect on the ACF formation and the enhancement of the removal of O^6-methylguanine from the colon mucosal DNA. Onoue *et al.* (1997) demonstrated a relationship between the intestinal microflora and the occurrence of 1.2-dimethylhydrazine-induced ACF using germfree, gnotobiotic and conventional F344 rats. The microflora of gnotobiotic rats was composed of four strains of *Bacteroides,* four of *Clostridium,* and two of *E coli.* The formation of ACF in gnotobiotic rats was greater than that in germfree and conventional rats. Further, following additive instillation of *Bifidobacterium breve* into gnotobiotic rats, the formation of ACF and its multiplicity were significantly reduced relative to gnotobiotic rats. It was suggested that the intestinal microflora plays an important role in colon carcinogenesis, with some intestinal bacteria behaving as promoters and others as anti-promoters.

4.7 Conclusion

Lactic acid bacteria are thought to promote health through the normalization of intestinal flora which has been disturbed by disease or drugs. The above-mentioned findings and other results have shown that lactic acid bacteria also have various other biological activities. The relationship between intestinal flora (including lactic acid bacteria) and systemic immunity as well as the relationship between intestinal flora and intestinal immunity are of particular interest. Comparisons of germfree and normal animals have shown that the intestinal flora is essential for proper development of the immune system. Compared with normal animals, germfree animals show poor development of the Peyer's patches, lack of plasma cells in lamina propria, and lower cytotoxicity of intraepithelial T lymphocytes. Peripheral lymphoid tissue also develops poorly as indicated by the low production levels of antibodies for T cell-dependent antigens and the low phagocytic and antigen-presenting activities of macrophages, which may lead to impairment of the systemic immune response. These findings suggest that the intestinal flora plays an important role in host immune system. Since oral administration of LC activates antitumour immunity and prevents carcinogenesis, lactobacilli in the intestinal flora may be involved in the development of the immune function. The lactic acid bacteria act as probiotics for human health. Some strains among lactobacilli have the potential to prevent development of cancer and infection by acting as immunomodulators. There needs to be more research into the various biological activities of lactic acid bacteria and possibility of protection against diseases in which the immune system is involved.

References

Arimochi, H., Kinouchi, T., Kataoka, K., Kuwahara, T. and Ohnishi, Y. (1997) Effect of intestinal bacteria on formation of azoxymethane-induced aberrant crypt foci in the rat colon. *Biochem. Biophys. Res. Commun.*, **238**, 753-7.

Asano, M., Karasawa, E. and Takayama, T. (1986) Antitumor activity of *Lactobacillus casei* (LC 9018) against experimental mouse bladder tumor (MBT-2). *J. Urol.*, **136**, 719-21.

Aso, Y., Akaza, H., Kotake, T., Tsukamoto, T., Imai, K., Naito, S. and the BLP Study Group (1995) Preventive effect of a *Lactobacillus casei* preparation on the recurrence of superficial bladder cancer in a double-blind trial. *Eur. Urol.*, **27**, 104-9.

Aso, Y., Akaza, H. and The BLP Study Group (1992) Prophylactic effect of *Lactobacillus casei* preparation on the recurrence of superficial bladder cancer. *Urol. Int.*, **49**, 125-9.

Boutron, M.C., Faivre, J., Marteau, P., Couillault, C., Senesse, P. and Quipourt, V. (1996) Calcium, phosphorus, vitamin D, dairy products and colorectal carcinogenesis: a French case--control study. *Br. J. Cancer*, **74**, 145-51.

Bueno de-Mesquita, H.B., Maisonneuve, P., Runia, S. and Moerman, C.J. (1991) Intake of foods and nutrients and cancer of the exocrine pancreas: a population-based case-control study in The Netherlands. *Int. J. Cancer*, **48**, 540-9.

Challa, A., Rao, D.R., Chawan, C.B. and Shackelford, L. (1997) *Bifidobacterium longum* and lactulose suppress azoxymethane-induced colonic aberrant crypt foci in rats. *Carcinogenesis*, **18**, 517-21.

Cook Mozaffari, P.J., Azordegan, F., Day, N.E., Ressicaud, A., Sabai, C. and Aramesh, B. (1979) Oesophageal cancer studies in the Caspian Littoral of Iran: results of a case-control study. *Br. J. Cancer*, **39**, 293-309.

Cramer, D.W., Harlow, B.L., Willett, W.C., Welch, W.R., Bell, D.A., Scully, R.E., Ng, W.G. and Knapp, R.C. (1989) Galactose consumption and metabolism in relation to the risk of ovarian cancer. *Lancet*, **2**, 66-71.

Davidkova, G., Popova, P., Guencheva, G., Bogdanov, A., Pacelli, E., Auteri, A. and

Mincheva, V. (1992) Endogenous production of tumor necrosis factor in normal mice orally treated with Deodan --a preparation from *Lactobacillus bulgaricus* "LB51". *Int. J. Immunopharmacol.*, **14**, 1355-62.

De Ambrosini, V.M., Gonzalez, S., Perdigon, G., Pesce de Ruiz Holgado, A.A. and Oliver, G. (1996) Chemical composition of the cell wall of lactic acid bacteria and related species. *Chem. Pharm. Bull. Tokyo.*, **44**, 2263-7.

Goldin, B.R. and Gorbach, S.L (1980) Effect of *Lactobacillus acidophilus* dietary supplements on 1,2-dimethylhydrazine dihydrochloride-induced intestinal cancer in rats. *J. Natl. Cancer Inst.*, **64**, 263-5.

Hashimoto, S., Nomoto, K., Matsuzaki, T., Yokokura, T. and Mutai, M. (1984) Oxygen radical production by peritoneal macrophages and Kupffer cells elicited with *Lactobacillus casei*. *Infect. Immun.*, **44**, 61-7.

Hashimoto, S., Seyama, Y., Yokokura, T. and Mutai, M. (1985) Cytotoxic factor production by Kupffer cells elicited with *Lactobacillus casei* and *Corynebacterium parvum*. *Cancer Immunol. Immunother.*, **20**, 117-21.

Hayashi, K. and Ohwaki, M. (1989) Antitumor activity of *Lactobacillus casei* (LC 9018) in mice: T cell subset depletion. *Biotherapy*, **3**, 1568-74.

Hayatsu, H. and Hayatsu, T. (1993) Suppressing effect of *Lactobacillus casei* administration on the urinary mutagenicity arising from ingestion of fried ground beef in the human. *Cancer Lett.*, **73**, 173-9.

Kampman, E., Giovannucci, E., van't Veer, P., Rimm, E., Stampfer, M.J., Colditz, G.A., Kok, F.J. and Willett, W.C. (1994c) Calcium, vitamin D, dairy foods, and the occurrence of colorectal adenomas among men and women in two prospective studies. *Am. J. Epidemiol.*, **139**, 16-29.

Kampman, E., Goldbohm, R.A., van den Brandt, P.A. and van't Veer, P. (1994b) Fermented dairy products, calcium, and colorectal cancer in The Netherlands Cohort Study. *Cancer Res.*, **54**, 3186-90.

Kampman, E., van't Veer, P., Hiddink, G.J., van Aken Schneijder, P., Kok, F.J. and Hermus, R.J. (1994a) Fermented dairy products, dietary calcium and colon cancer: a case-control study in The Netherlands. *Int. J. Cancer.*, **59**, 170-6.

Kato, I., Endo, K. and Yokokura, T. (1994) Effects of oral administration of *Lactobacillus casei* on antitumor responses induced by tumor resection in mice. *Int. J. Immunopharmacol.*, **16**, 29-36.

Kato, I., Tanaka, K. and Yokokura, T. (1999) Lactic acid bacterium potently induces the production of interleukin-12 and interferon-gamma by mouse splenocytes. *Int. J. Immunopharmacol.*, **21**, 121-131.

Kato, I., Yokokura, T. and Mutai, M. (1984) Augmentation of mouse natural killer cell activity by *Lactobacillus casei* and its surface antigens. *Microbiol. Immunol.*, **28**, 209-17.

Kato, I., Yokokura, T. and Mutai, M. (1985) Induction of tumoricidal peritoneal exudate cells by administration of *Lactobacillus casei*. *Int. J. Immunopharmacol.*, **7**, 103-9.

Kato, I., Yokokura, T. and Mutai, M. (1988) Correlation between increase in Ia-bearing macrophages and induction of T cell dependent antitumor activity by *Lactobacillus casei* in mice. *Cancer Immunol. Immunother.*, **26**, 215-21.

Kato, I., Yokokura, T and Mutai, M. (1983) Macrophage activation by *Lactobacillus casei* in mice. *Microbiol. Immunol.*, **27**, 611-8.

Kearney, J., Giovannucci, E., Rimm, E.B., Ascherio, A., Stampfer, M.J., Colditz, G.A., Wing, A., Kampman, E. and Willett, W.C. (1996) Calcium, vitamin D, and dairy foods and the occurrence of colon cancer in men. *Am. J. Epidemiol.*, **143**, 907-17.

Kulkarni, N. and Reddy, B.S. (1994) Inhibitory effect of *Bifidobacterium longum* cultures on the azoxymethane-induced aberrant crypt foci formation and fecal bacterial beta-glucuronidase. *Proc. Soc. Exp. Biol. Med.*, **207**, 278-83.

Masuno, T., Kishimoto, S., Ogura, T., Honma, T., Niitani, H., Fukuoka, M. and Ogawa,

N. (1991) A comparative trial of LC9018 plus doxorubicin and doxorubicin alone for the treatment of malignant pleural effusion secondary to lung cancer. *Cancer,* **68**, 1495-500.

Matsuzaki, T., Nagaoka, M., Nomoto, K. and Yokokura, T. (1990a) Antitumor effect of polysaccharide-peptidoglycan complex (PS-PG) of *Lactobacillus casei* YIT 9018 on Meth A. *Jpn. Pharmacol. Ther.,* **18**, 51-7 (In Japanese).

Matsuzaki, T., Shimizu, Y. and Yokokura, T. (1990b) Augmentation of antimetastatic effect on Lewis lung carcinoma (3LL) in C57BL/6 mice by priming with *Lactobacillus casei*. *Med. Microbiol. Immunol.*, **179**, 161-8.

Matsuzaki, T, Yokokura, T and Mutai, M. (1985) Anti-tumour activity of *Lactobacillus casei* on Lewis lung carcinoma and line-10 hepatoma in syngeneic mice and guinea pigs. *Cancer Immunol. Immunother.*, **20**, 18-22.

Matsuzaki, T, Yokokura, T and Mutai, M. (1987) Antimetastatic effect of *Lactobacillus casei* YIT9018 (LC 9018) on a highly metastatic variant of B16 melanoma in C57BL6J mice. *Cancer Immunol. Immunother.*, **24**, 99-105.

Matsuzaki, T, Yokokura, T and Mutai, M. (1988a) Antitumor effect of intrapleural administration of *Lactobacillus casei*. *Cancer Immunol. Immunother.*, **26**, 209-14.

Matsuzaki, T, Yokokura, T and Mutai, M. (1988b) The role of lymph node cells in the inhibition of metastasis by subcutaneous injection of *Lactobacillus casei* in mice. *Med. Microbiol. Immunol.*, **177**, 245-53.

Morotomi, M. and Mutai, M. (1986) *In vitro* binding of potent mutagenic pyrolyzates to intestinal bacteria. *J. Natl. Cancer Inst.*, **77**, 195-201.

Nagaoka, M., Muto, M., Matsuzaki, T., Nomoto, K. and Yokokura, T. (1990) Physico-chemical properties of polysaccharide-peptidoglycan complexes (PS-PG) of *Lactobacillus casei* YIT 9018. *Jpn. Pharmacol. Ther.,* **18**, 59-65 (In Japanese).

Nanno, M., Ohwaki, M. and Mutai, M. (1986) Induction by *Lactobacillus casei* of increase in macrophage colony forming cells and serum colony-stimulating activity in mice. *Jpn. J. Cancer Res.*, **77**, 703-10.

Nomoto, K., Yokokura, T., Tsuneoka, K. and Shikita, M. (1991) Radioprotection of mice by a single subcutaneous injection of heat-killed *Lactobacillus casei* after irradiation. *Radiat. Res.*, **125**, 293-7.

Ohotani, M., Miyanaga, N., Takeshima, H., Akaza, H., Koiso, K., Tobisu, K. and Kakizoe, T. (1993) Inhibitory effects of *Lactobacillus casei* on bladder carcinogenesis in mice. *J. Urol.*, **149**, 482A.

Okawa, T., Kita, M., Arai, T., Iida, K., Dokiya, T., Takegawa, Y., Hirokawa, Y., Yamazaki, K. and Hashimoto, S. (1989) Phase II randomized clinical trial of LC9018 concurrently used with radiation in the treatment of carcinoma of the uterine cervix. Its effect on tumor reduction and histology. *Cancer,* **64**, 1769-76.

Okawa, T., Niibe, H., Arai, T., Sekiba, K., Noda, K., Takeuchi, S., Hashimoto, S. and Ogawa, N. (1993) Effect of LC9018 combined with radiation therapy on carcinoma of the uterine cervix. A phase III, multicenter, randomized, controlled study. *Cancer,* **72**, 1949-54.

Onoue, M., Kado, S., Sakaitani, Y., Uchida, K. and Morotomi, M (1997) Specific species of intestinal bacteria influence the induction of aberrant crypt foci by 1,2-dimethylhydrazine in rats. *Cancer Lett.*, **113**, 179-86.

Perdigon, G., Alvarez, S. and Pesce de Ruiz Holgado, A.A. (1991) Immunoadjuvant activity of oral *Lactobacillus casei*: influence of dose on the secretory immune response and protective capacity in intestinal infections. *J. Dairy Res.*, **58**, 485-96.

Perdigon, G., Alvarez, S., Rachid, M., Aguero, G. and Gobbato, N. (1995) Immune system stimulation by probiotics. *J. Dairy Sci.*, **78**, 1597-606.

Perdigon, G., Nader de Macias, M.E., Alvarez, S., Oliver, G. and Pesce de Ruiz Holgado, A.A. (1987) Enhancement of immune response in mice fed with *Streptococcus thermophilus* and *Lactobacillus acidophilus*. *J. Dairy Sci.*, **70**, 919-26.

Perdigon, G., Nader de Macias, M.E., Alvarez, S., Oliver, G. and Pesce de Ruiz Holgado, A.A. (1990) Prevention of gastrointestinal infection using immunobiological methods with milk fermented with *Lactobacillus casei* and *Lactobacillus acidophilus*. *J. Dairy Res.*, **57**, 255-64.

Perdigon, G., Rachid, M., de Budeguer, M.V. and Valdez, J.C. (1994) Effect of yogurt feeding on the small and large intestine associated lymphoid cells in mice. *J. Dairy Res.*, **61**, 553-62.

Perdigon, G., de Macias, M.E., Alvarez, S., Oliver, G. and Pesce de Ruiz Holgado, A.A. (1986) Effect of perorally administered lactobacilli on macrophage activation in mice. *Infect. Immun.*, **53**, 404-10.

Perdigon, G., de Macias, M.E., Alvarez, S., Oliver, G. and Pesce de Ruiz Holgado, A.A. (1988) Systemic augmentation of the immune response in mice by feeding fermented milks with *Lactobacillus casei* and *Lactobacillus acidophilus*. *Immunology*, **63**, 17-23.

Popova, P., Guencheva, G., Davidkova, G., Bogdanov, A., Pacelli, E., Opalchenova, G., Kutzarova, T. and Koychev, C. (1993) Stimulating effect of Deodan (an oral preparation from *Lactobacillus bulgaricus* "LB51" on monocytes/macrophages and host resistance to experimental infections. *Int. J. Immunopharmac.*, **15**, 25-37.

Reddy, GV., Shahani, K.M. and Banerjee, M.R. (1973) Inhibitory effect of yogurt on Ehrlich Ascites tumor-cell proliferation. *J. Natl. Cancer Inst.*, **50**, 815-7.

Rowland, I.R., Rumney, C.J., Coutts, J.T. and Lievense, L.C. (1998) Effect of *Bifidobacterium longum* and inulin on gut bacterial metabolism and carcinogen-induced aberrant crypt foci in rats. *Carcinogenesis*, **19**, 281-5.

Sawamura, A., Yamaguchi, Y., Tohge, T., Nagata, N., Ikeda, H., Nakanishi, K.. and Asakura, A. (1994) Enhancement of immuno-activities by oral administration of *Lactobacillus casei* in colorectal cancer patient. *Biotherapy*, **8**, 1567-72 (in Japanese).

Sekine, K., Ohta, J., Onishi, M., Tatsuki, T., Shimokawa, Y., Toida, T., Kawashima, T. and Hashimoto, Y. (1995) Analysis of antitumor properties of effector cells stimulated with a cell wall preparation (WPG) of *Bifidobacterium infantis*. *Biol. Pharm. Bull.*, **18**, 148-53.

Sekine, K., Toida, T., Saito, M., Kuboyama, M., Kawashima, T. and Hashimoto, Y. (1985) A new morphologically characterized cell wall preparation (whole peptidoglycan) from *Bifidobacterium infantis* with a higher efficacy on the regression of an established tumor in mice. *Cancer. Res.*, **45,** 1300-7.

Sekine, K., Ushida, Y., Kuhara, T., Iigo, M., Baba-Toriyama, H., Moore, MA., Murakoshi, M., Satomi, Y., Nishino, H., Kakizoe, T. and Tsuda, H. (1997) Inhibition of initiation and early stage development of aberrant crypt foci and enhanced natural killer activity in male rats administered bovine lactoferrin concomitantly with azoxymethane. *Cancer Lett.*, **121**, 211-6.

Sekine, K., Watanabe-Sekine, E., Toida, T., Kasashima, T., Kataoka, T. and Hashimoto, Y. (1994) Adjuvant activity of the cell wall of *Bifidobacterium infantis* for *in vivo* immune responses in mice. *Immunopharmacol-Immunotoxicol.*, **16**, 589-609.

Shida, K., Makino, K., Morishita, A., Takamizawa, K., Hachimura, S., Ametani, A., Sato, T., Kumagai, Y., Habu S. and Kaminogawa, S. (1998) *Lactobacillus casei* inhibits antigen-induced IgE secretion through regulation of cytokine production in murine splenocyte cultures. *Int. Arch. Allergy Immunol.*, **115**, 278-87.

Simard, A., Vobecky, J. and Vobecky, J.S. (1991) Vitamin D deficiency and cancer of the breast: an unprovocative ecological hypothesis. *Can. J. Public Health.*, **82**, 300-3.

Tomita, K., Akaza, H., Nomoto, K., Yokokura, T., Matsushima, H., Honma, Y. and Aso, Y. (1994) influence of *Lactobacillus casei* on rat bladder carcinogenesis in mice. *Jpn. J. Urol.*, **85**, 655-63 (In Japanese).

Van't Veer, P., van Leer, E.M., Rietdijk, A., Kok, F.J., Schouten, E.G., Hermus, R.J. and

Sturmans, F. (1991) Combination of dietary factors in relation to breast-cancer occurrence. *Int. J. Cancer,* **47**, 649-53.

Watanabe, T. (1996) Suppressive effects of *Lactobacillus casei* cells, a bacterial immunostimulant, on the incidence of spontaneous thymic lymphoma in AKR mice. *Cancer Immunol. Immunother.*, **42**, 285-90.

Yasutake, N., Kato, I., Ohwaki, M., Yokokura, T. and Mutai, M. (1984a) Host-mediated antitumor activity of *Lactobacillus casei* in mice. *Gann,* **75**, 72-80.

Yasutake, N., Ohwaki, M., Yokokura, T. and Mutai, M. (1984b) Comparison of antitumor activity of *Lactobacillus casei* with other bacterial immunopotentiators. *Med. Microbiol. Immunol. Berl.*, **173**, 113-25.

Yokokura, T., Kato, I., Matsuzaki, T., Mutai, M. and Satoh, H. (1984) Antitumor activity of *Lactobacillus casei* YIT 9018 (LC 9018) –Effect of administration route. *Jpn. J. Cancer Chemother.*, **11**, 2427-33 (in Japanese).

Van't Veer, P., Dekker, J.M., Lamers, J.W., Kok, F.J., Schouten, E.G., Brants, H.A., Sturmans, F., Hermus, R.J. (1989) Consumption of fermented milk products and breast cancer: a case-control study in The Netherlands. *Cancer Res.*, **49**, 4020-3.

CHAPTER 5

Modification of Viral Diarrhoea by Probiotics

E. Isolauri

5.1 Acute diarrhoea

Acute infectious gastrointestinal diseases have been estimated to cause significant morbidity in infants and young children throughout the world. Rotavirus is recognised as the leading cause of these infections in children (Steinhoff 1980). Also other viruses such as intestinal adenoviruses, astroviruses, caliciviruses, Norwalk and Norwalk-like viruses and atypical rotaviruses can cause acute gastroenteritis.

In developing countries the annual death rate due to acute viral diarrhoea has been estimated as one million. Viral diarrhoea also causes significant morbidity in developed countries, although in these societies acute viral infections of the gastrointestinal tract are usually self-limiting diseases. The peak incidence of rotavirus diarrhoea in temperate countries occurs in winter, when most diarrhoeal diseases requiring hospitalisation are attributable to rotavirus infection.

The mucosae of the gastrointestinal tract form an important organ of host defence (Sanderson and Walker, 1993). In addition to its principal physiological function, digestion and absorption of nutrients, the intestinal mucosa provides a protective interface between the internal environment and the constant challenge from antigens from the external environment, also carrying defence mechanisms against viral diarrhoea. Protection against potentially harmful agents encountered by the enteric route is ensured by a number of non-immunological factors and immunological mechanisms.

5.2 Gut mucosal barrier

In order to establish infection the pathogen must circumvent the intestinal mucosal defence barrier (Table 5.1). Intestinal mucosal defence depends on a number of factors in both intestinal lumen and mucosa, which restrict colonisation by pathogenic bacteria in the gut, and interfere with the adherence of micro-organisms to the mucosal surface (Sanderson and Walker, 1993). The predisposition to acute

R. Fuller and G. Perdigon (eds.), Probiotics 3, 139–147.

gastrointestinal infectious diseases is associated with immaturity and dysfunction of the gut defence barrier.

Table 5. 1. Factors controlling antigen transport in the gut

Non–immunological	Immunological
Saliva	Secretory antibodies
Gastric acid	Peyer's patches
Intestinal microflora	Cells in lamina propria
Intestinal proteolysis	Intraepithelial lymphocytes
Peristalsis	
Mucus	
Epithelial membrane	

The immunological and non-immunological defence mechanisms act independently and cooperatively. Their interaction is particularly apparent during the postnatal development, when major maturational events occur such as appearance of mucosal proteins, digestive enzymes and the development of the intestinal microflora. Gastric acidity is an important defence against micro-organisms. Secretion of hydrochloric acid by gastric mucosa develops slowly during the first weeks of life, reaching the lower limit of normal for adults by three months of age (Grand *et al.*, 1976). Goblet cell mucus covering the epithelial surface of the gastrointestinal tract is an important physical barrier that interferes with intestinal attachment of luminal antigens and micro-organisms. Low proteolytic activity and lower mucous coat binding of antigens may partly explain increased intestinal permeability during the neonatal period. Maturational changes are also known to affect epithelial cell membranes. Studies in experimental animals have demonstrated greater microvillous membrane binding of cow's milk protein and cholera toxin postnatally than in adult animals. Lysosomal degradation provides a significant barrier to the passage of intact macromolecules across cells. Lysosomes contain acid hydrolases, such as lipases, proteases, nucleases and carbohydrases that break down all types of macromolecules. The breakdown in the immature intestine is less effective than in later life (Sanderson and Walker, 1993).

The gut-associated lymphoid tissue comprises an important element of the total immunological capacity of the host (Sanderson and Walker, 1993; Brandtzaeg, 1995). The unique mucosal immune system constitutes two arms of defence: immune exclusion performed by the secretory immunoglobulin system, and immune regulation pertaining to the state of specific hyporesponsiveness induced by prior oral administration of antigens. There are organised lymphoid tissues, which comprise Peyer's patches. In addition, lymphocytes and plasma cells are distributed throughout the lamina propria, while intraepithelial lymphocytes are located above the basal lamina, in the intestinal epithelium. Peyer's patches are aggregations of lymphoid follicles covered by a unique epithelium comprising cuboidal epithelial cells, very few goblet cells and specialised antigen sampling cells, the M cells. Antigen transport across this epithelium is characterised by rapid uptake and reduced degradation (Ducroc *et al.*, 1983).

Viruses and bacteria, which invade the cells of the small intestinal epithelium, stimulate the production of inflammatory cytokines, affecting phagocytosis together with the anti-inflammatory cytokines generating the IgA response. The net result is the eradication of the pathogen. IgA antibody production is abundant at mucosal surfaces. The secretory IgA antibodies in the gut are resistant to intestinal proteolysis and govern the common mucosal immune system including respiratory tract and lacrimal, salivary and mammary glands. Consequently, an immune response initiated in the gut-associated lymphoid tissue can affect immune response at other mucosal surfaces. The lymphocytes activated within the Peyer's patches disseminate *via* mesenteric lymph nodes, thoracic duct and bloodstream back to the lamina propria but also traffic between other secretory tissues.

5.3 Gut microflora

Microbial colonisation begins immediately after birth (Tannock, 1995). The maternal intestinal flora is a source of bacteria colonising the newborn's intestine. Colonisation is also determined by contact with surroundings. Facultative Gram-positive cocci (staphylococci, strepto-cocci and enterococci) and enterobacteria are the first bacteria to colonise the intestine during the first day of life, anaerobic colonisation occurs during the second day of life (Rotimi *et al.*, 1981; Yoshioka *et al.*,1983). Bifidobacteria then become the predominant species in intestinal flora of breast-fed and bottle-fed infants. Establishment of *Bacteroides* spp. occurs, depending on the study, in 30-80% of breast-fed infants during the first week. Colonisation with lactobacilli is less common during the first week (17-40%). After the initial bacterial ecosystem has established itself, the relative frequencies and levels of bacteria stay quite stable during the period of exclusive breast-feeding. After weaning, the composition of the microflora becomes more complex, resembling that of the adult flora, when the mucosal surfaces harbour more bacterial cells than the total cell count in the human body.

Normal gut microflora can prevent the overgrowth of potential pathogens in the gastrointestinal tract. These microbial antigens also elicit specific immune responses at local and systemic level. This has been explained by their capacity to bind to epithelial cells allowing antigen entry *via* enterocytes. The gut micrôflora bacteria includes a distinct type of IgA response (Mestecky *et al.*, 1999) which may allow the maintenance of the resident microbiota and provide immune responses in the gut-associated lymphoid tissue and control of its milieu. For the newborn intestinal colonisation acts as an effective antigenic stimulus for the maturation of the gut-associated lymphoid tissue (Moreau *et al.*,1978; Shroff *et al.*, 1995; Helgeland *et al* .,1996). The capacity to generate IgA-producing cells increases progressively during the establishment of the gut microflora.

5.4 The gut barrier dysfunction in acute diarrhoea

Rotaviruses invade the highly differentiated absorptive columnar cells of the small intestinal epithelium, where they replicate causing defective sodium and chloride transport. The invasion results in partial disruption of the intestinal mucosa with loss of microvilli and decrease in the villus/crypt ratio. Diarrhoea is mainly due to failure of the epithelium to differentiate during rapid migration to repair the disruption.

During gastrointestinal infection the gut microecologic balance is disturbed (Isolauri *et al.*,1994). Gastrointestinal infection results in partial disruption of the intestinal mucosa with increased intestinal permeability and aberrant absorption of intraluminal antigens (Isolauri *et al.*, 1993; Jalonen *et al.*, 1991). Heyman *et al.* (1987) studied macromolecular absorption *in vitro* in rotavirus-infected mice and demonstrated increased HRP absorption. They also concluded that the gut microflora affects gut permeability, because the disturbance in intestinal absorption of macromolecules was more severe and prolonged in germ-free mice than in conventional mice. Germ-free mice have also been shown to exhibit larger weight losses than conventional mice when infected with rotavirus.

The importance of the gut microflora in host resistance to rotavirus infection was confirmed in a clinical study in which the changes in the gut microecology were evaluated by measuring the bacterial enzyme profile in faeces during acute rotavirus diarrhoea in children (Isolauri *et al.*, 1994). During the diarrhoeal phase of rotavirus infection, urease levels increased significantly, indicating the overgrowth of specifically urease-producing bacteria. Urease has been considered a pro-inflammatory agent and the production of high concentrations of ammonia predisposes to sustained gut mucosal damage. Oral bacteriotherapy was shown to counteract the disorder.

5.5 The management of acute infantile diarrhoea

The clinical manifestations of acute gastrointestinal infection are due to water and electrolyte losses. The clinical characteristics of rotavirus infection include watery diarrhoea, fever and vomiting resulting in dehydration. Diarrhoeal deaths are frequently due to severe dehydration, or to protracted diarrhoea.

The current accepted guidelines for treatment of acute diarrhoea are based on correcting the dehydration by oral rehydration solutions (American Academy of Pediatrics,1996). In addition, immediately after the completion of oral rehydration full feedings of previously tolerated diet can be reintroduced (Sandhu *et al.*,1997). There is no need for elimination or restriction of milk or milk products.

In the search for an optimal treatment of acute viral diarrhoea, the gut mucosal barrier may be identified as a novel target (Table 5.2). In recent years, scientific interest has focused on dysfunction of this first line of host defence in various clinical conditions and the ways in which the barrier function could be strengthened by therapeutic means. One strategy has been based on the consumption of cultures of potentially beneficial micro-organisms as probiotics.

Table 5. 2. Goals of treatment in viral diarrhoea

Goal	Method	Effect
Correction of diarrhoeal dehydration	Oral Rehydration by ORS (Oral Rehydration Solutions)	Correction of fluid and electrolyte loss Weight gain Maintenance therapy
Nutritional repair	Not withholding of food when diarrhoea begins Rapid refeeding after rehydration in non-breastfed infants Continued breastfeeding	Prevention of nutritional repercussions Correction of nutritional state Weight gain
Cessation of diarrhoea	Specific probiotics	Early cessation of viral diarrhoea Shortening the duration of viral excretion Prevention of diarrhoea
Complete therapy	Introduction of probiotics In ORS	Reduction in the duration of diarrhoea and hospitalisation

5.6 Promotion of gut defence by probiotics

The criteria for a probiotic demand that the strain be of human origin, be safe in human use and resistant to acid and bile, and that it adheres to the intestinal mucosa and produces antimicrobial components (Salminen *et al.*, 1998).

The beneficial effects of probiotics have been attributed to their ability to promote the immunological and non-immunological defence barriers in the gut (Table 5.1): normalisation of increased intestinal permeability and altered gut microflora. They have also been shown to enhance humoral immune responses, and consequently to promote the intestine's immunological barrier. Probiotics have also been shown to stimulate non-specific host resistance to microbial pathogens, and thereby aid in immune elimination (Perdigón *et al.*,1988).

5.7 Probiotics in the treatment and prevention of acute diarrhoea in infants

Several clinical studies have investigated the use of probiotics as dietary supplements for the prevention and treatment of various gastrointestinal infections. In patients hospitalised for acute rotavirus diarrhoea, *Lactobacillus* strain GG as a fermented milk or as freeze-dried powder significantly reduced the duration of diarrhoéa compared with the placebo group given fermented-then-pasteurised milk product (Isolauri *et al.*, 1991). The result has been confirmed in studies carried out in a similar population (Kaila *et al.*, 1992; Majamaa *et al.*, 1995) as well as in different populations (Guandalini, in press). Moreover, probiotics have been shown to reduce the duration of rotaviral excretion (Saavedra *et al.*, 1994; Canani *et al.*, 1997). A reduction in the number of diarrhoeal episodes and the duration of diarrhoea was observed in infants given *Lactobacillus helveticus* and *Streptococcus thermophilus*-fermented formula (Brunser *et al.*, 1989) or *Lactobacillus acidophilus* and *Lactobacillus casei*-fermented milk (Gonzalez *et al.*, 1990) compared with a group given non-fermented formula or milk.

In more recent studies (Rautanen *et al.*,1998; Guandalini, in press), the early introduction of probiotic therapy has proven the greatest clinical benefit resulting in early cessation of diarrhoea, shorter duration of hospitalisation and prevention of protracted diarrhoea.

The preventive potential of the probiotic approach has also been demonstrated in a well-controlled clinical study. Saavedra *et al.* (1994) conducted a double-blind, placebo-controlled trial in hospitalised infants randomised to receive a standard infant formula or the same formula supplemented with *Bifidobacterium bifidum* and *Streptococcus thermophilus*. Over a 17-month follow-up, 31% of the patients given the standard infant formula, but only 7% of those receiving the probiotic-supplemented formula developed diarrhoea, and the prevalence of rotavirus shedding was significantly lower in those receiving probiotic-supplemented formula.

5.8 Conclusions

There is now good evidence that probiotic preparations have potential in the prevention and treatment of gastrointestinal infections. In particular, probiotic therapy has proven safe and effective in viral diarrhoea of infants and young children.

There is still a need for randomised placebo-controlled, double-blinded studies in in patients with specific intestinal infections. The precise mechanisms of action of candidate probiotic strains should be identified. The maintainance of a balanced intestinal microflora and effective gut barrier function during viral diarrhoea, may provide a novel therapeutic and preventive strategy for these conditions. Such an approach may offer the complete therapy for acute viral diarrhoea (Table 5.2).

5.9 Summary

The majority of cases of acute diarrhoea occur in children between 6 and 24 months of age in winter season, and most of them are caused by rotavirus. Symptoms of acute viral infections of the gastrointestinal tract appear 3 to 5 days after contact with the virus, and continue for 5 to 7 days. The clinical characteristics are watery diarrhoea accompanied by vomiting and fever. The main goal of treatment is correction of dehydration and maintaining hydration during the course of the usually self-limiting disease. This can be accomplished by well-balanced oral rehydration solutions. The second goal should be nutritional repair by reintroduction of full age-appropriate feedings immediately after rehydration. Scientists in several countries seek additional tools for the reduction of the diarrhoea. Probiotic micro-organisms have been shown to reinforce the gut defences. They have been shown to enhance humoral immune responses, and consequently to promote the intestine's immunological barrier. Probiotics have also been shown to stimulate non-specific host resistance during infection, and thereby aid in eradication of pathogens. The best-documented current therapeutic application is in the prevention and treatment of diarrhoeal diseases, in particular of viral origin. The probiotic approach could thus be a useful means of counteracting the disturbed microbial balance and impaired gut barrier function which accompanies acute viral diarrhoea.

References

Brandtzaeg, P. (1995) Molecular and cellular aspects of the secretory immunoglobulin system, *APMIS* **103**, 1-19.

Brunser, O., Araya, M., Espinoza, J., Guesry, P.R., Secretin, M.C. and Pacheco, I. (1989) Effect of an acidified milk on diarrhoea and the carrier state in infants of low socio-economic stratum, *Acta Paediatr. Scand.* **78**, 259-264.

Canani, R.B., Albano, F., Spagnuolo, M.I., Di Benedetto, L., Stabile, A. and Guarino, A. (1997) Effect of oral administration of Lactobacillus GG on the duration of diarrhea and on rotavirus excretion in ambulatory children, *J. Pediatr. Gastroenterol. Nutr.* **24**, 469.

Ducroc, R., Heyman, M., Beaufrere, B., Morgat, J.L. and Desjeux, J.F. (1983) Horseradish peroxidase transport across rabbit jejunum and Peyer's patches in vitro, *Am. J. Physiol.* **245**, G54-G58.

Grand, R.J., Watkins, J.B. and Torti, F.M. (1976) Development of the human gastrointestinal tract, *Gastroenterology* **70**, 790-810.

Gonzalez, S., Albarracin, G., *et al.* (1990) Prevention of infantile diarrhoea by fermented milk, *Microbiologie-Aliments-Nutrition* **8**, 349-354.

Helgeland, L., Vaage, J.T., Rolstad, B., Midtvedt, T. and Brandtzaeg, P. (1996) Microbial colonization influences composition and T-cell receptor V beta repertoire of intraepithelial lymphocytes in rat intestine, *Immunology* **89**, 494-501.

Heyman, M., Gorthier, G., Petit, A., Meslin, J.C., Moreau, C. and Desjeux, J.F. (1987) Intestinal absorption of macromolecules during viral enteritis: an experimental study on rotavirus-infected conventional and germ-free mice, *Pediatr. Res.* **22**, 72-78.

Isolauri, E., Juntunen, M., Rautanen, T., Sillanaukee, P. and Koivula, T. (1991) A human *Lactobacillus* strain (*Lactobacillus* GG) promotes recovery from acute diarrhea in children, *Pediatrics* **88**, 90-97.

Isolauri, E., Arvola, T., *et al.* (1993) Diet during rotavirus enteritis affects jejunal permeability to macromolecules in suckling rats, *Pediatr Res.* **33**, 548-553.

Isolauri, E., Kaila, M., Mykkänen, H., Ling, W.H. and Salminen, S. (1994) Oral bacteriotherapy for viral gastroenteritis, *Dig. Dis. Sci.* **39**, 2595-2600.

Jalonen, T., Isolauri, E., Heyman, M., Crain-Denoyelle, A.M., Sillanaukee, P. and Koivula, T. (1991) Increased ß-lactoglobulin absorption during rotavirus enteritis in infants: relationship to sugar permeability, *Pediatr. Res.* **30**, 290-293.

Kaila, M., Isolauri, E., Soppi, E., Virtanen, E., Laine, S. and Arvilommi, H. (1992) Enhancement of the circulating antibody secreting cell response in human diarrhea by a human lactobacillus strain, *Pediatr. Res.* **32**, 141-144.

Majamaa, H., Isolauri, E., Saxelin, M. and Vesikari, T. (1995) Lactic acid bacteria in the treatment of acute rotavirus gastroenteritis, *J. Pediatr. Gastroenterol. Nutr.* **20**, 333-339.

Mestecky, J., Russell, M.W. and Elson, C.O. (1999) Intestinal IgA: novel views on its function in the defence of the largest mucosal surface, *Gut* **44**, 2-5.

Moreau, M.C., Ducluzeau, R., Guy-Grand, D. and Muller, M.C. (1978) Increase in the population of duodenal IgA plasmocytes in axenic mice monoassociated with different living or dead bacterial strains of intestinal origin, *Infect. Immun.* **21**, 532-539.

Perdigón, G., Nader de Macías, M.E., Alvarez, S., Oliver, G and Pesce de Ruiz Holgado, A. (1988) Systemic augmentation of the immune response in mice by feeding fermented milks with *Lactobacillus casei* and *Lactobacillus acidophilus*, *Immunology* **63**,17-23.

Rautanen, T., Isolauri, E., Salo, E. and Vesikari, T. (1998) Management of acute diarrhoea with low osmolarity oral rehydration solutions and Lactobacillus strain GG, *Arch. Dis. Child.* **79**, 157-161.

Rotimi, V.O. and Duerden, B.I. (1981) The development of the bacterial flora in normal neonates, *J. Med. Microbiol.* **14**, 51-62.

Saavedra, J.M., Bauman, N.A., Oung, I., Perman, J.A. and Yolken, R.H. (1994) Feeding of *Bifidobacterium bifidum* and *Streptococcus thermophilus* to infants in hospital for prevention of diarrhoea and shedding of rotavirus, *Lancet* **344**, 1046-1049.

Salminen, S., Bouley, C., Boutron-Ruault, M.C., *et al.* (1998) Functional food science and gastrointestinal physiology and function, *Br. J. Nutr.* **80**, S147-S171.

Sanderson, I.R. and Walker, W.A. (1993) Uptake and transport of macromolecules by the intestine: possible role in clinical disorders (an update), *Gastroenterology* **104**, 622-639.

Sandhu, B.K., Isolauri, E., Walker-Smith, J.A. *et al.* (1997) Early feeding in childhood gastroenteritis. A multicentre study on behalf of the European Society of Paediatrc Gastroenterology and Nutrition (ESPGAN) working group on acute diarrhoea, *J. Pediatr. Gastroenterol. Nutr.* **24**, 522-527.

Shroff, K.E., Meslin, K. and Cebra, J.J. (1995) Commensal enteric bacteria engender a self-limiting humoral mucosal immune response while permanently colonizing the gut, *Infect. Immun.* **63**, 3904-3913.

Steinhoff, M.C. (1980) Rotavirus: the first five years, *J. Pediatr.* **96**, 611-622.

Tannock, G.W. (1995) *Normal microflora. An introduction to microbes inhabiting the human body*, Chapman and Hall, London: pp 1-36.

Yoshioka, H., Iseki, K. and Fujita, K. (1983) Development and differences of intestinal flora in the neonatal period in breast-fed and bottle-fed infants, *Pediatrics* **72**, 317-321.

CHAPTER 6

Modulation of the Immune Response of the Immunosuppressed Host by Probiotics

G Perdigón and G Oliver

6.1 Introduction

An immunocompromised host is an immunodeficient host. The immunodeficiency disorders can be primary (genetically determined) which is rare occurring with a frequency of aproximately 1/50,000 or secondary induced by malnutrition, tumour growth, drug therapy (such as in autoimmunity or allergic illness) or by the strong immunosuppression associated with organ transplantation. In the immunosuppressed host the disorders may affect one or more components of the immune system including T and B cells and natural killer (NK) lymphocytes as well as phagocytic cells and the humoral immune response. The immunodeficiency is characterized by an increase in the suceptibility to infection, malignancy or defective tumour immunosurveillance.

The immune system has evolved a very sophisticated set of responses designed to protect against infectious microbes. The knowledge of the cellular and molecular component of these reactions has opened up oportunities for new forms of treatment. This often involves biological agents derived from the immune system which are administered as adjuvant therapy to eliminate residual cancer cells, or to improve the immune state of the host after chemotherapy or radiotherapy. It is unlikely that such procedures can induce a full remission of the process. However, treatment for a short time may give a long-term effect.

The major group of these therapies covers the immunotherapy using cellular or antibody therapeutics. The potential for therapeutic application through other substances is open to question.

In this chapter we discuss the possible use of lactic acid bacteria (LAB) or yoghurt for the immunosuppressed host suffering secondary immunodeficiency. We focused our study on malnutrition and immunosuppression induced by drugs or by tumour growth.

R. Fuller and G. Perdigon (eds.), Probiotics 3, 148–175.

6.2 Malnutrition

6.2.1 Introduction

The increasing recognition that the intestinal tract is a major immunological organ has led to intensification of the study of the complex interrelationships between food that is ingested, the body's general state of nutrition and its immunological status (MacDermot, 1993).

The clear association between malnutrition, infection and impairment of the immune response is well known. The precise interrelationships are not yet clear. It is certainly true that recurrent infections may result in severe malnutrition and in the same way malnutrition is often complicated by viral or bacterial infections (Abraham and Ogra, 1993). The involvement of mucosal lymphoid tissue in the host defence mechanisms has been extensively studied over the last two decades. However, factors such as malnutrition, infection and mucosal injury can produce major changes in the intestinal environment. Nutritional deficiences, especially protein-energy malnutrition (PEM) impair immunological response and increase suceptibility to infection (Chandra and Wadhwa, 1993). Systemic cell-mediated immunity is decreased in protein-energy malnutrition as judged by the reduced number and function of thymus lymphocytes, the delayed cutaneous hypersensitivity reactions, cytokine production and the reduced number of intraepithelial lymphocytes (IEL).

There is a reduction in secretory immunoglobulin A (S-IgA), as well as the antibody response and antibody affinity following viral vaccine administration. The process of phagocytosis is also affected in PEM. Complement is an essential opsonin, and the levels and activity of most complement components are decreased. Macrophage migration is also altered as well as the receptor's expression. Lymphoid tissues show a significant atrophy, in particular the size of thymus is small. Histologically there is a loss of corticomedullary differentiation and fewer lymphoid cells. The reduction of thymic factor affects the spleen where there are T lymphocytes. There is also a loss of lymphoid cells and in the lymphoid node, the thymus dependent areas show depletion of lymphoid cells.

Considerable work in animals deprived of one dietary component have confirmed the crucial role of several vitamins and trace elements in immunocompetence. The best studied were zinc, iron, vitamin B_6, vitamin A, copper and selenium. Iron is needed by neutrophils and lymphocytes for optimal function, so the bactericidal capacity is reduced by iron deficiency. Zinc is critical to the biological activity of thymic factors and the 80% of such activity is lost when zinc is chelated. Vitamin B deficiency results in decreased lymphocyte stimulation in response to mitogens such as phytohaemagglutinin A (PHA) (Chandra and Wadhwa, 1993).

The malnourished host has an impairment of intestinal barrier functions, indicating that the intestine may become increasingly permeable to the absorption of dietary and other environmental antigens (Lunn *et al.*, 1991). This also suggests that in malnutrition there is bacterial translocation by the normal microflora. The bacteria translocate from the intestine to the mesenteric lymph node, liver, spleen and blood (Backer and Backer, 1993). The early enteral feeding prevents the increase of the intestinal permeability and maintains gut mucosal integrity. Malnutrition induces a mucosal atrophy (Sullivan *et al.*, 1991). It has been hypothesized that an increase in the lumenal contents is important to avoid the progressive decrease in villus size from the duodenum to the ileum. Thus not only the parenteral, but the enteral feeding is necessary to improve intestinal barrier and mucosal immune function in the malnourished host. Although both parenteral and enteral forms of nutrition can be effective the exclusive use of the parenteral form does not prevent the gut atrophy or the bacterial translocation; thus the enteral nutrition would be the most advisable in the renutrition process.

It was demonstrated that after renutrition the Peyer's patches increased in size and increased the number of receptors and markers on the T lymphocytes surface (Roux and Lopez, 1987; Roux *et al.*, 1983).

It was well demonstrated that the presence of a number of growth factors and hormones in the milk of various species including human and bovine (Koldovsky, 1989; Kong *et al.*, 1992) together with the low proteolytic activity in the gastrointestinal tract, suggest its potential use in the renutrition process. In the same way in fermented milk such as yoghurt, the peptides released in the fermentation process are functional and can produce an effect in the digestive tract, or elsewhere in the body after passing into the circulatory system (Tirelli *et al.*, 1997) where they can exert an immunomodulatory effect (Kayser and Meise, 1996). This will be extensively reviewed in another chapter of this book.

Taking into account the above consideration we analyzed the effect of *Lactobacillus casei* as an oral adjuvant and of yoghurt on the immunosuppressed host by PEM malnutrition before and after milk renutrition. We studied the effect of these probiotics on the improvement of a) the systemic and mucosal immune response, b) bacterial translocation, c) the recovery of the histological structure of the villi and microvilli of small intestine and d) resistance to *Salmonella typhimurium* infection.

6.2.2 *Effect of probiotics on the systemic and mucosal immune response*

In previus studies we demonstrated, using mice as the experimental model, that *Lactobacillus casei* CRL 431 could be used as an oral adjuvant; in a normal host it was able to increase the systemic and mucosal immune response (Agüero *et al.*, 1996; Perdigón *et al.*, 1995 a). We also demonstrated the enhancement of the immune system when yoghurt was included in the diet (Perdigón *et al.*, 1995 b). Considering these previous works we analyzed the effect of these probiotics on malnutrition. The aim was to determine if the probiotic's affect on the unbalanced intestine was similar to that found in a normal host.

Our experimental model was malnourished mice after the weaning . They were given a protein-free diet during 20 days, resulting in a weight loss of about 40% compared with the well- nourished group. The groups of malnourished mice were given *L. casei* or yoghurt for 2 days. Another group was fed with milk for 7-14 days and then received *L. casei* or yoghurt for 2 days. We determined 1) the recovery in the body weight, 2) haematological values from peripheral blood, 3) phagocytic activity of peritoneal macrophages as a measure of the systemic immune response, 4) the number of IgA^+ cells on a histological slice of small intestine and 5) $CD4^+$ and $CD8^+$ T cells in the small intestine. This last determination was only performed in the malnourished groups treated with *L. casei* or yoghurt but not in the refed group (Agüero *et al.*, 1996).

We observed 1) that yoghurt but not *L. casei* improved the body weight compared to the malnourished control. Milk refeeding was also effective after 14 days. These results are shown in Table 6.1.

Table 6.1. Effect of different treatments on body weight of malnourished mice

	Wellnour.	Malnour	Malnour + *L. c.* 2d	Malnour + Yoghurt 2d	Refeeding milk 14 d.	Refeeding milk 14 d + *L. c.* 2d
Weight (g)	25 ± 2	12 ± 1	12 ± 2	$20^* \pm 3$	$21^* \pm 2$	$22^* \pm 3$

Significant differences * $P < 0.01$, were found in the malnourished group treated with yoghurt and also in those refed with milk and milk plus *L. casei* . Values are mean of n = 10 ± S.D. Wellnour = wellnourished, Malnour.= Malnourished.

2) When we determined the effect on the haematological response, we observed that after malnutrition the number of leucocytes decreased but rapidly increased when the animals received *L. casei* or yoghurt or when they were refed. See Table 6.2.

Table 6. 2. Effect of probiotic treatment on the haematological response of malnourished mice

	Hematocrit (%)	Leucocytes/ul
Wellnourished	55 ± 4.8	4,800 ± 210
Malnourished	46 ± 5.2	2,800 ± 610
Malnourished +*L.casei* 2 d	48 ± 6.0	3,400 ± 600
Malnourished+yoghurt 2 d.	50 ± 5.0	4,000* ± 400
Refeeding milk 14 d	52* ± 2.0	4,300* ± 250
Refeeding milk 14d.+*L.c* 2 d	53* ± 3.0	4,400* ± 300

Values are mean of 5 determination ± S.D. * Significant differences, $P < 0.05$ compared to the malnourished control.

3) When we measured the effect of the probiotics on the phagocytic capacity of peritoneal macrophages, we found a marked increase in this activity in the refed group treated with *L. casei* and in the malnourished one treated with yoghurt where the values reached those obtained with the wellnourished control (Table 6.3).

Table 6. 3. Phagocytosis of peritoneal macrophages from malnourished mice with *L. casei* or yoghurt

	Wellnour.	Malnour.	Malnour. + *L. c.* 2d	Malnour. + yoghurt 2d	Malnour. Milk 14 d.	Malnour.+ milk 14 d + *L. c.* 2d
Phagocytosis (%)	20 ± 2	10 ± 1	10 ± 3	19*± 2	17*± 2	25*± 3

Each experimental group consisted of 6 mice. Values are the mean ± S.D. Significant difference $P < 0.05$ related to the malnourished control.

4) When we analyzed the IgA cells associated with the lamina propria of the small intestine we saw that in the: *L. casei* and yoghurt and the refeeding group, the values obtained were near those of wellnourished animals, the effect being greatest in the groups treated with yoghurt. However, $CD4^+$ or $CD8^+$ T cells in all groups were slightly increased compared with the malnourished group. Although, yoghurt showed a slight increase compared with the control malnourished group, the values were not significant. See Table 6.4.

Table 6. 4. Number of IgA$^+$, CD4$^+$, and CD8$^+$ present in the small intestine of malnourished mice treated with *L. casei* or yoghurt.

Cells	Wellnour	Malnour.	Malnour.+ *L. casei* 2d	Malnour. + Yoghurt 2d	Malnour. + milk 14 d.	Malnour. + milk 14 d. + *L. c.* 2d
IgA$^+$	83 ± 5	35 ± 6	75*± 5	86*± 2	70*± 5	83*± 4
CD4$^+$	49 ± 5	20 ± 4	22 ± 3	29 ± 4	ND	ND
CD8$^+$	38 ± 5	23 ± 4	24± 4	27 ± 3	ND	ND

Results are expressed as the number of cells/10 villi. Values are means of n = 6 ± S.D. * Significant difference P < 0.01 as regard malnourished control. ND = no determined.

6.2.3 Effect on the intestinal microflora and bacterial translocation

As was mentioned before malnutrition can lead to alteration in the intestinal microflora and the gastrointestinal barrier function that may contribute to bacterial translocation from the intestine to other organs such as liver, spleen or into the blood.

We studied the strict and facultative anaerobes present in the small and large intestines. We did not identify the different species. We also determined for those two groups of microorganisms bacterial translocation to the liver or spleen. We saw that the number of strict anaerobes in both sites were greatly decreased in the malnourished animals and improved when yogurt was included in the diet; *L. casei* was not effective.

In the refed animals treated only with milk or milk plus *L. casei* the improvement was achieved reaching normal values after 7 days of treatment. Milk and yoghurt administration inhibited the bacterial translocation. (Perdigón *et al.*, 1995 a; Perdigón *et al.*, 1995 b) (Table 6.5).

Table 6.5. Effect of probiotic on the intestinal flora and bacterial translocation in malnourished animals

	Welln Anaerobes Fac.	Welln Anaerobes Strict	Maln. Anaerobes Fac.	Maln. Anaerobes Strict	Maln.+ *L. c.* 2d Anaerobes Fac.	Maln.+ *L. c.* 2d Anaerobes Strict	Maln.+Yog 2d Anaerobes Fac.	Maln.+Yog 2d Anaerobes Strict	Maln. + milk 7 d Anaerobes Fac.	Maln. + milk 7 d Anaerobes Strict	Mal.+ milk 7d.+*L. c.* 2d Anaerobes Fac.	Mal.+ milk 7d.+*L. c.* 2d Anaerobes Strict
Small Intestine	9.8	5.7	8.8	1.5	8.5	2	9*	5.3*	9.3*	5.2*	9.8*	5.8*
Large Intestine	11	13	10	3.0	10	5	11*	9.0*	11*	12*	12*	13*
Bacterial translocation	-		+		+		-		-		-	

Results are expressed as $\log_{10}$ number bacteria/organ. Values are mean of 5 determinations. * Significant differences $P < 0.05$ compared with the malnourished control.

6.2.4 Histological and ultrastructural studies

We determined by histological slices of the small intestine, the recovery of the length of the villi and the increase in the number of the globet cells. We performed ultrastructural studies to examine by transmission and scanning electron microscopy the height of microvilli, the improvement of the epithelial cells and the restoration of mucus production identified by the electrodense layer on the microvilli.

We demonstrated by histological observation a recovery of intestinal villi as measured by the size and number per area and an increase in the number and activity of globet cells in the malnourished animals treated with yoghurt; *L. casei* induced only a slight improvement. The refeeding with milk produced a marked recovery in the intestinal structure; the effect was more evident when *L. casei* was administered. By electron microscopy we saw an enhancement in the height of the microvilli, specially when yoghurt was administered. However, the effect was most evident in the malnourished animal after refeeding with milk plus *L. casei.* We observed improvement of the epithelial cells without cytoplasmic oedema and with prominent rugose endoplasmic reticulum. These extended cisternums suggest an important synthesis of protein. There was a recovery in the layer of mucus. (Allori *et al.*, 1999).

6.2.5 Effect on the prevention against Salmonella typhimurium infection

The association between malnutrition and infection is a well-established fact and PEM results in an increased risk of gastrointestinal infection.

We determined the effect of *L. casei* and yoghurt on the resistance to *Salmonella typhimurium* infection. In the refed animals we also studied the preventive effect of the probiotics against *E. coli* infection.

We demonstrated that the probiotic administration to the malnourished animals without refeeding was not effective in the protection against *Sal. typhimurium* infection, even in the case of yoghurt where we observed an improvement in the mucosal immune system (Perdigón *et al.,* 1995 a). The effectiveness of *L. casei* was observed in the refed animals. The protective effect was more marked against *E. coli* infection (See Table 6.6).

Table 6.6. Effect of probiotics on resistance to enteropathogens in malnourished mice

Enteropathogens	Wellnour.	Malnour	Malnour + *L. c.* 2d	Malnour.+ Yoghurt 2d	Malnour + milk 14 d	Malnour +milk 14d. + *L.c.* 2d
Sal. typhimurium	3.5 ± 1.6	3.8 ± 1.7	4.0 ± 1.9	3.0 ± 1.8	2.3 ± 1.1	1.2 ± 0.5
E. coli	3.0 ± 1.0	3.2 ± 1.2	ND	ND	1.2 ± 1.0	0

Results are expressed as log_{10} number bacteria/organ (liver). Values are the mean of n = 6 ± S.D. After malnutrition and the different treatments, the animals were challenged with the pathogens. The colonization assays were performed on day 7 after *Salmonella typhimurium* infection (2 x 10^7cells) and on day 5 after *E. coli* challenge.

The nutritional properties of yoghurt are unquestionable as is the immunomodulatory effect. In other studies lactic acid bacteria such as *Lactobacillus rhamnosus* strain GG and *L. casei* CRL 431 have been proved to be immunostimulatory in the normal host (animal and human) and the malnourished animal (Boudraa *et al.*, 1989; Spector and Hadden, 1988).

We have also observed the importance of the yoghurt feeding to the malnourished host. However, the use of LAB as an oral adjuvant in the host immunosuppressed by malnutrition would only be advisable after enteral renutrition, when the physiological barrier of gut has recovered.

6.3 Immunosuppression by drugs: corticoid and antibiotic therapy

6.3.1 Introduction

Immunodeficiency resulting from immunosuppressive therapy by corticoids, produces profound defects which are more evident in cellular than in humoral immunity (Spector and Hadden, 1988). However, the corticoid therapy is extensively used in allergic or autoimmune illness cancer treatment and also in infectious diseases.

The immunosuppression induced by corticoid therapy is not antigen specific and its effect is not only on the systemic and mucosal immune response (inflammatory, cellular, humoral) but, can act on other systems inducing secondary effects in the host such as osteoporosis, obesity, gastric haemorrage. One of the most important pharmacologic effects of corticoid is the diminution in the number of leucocytes in peripheral blood, especially T and B lymphocytes (Claman, 1983; Munck and Crabtree, 1981) and on the thymus which suffers an involution by increase in the mechanisms of cellular apoptosis (Cohen and Duke, 1984). On the other hand, sex hormones such as estradiol and progesterone are glucocorticoids that can regulate uterine and cervicovaginal levels of IgA, IgG and secretory component (Sullivan and Wira, 1983 a; b). Thus at physiological concentrations the corticoids maintain the homeostasis but, not when they are used at high concentrations such as those during therapy. Dexamethasone also affects the mucosal immunity inducing lower levels of IgA in the secretion (Wira and Prabhala, 1993). Patients undergoing corticoid therapy frequently are infected with common bacterial pathogens such as *Salmonella,* or *Streptococcus* or oportunistic microorganisms such as *Candida albicans*.

The immune therapy has evolved as a method for restoring the normal immune response particulary in the immunocompromised host. Several adjuvant substances (e.g. aluminium salts, liposomes, immunostimulating complexes (ISCOMs) muramyl dipeptides) have been developed (Lise and Audibert, 1989) for restoration of the immunosuppressed host but with limited clinical success.

It is well known that the indigenous intestinal microflora of human and animals provides a barrier of defence for the host (Fuller, 1997). The protective effect of the intestinal flora was determined by studies in germ-free or antibiotic treated experimental animals (Nardi *et al.*, 1990). The disruption of the ecological balance in the gastrointestinal (GI) tract by oral antibiotic allows both bacterial overgrowth and translocaction of these bacteria from the GI tract to other organs such as liver (Berg *et al.*, 1988; Berg, 1981). Bacterial translocation could be a first step in the development of disease by opportunistic microorganisms of the normal flora. Antibiotic treatment is often accompained by diarrhoea and other gastrointestinal disturbances; pseudomembranous colitis is related to an overgrowth of toxin-producing strains of *Clostridium difficile* in the large intestine (Corthier, 1997). Antibiotic treatment induces a partial destruction of the intestinal microflora, and at the end of this treatment the important functions of microflora such as colonization resistance to pathogen are not easily restored. The search for new treatments has suggested the prophylactic use of preparations containing living microorganisms. Several studies have examined the proposal that fermented dairy products containing lactobacilli or other lactic acid bacteria could be used as dietary supplements in various gastrointestinal infections (Gotz *et al.*, 1979; Siitonen *et al.*, 1990; Borgia *et al.*, 1982]. *Saccharomyces boulardii* has already proved to be useful in control of *C. difficile* diarrhoea (Buts *et al.*, 1993).

The immunopotentiating capacity of lactic acid bacteria (Salminen and Deighton, 1992) and their beneficial effect on the host allow their use as prophylatic or therapeutic agents in an immunodeficient host.

Considering the above studies, we analyzed in an immuno-suppressed mouse-model the reversion of this immunosuppression. We focused our study on the sytemic mucosal immune response and on the role of the LAB in the protection against opportunistic microbial infections.

6.3.2 Effect of LAB in corticoid immunosuppressed mice

We determined whether or not LAB administration was able to reverse immunosuppression. Their effectiveness on the nonspecific or specific immune response and their possible use in immunodeficiency to prevent infection with the oportunistic microorganism *C. albicans* was examined.

Our experimental model was mice immunosuppressed by a single injection of a dexamethasone (60 mg/kg). This dose allowed us to maintain the immunosuppression up to the 22nd day after corticoid inoculation. The LAB assayed were *L. casei*, *L. acidophilus*. *L. delbrueckii* ssp. *bulgaricus* and *S. thermophilus* which were orally administered on 7th and 8th day after dexamethasone injection. After LAB administration we evaluated: 1) haematological values and spleen and thymus weights, 2) nonspecific and specific immune response, 3) resistance to *C. albicans* infection.

6.3.3 Effect on haematological values and spleen and thymus weights

We observed an increase in the number of leucocytes when the LAB were administered; with exception of *S. thermophilus* the values obtained were close to the non-suppressed control. As regard the lymphoid organs weights, LAB feeding recovered spleen weights but, not the thymus weights (Table 6.7).

Table 6.7. Haematological values, spleen and thymus weights of immuno-suppressed mice treated with LAB

Mice	Leucocytes (mm^3)	Spleen (mg)	Thymus (mg)
Normal control	5.8 ± 1.7	100 ± 10	6.0 ± 2.0
Immunosuppressed (I.S.)	4.2 ± 1.4	48 ± 3.0	2.9 ± 2.0
I.S. + *L. casei*	5.7 ± 2.0	100 ± 3.0	3.0 ± 2.0
I.S.+ *L. acidophilus*	5.5 ± 2.0	91 ± 4.0	2.8 ± 1.0
I.S. + *L. bulgaricus*	5.7 ± 1.4	110 ± 2.0	2.8 ± 2.0
I.S. + *S. thermophilus*	4.3 ± 1.6	92 ± 5.0	2.7 ± 1.0

Values are mean of n = 6 ±S.D. Normal control are animals without dexamethasone injection.

6.3.4 Effect on the nonspecific and specific immune response

The nonspecific response was studied by comparing the phagocytic activity of peritoneal macrophage. We showed that the lactobacilli but not *S. thermophilus* were able to reverse the immunosuppression. The effect was most marked when *L. delbrueckii* ssp. *bulgaricus* was administered, the value reached those of the normal control mice. The specific immune response was measured for the antigen sheep red blood cells (SRBC) by the asasy of plaque forming cells (PFC) using spleen cells. The treatment with *L. casei* and *L. delbrueckii* ssp. *bulgaricus* but, not *L. acidophilus* and *S. thermophilus* increased the specific immune response, the values obtained were still higher than those of the normal control. (See Table 6. 8). These results have been published (Petrino *et al.*, 1996).

Table 6.8. Phagocytosis and Plaque forming cells (PFC) assays in immunosuppressed mice with and without LAB treatment.

Mice	Phagocytosis (%)	N° PFC/10^6 spleen cells
Normal control	19 ± 2	243 ± 12
Immunosuppressed (I.S.)	10 ± 2	134 ± 10
I.S. + *L. casei*	18* ± 2	280* ± 15
I.S. + *L. acidophilus*	15 ± 1	159 ± 9
I.S. + *L. bulgaricus*	20* ± 2	300* ± 15
I.S.+*S. thermophilus*	10 ± 1	127 ± 5

Phagocytosis and PFC assays were performed on day 14 post-corticoid injection. Values are mean of n = 5 ± S.D. * Significant difference P < 0.01 related to the I.S. control

6.3.5 Protective effect of LAB against Candida albicans in the immuno-suppressed mice

In this study LAB were administerd on days 4 and 5 post corticoid inoculation. Colonization assays in liver, spleen and kidney were performed on day 10 after *C. albicans* infection. We demonstrated that only *L. casei* and *L. delbrueckii* ssp. *bulgaricus* were able to control *C. albicans* infection. The values were significantly lower than those obtained in the untreated immunosuppressed mice (Petrino *et al.*, 1995).

6.4 Effect of LAB on the immune cells associated with the gut and bacterial translocation in mice with antibiotic therapy

The indigenous microflora maintains the intestinal barrier and the multiple functions of the gut. We studied the effect of several LAB orally administered to mice treated with ampicillin which is the main antibiotic administered in most infections. We focused our study on the immune cells associated with gut mucosa and the importance of LAB administration in the avoidance of bacterial translocation.

Mice received 75 mg/Kg ampicillin orally during 3 consecutive days. After antibiotic treatment LAB were administered for 2 days.

6.4.1 Effect of LAB on the immune cells associated with the gut

Ampicillin induced a decrease in the number of immune cells associated with the lamina propria of small intestine. The effect was greatest for lymphocytes and plasma cells. We have shown that these cells increased when lactobacilli were administered. *L. casei* also showed a slight increase in eosinophils. *S. thermophilus* was not effective and induced an inflammatory response with oedema of the villi. The IgA^+ cells on the gut mucosa are also reduced by ampicillin treatment but increased when lactobacilli were administered, reaching values similar to the normal control.

S. thermophilus was not effective in the enhancement of gut mucosal immunity (See Table 6.9).

Table 6. 9. Effect of LAB administration on IgA cells in mice treated with ampicillin

Mice	N° IgA/10 villi
Normal control	80 ± 5
Immunosuppressed (I.S.)	45 ± 3
I.S. + *L. casei*	83* ± 2
I.S. + *L. acidophilus*	80* ± 2
I.S. + *L. bulgaricus*	85* ± 3
I.S. + *S. thermophilus*	48 ± 1

IgA^+ cells were determined on day 4 after ampicillin treatment. Normal controls are mice untreated with ampicillin. Values are mean of n = 4 ± S.D. * $P < 0.01$ related to the control (IS) treated with ampicillin.

6.4.2 Effect of LAB on bacterial translocation in mice treated with ampicillin

Ampicillin treatment induced liver translocation of enterobacteria, strict and facultative anaerobes. This bacterial translocation which was reversed when *L.casei*, *L. delbrueckii* ssp. *bulgaricus* and *L. acidophilus* were administered may be due to the improvement of the intestinal microflora induced by the lactobacilli. *S. thermophilus* did not reverse the bacterial liver translocation (Petrino *et al.*, 1997).

The implication of these finding in mice with experimental mucosal immunosuppression by ampicillin for humans is still not clear. The immunocompetence in mice would be correlated with the improvement of the intestinal microflora. Similary one may speculate that the secondary immunodeficiency of patients coupled with poor nutritional status or extensive antibiotic therapy, may result in an altered intestinal microflora increasing the suceptibility to infection by pathogenic or non-pathogenic microorganisms. The use of LAB could have some benefit in alleviating symptoms however, their use in human beings as a treatment for avoiding bacterial translocation is still limited. The most severe immunocompromised hosts are those patients with the acquired immunodeficiency syndrome (AIDS) and there is not scientific evidence to prove that LAB could be used as adjuvant agents to improve the immune response or in the prevention of infection with opportunistic microorganisms.

Several studies confirm the effective utilization of selected *Lactobacillus* species for the improvement of the intestinal microenvironment in antibiotic therapy. Bacterial overgrowth can also result from clinical situations such as cancer, transplantation, heart or brain surgeries. The probiotic therapy should be devised carefully using selected LAB species chosen to exibit beneficial effects on the host without inducing adverse side effects.

Similary the immunosuppression can be induced by corticoid therapy. Even though some LAB can reverse the immunosuppressed state, corticoid therapy in transplantation or neoplastic diseases is necessary as a mechanism for limiting damage mediated by the immunopathological process.

Thus for therapeutic purposes in immunodeficiency induced by drugs the use of LAB must be considered not only as a means of reversing the immunodeficiency but also of re-establishing immune regulation. Work is still neccesary to understand the mechanisms by which LAB can produce immunoregulation.

6.5 Immunodeficiency Induced by Cancer

6.5.1 Introduction

Cancer involves a fundamental process including disordered cell replication, cell death and disorganisation of organ structure. Cancer is similar to other chronic diseases, such as coronary heart disease and infectious and deficiency diseases in that food and nutrition are important factors in its pathogenesis. However, cancer is different from other diseases due to the changes in the genetic information coded in the DNA of cells. This does not mean that cancer is an inherited disease, although a small proportion of cancers result directly from the inheritance of predisposing genes. DNA damage provides an escape from the mechanisms that are usually in place to protect the organisms from the growth and spread of such cells. These protective mechanisms are both internal (the body's own system) and external (the environment including food and nutrition).

Molecular and cell biologists are interested in events taking place in the cell, physicians and surgeons treat the disease by focusing on the specific organ involved. In contrast, the cancer epidemiologist takes account of the differences in the patterns of , and risks for specific cancer across whole populations, and attemps to identify the underlying cause of these differences, whether they exist in relation to factors such as dietary habits, drug use, ethnicity, geography, etc.

The term neoplasm is used to defined cancer as new growths that were contrary to nature. The ability of neoplasms to migrate to other tissues or organs and form additional tumour destroys surrounding tissue, induces increased blood vessel formation to supply nutrients to the multiplying cancer cells and eventually may spread to distant tissues (metastasis).

A cancer occurs only in cells that are replicating; the pattern of cancer is quite different in children and adults. In early life, the brain, nervous system, bones, muscles and connective tissue are still growing, cancer is much more common in these tissues in children than in the fully developed epithelial lining. Leukaemias and lymphomes occur early or late in the life.

The fact that each cancer arises from a single cell provides evidence that once the abnormal arises, this capacity is transmited to the daughter cells. This shows that cancer is a disease that fundamentally involves the structure and function of DNA.

DNA can be damaged at any time in life by agents in the environment such as radiation and substances (synthetic or natural) in our food, water, air. It is clear that the individuals are capable of eliminating this damage and its consequences, only those exposed to constant high levels of DNA damaging agents for prolonged periods are at a particular high risk of cancer. Studies on the aetiology of cancer have focused on three agents: viruses, radiation and chemicals. For dietary patterns the epidemiologist tends to separate the specific causes of cancer.

How is the diet involved in the cancer process? It is thought than food and nutrition affect cancer risk because, the diets may contain specific carcinogenic substances. However, the role of food and nutrition in the modification of the cancer process is much more complex, and the specific mechanisms by which individual constituents of diet affect the cancer process are often not fully understood.

The mechanisms of chemical carcinogenesis have been studied extensively in animal models. Briefly the cancer process has at least three stages: initiation, promotion and progession (Harris, 1991; 1993; Pitot and Dragan, 1994). In experimental systems it is possible to ensure that initiation, promotion and progression are the consequence of exposure to specific, sequential and ordered agents. For humans or non-experimental animals none of these conditions is likely to occur.

6.5.2 Role of food and nutrition

The modifying effects of diet upon cancer induced in animals by carcinogens has been demonstrated (Poirier, 1987). The interest in the interaction between dietary constituents and cancer-causing agents and the beneficial effect of nutrition was also extensively analysed. It was shown that essential nutrients can inhibit chemically induced tumours. For example vitamin A (retinol) inhibited carcinoma formation in epithelial tissues and riboflavin inhibited liver cancer caused by azodyes in rats (Poirier *et al.*, 1986). The nutrients showing modulatory effects in experimental cancer include: macronutrients (carbohydrates, protein and fibre), vitamins (folic acid , riboflavin, β carotene, vitamin B 12) and minerals (selenium, zinc, magnesium and calcium).

Carcinogenesis, particulary in relation to the interaction with diet includes a series of events: 1. Initiation: exposure to the agent and metabolism of its interaction between the agent and the cell constitutents (especially DNA). 2. Promotion: repair of the DNA damage, death of the cell or persistence and replication of a clone of abnormal cells within the tissue or growth of this abnormal clone into a focus of pre-neoplastic cells. 3. Progression: growth of the tumour and its spread to other parts of the body.

The host's susceptibility and its defences throught of the immune system interacting with the tumour can modify every stage of this process.

One of the roles of the diet could be the detoxification of metabolites by conversion to stable metabolites that can be excreted. The dietary components can impede carcinogenesis by: 1) blocking the metabolic activation that is controlled by enzymes that catalyse oxidation or conjugation reactions, 2) increasing metabolic detoxification by similar process or 3) providing an alternative target for the electrophilic metabolites (Wattenberg, 1992; Steinmetz and Potter, 1991). An increase in detoxification enzymes induced by dietary components tends to decrease overall metabolic activation of carcinogens and carcinogenesis in experimental animals, it is still not clear whether reduction in human carcinogenesis occurs. The binding of carcinogen to proteins, not DNA, generally accounts for the vast majority of carcinogen residues bound to molecules with high specifity. Blood proteins such as serum albumin and haemoglobin often trap electrophoretic metabolites of carcinogens. For serum albumin, this may occur in the liver, as a result of its abundance in this organ. Albumin may be an imporant detoxification agent. If the carcinogens bind nucleic acids of DNA or RNA this involves macromolecular damage that is critical in the initiation and promotion of the neoplastic process (Meuth, 1989).

Genetic damage can occur anywhere in the genome. Damage to proto-oncogens and tumour suppressor genes (genes that control DNA repair) is the most important. Proto-oncogens are genes containing almost identical DNA sequences to those found in DNA tumour viruses. By mutation of its DNA an over expression of the gene results in a protein that is abnormal and can transmit signals to the cell to replicate leading to uncontrolled cell growth. Oncogens or proto-oncogens are crucial to the control of normal cell replication. The nature of the protein that they code are: protein kinases, the G proteins and growth factors (Anderson *et al.*, 1992). It has been shown that in different cells and tissue types the coordinated activation or over expression of more than one oncogen (for example ras and myc) is often required to confer the full potential for neoplastic growth. Carcinogens can induce mutation of the ras family of oncogens. Tumour suppressor genes Rb, p53, APC produce a heterogenous group of proteins that prevent the cell from reproducing. If they lose their function there is a higher risk of specific tumour development.

How can both macro and micronutrients and other biactive constituents of the diet alter the various stages of carcinogenesis?

Although a larger number of important animal experimental studies (Birt *et al.*, 1992, Newberne and Rogers, 1986; Newmark and Lipkin, 1992) have examined the role of diet in the modulation of tumour promotion, relatively few studies have examined modulation of initiation by diet.

However, we can not generalize the mechanisms of nutritional modulation of the early stages of carcinogenesis because there are other biochemical and pharmacological factors involved in the molecular pathogenesis of this disease. There are no data to suggest that any dietary exposure is related directly to the efficiency of the process of DNA repair. There are also no established dietary agents that alter the *in vivo* apoptosis pathway. However, there are data that suggest that volatile short-chain fatty acids (produced in the colon by fibre or carbohydrate fermentation) may induce apoptosis in colon cancer cell lines under *in vitro* conditions (Hague *et al.*, 1995). The effect of diet on experimental tumour promotion showed that some nutrients such as selenium and vitamin D can have a protective effect, but the efficacy of specific nutrients in delaying the progression of precancerous lesions is not always effective. The promotion and progression are frequently accompanied by decreased or increased levels of oxidative damage in the target tissues (Notani and Jayant, 1987). As was mentioned before, the binding of the carcinogens to

DNA is the main step in promoting tumour growth. However, many chemicals can provide a hormonal stimulus or depress the immune response and induce cell proliferation. It is imporant to note that no single genetic mechanism can account for all the steps in carcinogenesis in a single tissue. It is possible that a number of mechanisms even in the same tissue and with the same agents take place in the transition from normal to transformed cells and cancer. The role of food and nutrition in the progression of tumour is not yet clear.

Later in the cancer process when DNA damage is again central, vegetables, fruits and may be dairy products can provide folate which is a major source of physiological methyldonors reducing the likelihood of DNA hypomethylation and chromosome breakage. Colon fibre fermented in the colon by the bacteria of the normal microflora produces volatile fatty acids that increase the probability that abnormal cells undergo programmed cell death (apoptosis). Antioxidants may reduce the generation of oxygen radicals that could play a role in the later stages of the cancer during the gross disorganization of DNA. Through such chemical changes the constituents of diet and specific foods have a role in all the stages of the cancer process.

Although the link between food, nutrition and cancer exists, the methods used to assess this linkage and identify the mechanism are not always valid because, they were performed in animal models or in *in vitro* studies.

The main advantages of animal studies is that the laboratory conditions can be controlled (it is impossible in human studies) and the genetic variability between individuals can be avoided. Animal studies also have limitations because in order to obtain statistically significant results carcinogens and nutrients are both commonly administered to animals in higher dose than in real life. However, animals studies may allow identification of specific dietary factors that modify cancer incidence and can help to identify biological pathways by which dietary factors modify cancer risk. *In vitro* studies can also help to explain biological mechanisms of action. However, their results cannot and should not be extrapolated directly to human beings. Important human carcinogens are not mutagenic and they do not cause mutations in mammalian cells. Thus false negative or false positives results will be obtained. However, the sensitivity of such tests have contributed to the knowledge of carcinogenesis. Microbial mutagen testing data may guide and support epidemiological studies, but do not provide good evidence on human cancer risk and should be interpreted with more caution than animal data.

6.5.3 Milk and dairy products in cancer

There are many studies on the association between dairy product and risk of cancer of the mouth and pharynx (Notani and Jayant, 1987; Mc Laughlin *et al.*, 1988; La Vecchia *et al.*, 1991). Cheese has been associated with both a statistically significantly decrease and increase risk for cancer of the pharynx (Fransceschi *et al.*, 1990). Buttermilk also showed a protective effect against those cancers, this effect was not observed from studies on milk (Zheng *et al.*, 1992). Mc Laughlin *et al* (1988) found no association between milk and cancer of mouth, conversely this author found an increased risk for higher consumption of dairy product. In larynx cancer dairy products have shown protective association (Notani and Jayant, 1987). In the studies to examine the association between risk of oesophageal cancer and the consumption of milk or dairy products there is no statistically significant protective effect relating to those foods (Tuyns *et al.*, 1987). The protective effect of dairy products has been related to the riboflavin, zinc and perharps calcium present in these products. Deficiencies in riboflavin and zinc have been associated with oesophageal cancer.

In lung cancer there is evidence that a diet high in vegetables and fruit rich in carotenoids, but not dairy products, are protective. As regards liver cancer, La Vecchia *et al.* (1988) reports a decreased risk of cancer with higher milk intake, but other studies (Fukuda *et al.*, 1993; Hising *et al.*, 1991) did not find a relationship between milk consumption and liver cancer. In colon cancer there are studies that have reported no association between any dairy food and risk of colon-rectal cancer (Manousos *et al.*, 1983; Lee *et al.*, 1989; Bostick *et al.*, 1994) and there are others that show protective association between cultured milks or yoghurt and colon cancer (Kampman *et al.*, 1994; Macquart *et al.*, 1986). Cheese has been reported to be associated with a high risk of colon and rectal cancer (Bidoli *et al.*, 1992; Tuyns *et al.*, 1988). In breast cancer several studies showed protective and nonprotective effects against breast cancer (Kato *et al.*, 1992; Katosouyanni *et al.*, 1986). In the positive cases the protection against chemically induced tumours in animals has been atributed to the calcium and conjugated linoleic acid present in the dairy product. There was an association between milk or dairy product and risk of ovary and cervical cancer (Ziegler *et al.*, 1990). In bladder cancer the studies on the effect of dairy products gave variable results (Chyou *et al.*, 1993; Mils *et al.*, 1991).

In spite of all of this research, the different results obtained do not demonstrate a definite link between diets high in milk and dairy products, and the risk of several cancers. However, milk and dairy products (cheese, yoghurt) are good sources of protein, vitamin D., B12, calcium and riboflavin all of which are involved in the decreasing of risk of several cancers. Yoghurt also can activate the immune system (De Simone *et al.*, 1986. 1989; Pereyra *et al*, 1989).It may be that the consumption of these products is responsible for the diminished risk of cancer, or cancer prevention.

As was mentioned the mechanism involved in cancer growth is very complex and the normal control of vigilance exerted by the immune system is not functional. The immunodepression caused by carcinogens involves the cellular immune response and cytokine production by immune cells as well as the humoral response. Thus the studies on cancer prevention should be more important than the therapeutic ones, avoiding the initiation process of cancer. The immunotherapy has been shown to be effective especially in avoidance of the promotion of cancer. The use of adjuvants such as lactic acid bacteria cultures or yoghurt have been shown to have immunopotentiating capacity and also antimutagenic capacity. These properties of LAB are extensively reviewed in an other chapter of this book. However, here we want to describe the effect of one *Lactobacillus* and yoghurt as inhibitors in the promotion or initiation of two cancers: fibrosarcoma and carcinoma respectively. We will demonstrate how these treatments can reverse the immunosuppression caused by the carcinogens and indicate the mechanisms involved.

6.5.4 Study of the effect of L. casei and yoghurt on the immuno-suppression induced by chemical carcinogens.

We analyzed the effect of oral administration of *L. casei* used as an immunomodulator on the promotion of a fibrosarcoma. We determined the immunosuppression obtained by the growth of a fibrosarcoma induced by methylcholantrene and the effect of *L. casei* on the inhibition of the tumour growth and the improvement of the immune system. We also studied the effect of yoghurt on the inhibition of the induction of an intestinal carcinoma induced with 1-2 dimethylhydrazine and on the immune system compared to the effect of carcinogen.

In the studies using *L. casei* as immunomodulator, we determined 1) the inhibition of tumour growth, 2) level of the enzyme alkaline phosphatase as marker of inflammation and haematological values, 3) β-glucuronidase histochemical activity and phagocytic capacity of peritoneal macrophages and 4) cytotoxic effects of serum on tumour cells.

We demonstrated (Perdigón *et al.*, 1993 a; Perdigón *et al.*, 1995 c; Perdigón *et al.*, 1993 b) the importance of the dose of *L. casei* in the inhibitory effect on the fibrosarcoma growth. The better effect was obtained at low doses (Table 6.10).

Table 6.10. Effect of *L. casei* dose on the inhibition of tumour promotion

L. casei dose (cells)	Tumour weight (g)	N° animals with Tumour/total	% Tumour growth	Tumour growth inhibition (%)
$2.4x10^9$	0.755±0.3*	18/55	32*	68*
$6.0x10^9$	3.365±0.1	22/33	66	33
$8.4x10^9$	3.550±0.2	29/37	79	21
Control	2.019±0.3	38/50	76	-

Values are mean of animal numbers ± S.D. * significant difference from the control group. P < 0.01. Tumour weights were measured after 40 days post tumour cells inoculation.

When we analyzed the diminution in the level of alkaline phosphatase and the haematological values of peripheral blood, we observed a significant decrease in the levels of enzyme at a dose of 2,4 x 10^9 cells in relation to the mice bearing tumour untreated with *L. casei*. Values were similar to those obtained in the feeding control without tumour inoculation. As regards the haematological values at the low dose of *L. casei* (2.4 x 10^9 cells) on day 12 post tumour inoculation, we had a diminution in the number of total leukocytes which were close to the control animal with no tumour.

In the study on the phagocytic activity, we observed that the activity of peritoneal macrophages measured by phagocytosis, and the activity of β-glucuronidase, were increased in the mice bearing tumour treated for 2 day with *L. casei* (2.4 x 10^9 cells). Phagocytosis values were similar to the normal control and the activity of β-glucuronidase was significantly increased. See Table 6.11.

Table 6.11. Phagocytosis percentage and β-glucuronidase activity of peritoneal cells

L. casei dose (cells)	% Phagocytosis 12 d. post tumour inoculation	β glucuronidase activity (% postitive)
$2.4x10^9$	22±2*	90*±5
$6.0x10^9$	12±2	48±5
$8.4x10^9$	7±1	40±8
Untreated tumour control	5±2	10±7
Normal control	23±1	40±5

Values are mean of n = 5 determinations ±S.D. * Significant difference as regard untreated control mice. P < 0.01. Normal control are animals without tumour.

When we analyzed the cytotoxic activity of the peritoneal macrophages in the tumour cells, we observed an enhanced activity when the animals bearing tumour were treated with *L. casei* at a dose of 2.4 x 10^9 cells. (See Table 6.12).

Table 6.12. Effect of *L. casei* on the cytotoxic activity of peritoneal macrophages in immunosuppressed mice bearing tumour

L. casei dose (cells)	% cytotoxicity
2.4×10^9	$40 \pm 2^*$
6.0×10^9	$36 \pm 1^*$
8.4×10^9	$34 \pm 1^*$
Untreated tumour control	18 ± 2
Normal control	25 ± 1

Values are mean of n=6 ± S.D. Cytotoxic assays were performed on day 6 after tumour inoculation. * Significant difference $P < 0.01$ compared with both controls.

In these experiments we demonstrated that *L. casei* was effective in the inhibition of tumour promotion. However, its effect was dose dependent. We also showed that *L.casei* increased the immune response which was diminished by tumour growth. The effect observed with the high dose could be due to the autoregulation of immune mechanisms as consequence of an over stimulation. In appropiate doses oral administration of *L. casei* might induce release of cytokines that can act at sites distant from the gut.

To evaluate the effect of yoghurt on the inhibition of tumour initiation and on the immunosuppression caused by carcinogen (DMH) administration (Valdez *et al.*, 1997; Perdigón *et al.*, 1998), we determined: 1) tumour incidence by histological studies, 2) number of peripheral blood leukocytes, 3) number of IgA^+, IgG^+ B cells, $CD4^+$, $CD8^+$ T cells associated to large intestine, 4) cytotoxic and phagocytic activity of peritoneal macrophages and phagocytic capacity of macrophages associated with the large intestine.

When we analyzed the tumour incidence at week 20 after carcinogen inoculation, we saw that 70% of control mice developed intestinal tumour but, no tumours were detected in mice given yoghurt for 7 and 10 consecutive days (this procedure was repeated every 10 d). In this case, we only observed an infiltration of lymphoid cells. As regards the number of leukocytes on week 20, the values obtained in the group treated with the carcinogen and yoghurt were similar to those observed in mice without any treatment. When the carcinogen was administered the values on week 20 were twice those of normal control.

The B and T cells associated with large intestine on week 20 after carcinogen treatment showed an increase in the number of IgA$^+$ compared with the control. Values for IgG$^+$ cells were close to the control. CD4$^+$ was increased in the mice treated with DMH plus yoghurt and CD8$^+$ T cells were increased in the group with DMH related to the normal control (Perdigón *et al.*, 1996; 1998). (Table 6.13).

Table 6. 13. Effect of tumour induction and dietary yoghurt on the number of B and T lymphocytes in the large intestine

Group of animals	IgA$^+$ secreting cells (N°/10 villi)	IgG$^+$ secreting cells (N° /10 villi)	CD4$^+$ T cells (N°/10 villi)	CD8$^+$ T cells (N°/10 villi)
Carcinogen control (week 20th)	20±2	100±8*	35*±3	80*±4
Carcinogen+Yoghurt 7d	50*±6	30±3	48±2	20±3
Normal controls	30±3	20±2	30±2	18±3

Values are means for n = 5 ± S.D. * Significant difference as regard normal controls P < 0.01. The immunofluorescence tests were performed on week 20th after DMH inoculation.

The phagocytic activity of peritoneal macrophage was measured by detection of β- glucuronidase enzyme by the histochemical test.

Cytotoxic activity was measured against the tumour cells using MTT (tetrazolium salt) colorimetric assay. The phagocytic activity of the macrophage associated with the large intestine was determined on histological slices by the assay of iron dextran uptake (Bugelski *et al.*, 1987). We observed an increase in the phagocytic and cytotoxic activity of the peritoneal macrophages on week 20 in the mice treated with carcinogen and yoghurt. The ability of macrophage-associated intestinal mucosa to phagocytose iron dextran was significantly increased in the group given yoghurt compared with the tumour control group in which the phagocytic activity of macrophages was similar to those found in the normal control. (Table 6.14)

Table 6. 14. Effect of yoghurt on phagocytic and cytotoxic activity

	Peritoneal Macrophages		Intestinal Macrophages
Groups of animals	% β-glucuronidase possitive	Cytotoxicity (%)	Positive for iron dextran uptake
Control (without treatment)	36±1.2	56±1.1	+
DMH control (treated only with carcinogen)	50±1.3*	66±2.4	+
Treated with DMH and fed with yoghurt (10 d.)	57±3.8*	78±1.5*	+++

The assays were performed on week 20 after carcinogen inoculation. Values are mean n = 5 ± S.D. * Signifcant differences $P < 0.01$ related to the normal control.

We demonstrated that feeding yoghurt inhibited tumour initiation and reversed the immunosuppression caused by the carcinogen. We also demonstrated that in the group of animals given yoghurt, the markers of the inflammatory immune response (IgG^+ B cells, $CD8^+$ T cells) were diminished but, the IgA values were increased. This IgA^+ increase suggested that yoghurt could contribute to limiting the inflammatory response because IgA is considered to be an immune barrier in colonic neoplastic disease (Issacson, 1982). The increase in the peritoneal macrophage activity and also in the activity of macrophages present in the large intestine would mean that yoghurt induced a reversion of the immunosuppression. Thus it is possible that yoghurt maintains an systemic immune response adequate to eliminate cells transformed by the carcinogens. We suggest that one of the mechanisms by which yoghurt inhibits the initiation and promotion of tumour is through a marked reduction in the inflammatory immune response. Another possibility would be that yoghurt favoured the apoptosis mechanisms. Work in progress would seem to demonstrate that this last mechanism is involved.

6.6 Conclusion

We demonstrated the importance of LAB or yoghurt administration for the immunosuppressed host. They were able to reverse this state in malnutrition, the effect being more marked after milk renutrition. Some LAB might reverse the immunosuppression by drugs and prevent oportunistic infection, but their use is not advised when the corticoid therapy is administered as the immunosuppressor (e.g. autoimmune diseases, transplants).

Yoghurt and lactobacilli can inhibit the initiation and promotion of tumours and also reverse the immunosuppression induced by the chemical carcinogens. These approaches offer the prospect for use of LAB or yoghurt in HIV infection, to alleviate the symptoms of this illness and also to provide protection against infection.

Acknowledgements

The authors whish to thank Dr. Marta Medici for typing the manuscript, and also the coworkers from the Immunology Department at CERELA and of the Immunology Laboratory at the Microbiology Institute of Tucuman University. This research was supported by grants from CONICET PIP 5011/97, CIUNT 96/98 and 98/2000.

References

Abraham, R. and Ogra, P. (1993) Effect of intestinal microenviroment on mucosal immune response to viruses. In *Immunophysiology of the Gut* (eds. A. Walker, P. Harmatz and B. Wershil.), Academic Press, Inc. San Diego, USA, pp. 373-388.

Agüero, G., Sanchez, S., Fernandez, S., Allori, C., P.de Ruiz Holgado A. and Perdigón G. (1996) Administration of yoghurt or *Lactobacillus casei* to malnourished mice: comparative effect on lymphoid cells and mucosal reconditioning of the intestine, *F. Agricult. Immunol*, **8**, 229-238.

Allori, C., Agüero, G., P.de Ruiz Holgado, A., M.de Nader, O. and Perdigón, G. (1999,in press) Gut mucosa morphology and microflora after renutrition with milk and administration of *L. casei*. *J. Food Prot.* **62**.

Anderson, M., Reynolds, S., You, M., Maronpot, R. (1992) Role of proto-oncogens activation in carcinogenesis, *Environ. Health Persp.*, **98**, 13-24.

Backer, S. and Backer, R. (1993) Enteric versus parenteral feeding and mucosal function. In *Immunophysiology of the Gut*, (eds. A. Walker, P. Harmatz and B. Wershil)Academic Press, Inc. San Diego, USA, pp. 401-414.

Berg, R. (1981) Promotion of the translocation of enteric bacteria from the GI tracts of mice by oral treatment with penicillin, clindamycin or metronidazole, *Infect. Immun.*, **33**, 854-871.

Berg, R., Wommark, E. and Deitch, E. (1988) Immunosuppression and intestinal bacterial overgrowth synergistically promote bacterial translocation. *Archives of Surgery*, **123**, 1359-1364.

Bidoli, E., Franceschi, S. and Talamini, R. (1992) Food consumption and cancer of the colon and recturm in north-eastern Italy, *Int. J. Cancer* **50**, 223-229.

Birt, D., Kris, E., Choe M. and Pelling, J. (1992) Dietary, energy, and fat effects on tumour promotion, *Cancer Res.*, **52**, 2035 s-2039 s.

Borgia, M., Sepe, N., Brancato, V. and Borgia, R. (1982) A controlled clinical study on *Streptococcus faecium* preparation for the prevention of side reactions during long term antibiotic therapy, *Curr. Ther. Res.* **31**, 265-271.

Bostick, R., Potter, J., Kushi, L., Sellers, T., Steinmetz, K., McKenzie, D., Gapstur, S. and Folsom, A. (1994) Sugar, meat, and fat intake and non-dietary risk factors for colon cancer incidence in lowa women (United States), *Cancer Res.* **5**, 38-52.

Boudraa, G., Touhami, M., Pochart., P., Soltana, R., Mary, J and Desjeux, J., (1989) Effets comparés du yaourt et du lait sur la diarrhée persistante du nourrisson et de l'enfant: résultats préliminaires. In *Les laits Fermentés. Actualité de la Recherche*, John Libbey Eurotext Ltd., pp. 229-232.

Bugelski, P., Corwin, S., North, S., Kirsh, R., Nicolsanarid, G. and Poste, G. (1987) Macrophage content of spontaneous metastases at different stages of growth. *Cancer Res.* **47**, 4141-4145.

Buts, J., Corthier, G. and Delmée, M. (1993) *Saccharomyces boulardii* for *Clostridium difficile* associated enteropathies in infants, *J. Pediatr. Gastroenterol.* **16**, 419-425.

Chandra, R. and Wadhwa, M. (1993) Nutritional deficiences and intestinal mucosal immunity. In *Immunophysiology of the Gut*, (eds. A. Walker, P. Harmatz and B. Wershil), Academic Press, Inc. San Diego, USA, pp. 389-399.

Chyou, P., Momura, A. and Stemmermann, G. (1993) A prospective study of diet, smoking, and lower urinary tract cancer, *Ann. Epidemiol.* **3**, 211-216.

Claman, H. (1983) Glucortids I anti-inflammatory mechanisms. II the clinical response. *Hosp. Pract*, **18**, 123-135.

Cohen, J. and Duke, R. (1984) Glucocorticoid activation of a calcium dependent endonuclease in thymocyte nucleid lead to cell death, *J. Immunol.* **132**, 38-43.

Corthier, G. (1997) Antibiotic-associated diarrhoea: treatments by living organisms given by the oral route (probiotics). In *Probiotics 2: Applications and Practical Aspects.* (ed. R. Fuller) Chapman and Hall, London, pp. 40-64.

De Simone, C., Bianchi Salvadori, B., Jirillo, E., Baldinelli, L., Di Fabio, S. and Vesely, R. (1989) Yogurt and the immune response. In *Les laits Fermentés. Actualité de la Recherche*, John Libbey Eurotext Ltd., pp. 63-67.

De Simone, C., Bianchi-Salvadori, R., Negri, R., Ferrazi, M., Boldinelli, L. and Vessely, R. (1986) The adjuvant effect of yogurt on production of gamma-interferon by Con A- stimulated human peripheral blood lymphocytes, *Nutr. Rep. Intern*, **33**, 419-433.

Fransceschi, S., Bidoli, E., Baron, A. and LaVecchia, C. (1990) Maize and risk of cancers of the oral cavity, pharynx and esophagus in northern Italy, *JNCI*, **82**, 1407-1411.

Fukuda, K., Shibata, A., Hirohata, I., Tanikawa, K., Yamaguchi, G., and Ishii, M. (1993) A hospital-based case-control study on hepatocellular carcinoma in Fukuoka and Saga prefectures, Northerm Kyushu, Japan, *Jpn. J. Cancer Res.* **84**, 708-714.

Fuller, R. (1997) Introduction . In *Probiotics 2: Applications and Practical Aspects*, (ed. R.Fuller), Chapman and Hall, London, pp. 1-9.

Gotz, V., Romankiewics, J., Mose, J. *et al.* (1979) Prophylaxis against ampicillin-associated diarrhoea with a *Lactobacillus* preparation, *Am. J. Hosp. Pharm.*, **36**, 754-757.

Hague, A., Elder, D., Hicks, D. and Paraskeva, C. (1995) Apoptosis in colorectal tumour cells: induction by the short chain fatty acids butyrate, propionate and acetate and by the bile salt deoxycholate, *Int. J. Cancer*, **60**, 400-406.

Harris, C. (1991) Chemical and physical carcinogenesis: advances and perspectives for the 1990's, *Cancer Res.* (Suppl) **51**, 5023 s-5044 s.

Harris, C. (1993) At the crossroads of molecular carcinogenesis and risk assessment, *Science*, **262**, 1980-1981.

Hising, A., Guo, W., Chen, J., Stone, B., Blot, W. and Fraumeni, C. (1991) Correlates of liver cancer mortality in China, *Int. J. Epidemiol.* **20**, 54-59.

Issacson, P. (1982) Immunoperoxidase study of the secretory immunoglobulin system in colonic neoplasia, *J. Clin. Pathol.* **35**, 14-25.

Kampman, E., Goldbohm, A., van den Brandt, P. and van't Veer, P. (1994) Fermented dairy products, calcium and colorectal cancer in the Netherlands cohort study, *Cancer Res.* **54**, 3186-3190.

Kato, I., Miura, S., Kasumi, F., Iwase, T., Tashiro, H. et al. (1992) A case-control study of breast cancer among japanese women: with special reference to family history and reproductive and dietary factors, *Breast Cancer Research Treatment,* **24**, 51-59.

Katosouyanni, K., Trichopoulos, D. and Boyle, P. (1986) Diet and breast cancer: a case-control study in Greece, *Int J. Cancer* **38**, 815-820.

Kayser, H. and Meise, H. (1996) Stimulation of human peripheral blood lymphocytes by bioactive peptides derived from bovine milk proteins, *FEBS Letters*, **383**, 18-20.

Koldovsky, O. (1989) Hormones in milk: their possible physiological significance for the neonate. In *Gastroenterology and Nutrition in Infancy,*(ed. E. Lebenthal), Raven Press, New York, pp. *97-119.*

Kong, W., Koldovsky, O. and Rao, R. (1992) Appearance of exogenous epidermal growth factor in liver, bile and intestinal lumen of suckling rats, *Gastroenterology*, **102,** 661-667.

LaVecchia, C., Negri, E. and D'Avanzo, B. (1991) Dietary indicators of oral and pharyngeal cancer, *Int. J. Epidemiol.*, **20**, 39-44.

LaVecchia, C., Negri, E., Decarli, A., D'Avanzo, B. and Franceschi, S. (1988) Risk factors for hepatocellular carcinoma in northern Italy, *Int. J. Cancer*, **42**, 872-876.

Lee, H., Gourley, L. and Duffy, S. (1989) Colorectal cancer and diet in an Asian population a case control study among Singapore Chinese, *Int. J. Cancer*, **43**, 1007-1016.

Lise,L.and Audibert, F. (1989) Immunoadjuvants and analogs of immunomodulatory bacterial structures, *Current Opinion in Immunology*, **2**, 269-274.

Lunn, P.G., Northrop-Clewes, C. and Downes, R. (1991) Intestinal permeability, mucosal injury and growth faltering in gambian infants, *Lancet* **338**, 907-910.

Mac Dermott, R. (1993) Effect of nutritional factors and the microenviroment on mucosal immune function. In *Immunophysiology of the Gut*, (eds. A. Walker, P.Harmatz and B. Wershil), Academic Press, Inc. San Diego, USA, pp. 365-371.

Macquart-Moulin, G., Riboli, E. and Cornje, J. (1986) Case-control study on colorectal cancer diet in Marseilles, *Int, J. Cancer* **38**, 183-191.

Manousos, O., Day, N., Trichopoulos, D. (1983) Diet and colorectal cancer: A case-control study in Greece, *Int. J. Cancer*, **32**, 1-5.

McLaughlin, J., Gridley, G., and Block, G. (1988) Dietary factors in oral and pharyngeal cancer, *J. Natl. Cancer Inst.*, **80**, 1237-1243.

Meuth, M. (1989) The molecular basis of mutations induced by deoxynucleotide triphosphate pool imbalances in mammalian cells, *Exp. Cell Res.*, **181**, 305-316.

Mils, P., Beeson, W., Phillips, R. and Fraser, G. (1991) Bladder cancer in a low risk population: results from the adventist health study, *Am. J. Epidemiol.* **133**, 230-239.

Munck, A. and Crabtree, G. (1981) Glucocorticoid induced lymphocyte death. In *Biology and Pathology*, (eds. I. Bowen. and R. Lockshin), Chapman and Hall, New York pp. 329-359.

Nardi, R., Vierira, E. and Crocco-Alfonso, L. (1990) Experimental salmonellosis in conventional and germ-free mice. Bacteriological and immunological aspects. *Program and Abstracts 10th Symposium on Gnotobiology*, pp. 27-34.

Newberne, P. and Rogers, A. (1986) The role of nutrients in cancer causation . In *Diet, Nutrition, and Cancer*, (ed. Y. Hayashi), Japan Scientific Press, pp. 205-222.

Newmark, H. and Lipkin, M. (1992) Calcium, Vitamin D and colon cancer, *Cancer Res.* **52**, 2067 s- 2070 s.

Notani, P. and Jayant, K. (1987) Role of diet in upper aerodigestive tract cancers, *Nutr. Cancer*, **10**, 103-113.

Perdigón, G., Agüero, G., Alvarez, S., Gaudioso de Allori, C. and P.de Ruiz Holgado, A. (1995 a) Effect of viable *Lactobacillus casei* feeding on the immunity of the mucosae and intestinal microflora in mal-nourished mice, *Milchwiss.* **50**, 251-256.

Perdigón, G., Alvarez, S., Rachid, M., Agüero, G. and Gobbato, N. (1995 b) Immune system stimulation by Probiotics, *J. Dairy Sci..* **78**, 1597-1606.

Perdigón, G., Alvarez, S., Valdez, J. and Rachid, M. (1996) Effect of feeding *Lactobacillus casei, Lactobacillus acidophilus* and yogurt on the secretory immune system. In *Proceedings: "Yogurt: Myth versus Reality" Conference*, (ed. D. Curtis)

Published in the United States of America by National Yogurt Association, pp. 65-76.

Perdigón, G., B.B.de Jorrat, M. E., Petrino, S. de, and Rachid, M. (1993 a) Antitumour activity of orally administered *Lactobacillus casei*: Significance of its dose in the inhibition of a fibrosarcoma in mice, *F. Agricult. Immunol.* **5**, 39-49.

Perdigón, G., B.B.de Jorrat, M.E., Valdez, J., Budeguer, M. de and Oliver, G. (1995 c) Cytolytic effect of the serum of mice fed with *Lactobacillus casei* on tumour cells, *Microbiol. Alim. Nutr.* **13**, 15-24.

Perdigón, G., Medici, M., B.B.de Jorrat, M.E., Valverde de Budeguer, M. and Pesce de Ruiz Holgado, A. (1993 b) Immunomodulating effects of lactic acid bacteria on mucosal and tumoral immunity, *Int. J. Immunotherapy* **IX**, 29-52.

Perdigón, G., Valdez, J. and Rachid, M. (1998) Antitumour activity of yogurt: study of possible immune mechanisms, *J. Dairy Res.* **65**, 129-138.

Pereyra, B., Falcoff, R., Falcoff, D. and Lemmonier, D. (1989) Production d'interférons chez la souris par les bactéries lactiques du yaourt. In *Les laits Fermentés. Actualité de la Recherche*, John Libbey Eurotext Ltd., pp. 69-76.

Petrino, S. de, B. B. de Jorrat, M. E., Mesón, O. and Perdigón, G. (1995) Protective ability of certain lactic acid bacteria against an infection with *Candida albicans* in a mouse immunosuppression model by corticoid, *Fd. Agricult. Immunol.*, **7**, 365-373.

Petrino, S. de, B. B.de Jorrat, M.E., de Budeguer, M. and Perdigón, G. (1997) Influence of the oral administration of different lactic acid bacteria on intestinal microflora and IgA-secreting cells in mice treated with ampicillin, , *Fd. Agricult. Immunol.*, **9**, 265-275.

Petrino, S. de, B.B. de Jorrat, M.E. and Perdigón, G. (1996) Effect of different lactic acid bacteria on immune response in corticoid immunosuppressed mice. *Microbiol. Alim. Nutr.*, **14**, 227-236.

Pitot, H., Dragan, Y. (1994) The multistage nature of chemically induced hepatocarcinogenesis in the rat, *Drug Metab.Rev.* **26**, 209-220.

Poirier, L. (1987) Stages in carcinogenesis: alteration by diet, *J. Clin. Nutr.* **45**, 185-190.

Poirier, L., Newberne, P. and Pariza, M. (1986) *Essential Nutrients in Carcinogenesis*, New York: Plenum Press.

Roux, M. and Lopez, M. (1987) Impairment of IgA expression and cell mediated immunity observed on Peyer's patch protein-depleted rats at weaning and then fed on 20% casein, *Recent Adv. Exp. Med. Biol.*, **216 A,** 847-855.

Roux, M., Slobodianik, N., Cosaninsky, R., Langini, S. and Sanahuja, Y. (1983) Effect of severe protein deficiency on the expression of surface and intracellular markers of lymphoid organs in growing rats, *Comunicaciones Biológicas*, **2**, 175-181.

Salminen, S. and Deighton, M. (1992) Lactic acid bacteria in the gut in normal and disordered states. In *Digestive Diseases* (eds. T. Chen, N. East Orange) Karger, Basel, pp. 227-238.

Siitonen, S., Vapaatalo, H., Salminen, S. *et al.* (1990) Effect of *Lactobacillus* GG yogurt in prevention of antibiotic associated diarrhoea, *Am. Med.* **22**: 57-59.

Spector, S. and Hadden, J. (1988) Immunopharmacology basis of immunotherapy to correct T cell deficiences. In *Advances in Immunomodulation*, (eds. B. Bizzini and S. Bonasar), Pythagorz Press, Rome-Milan, Italy, pp. 363-370.

Steinmetz, K. and Potter, J. (1991) A review of vegetables, fruit, and cancer II: Mechanisms, *Cancer Causes Control*, **2** 427-442.

Sullivan, D. and Wira C. (1983 a) Variations in free secretory component levels in mucosal secretions of the rat, *J. Immunol.*, **130**, 1330-1335.

Sullivan, D. and Wira, C. (1983 b) Hormonal regulation of immunoglobulins in the rat uterus: uterine response to multiple estradiol treatment, *Endocronology*, **112**, 260-268.

Sullivan, P.B., Marsh, M., Mirakian, R., Hill, S., Mila, P. and Neale, G. (1991) Cronic diarrhea and malnutrition: Histology of the small intestinal lesion, *J. Pediatric Gastroenterol. Nutr.*, **12**, 195-203.

Tirelli, A., De Noni, I. and Resmini (1997) Bioactive peptides in milk products, *Ital. J. Food Sci.*, **2**, 91-98.

Tuyns, A., Kaaks, R. and Haelterman, M. (1988) Colorectal cancer and the consumption of foods: a case-control study in Belgium, *Nutr. Cancer* **11**, 189-204.

Tuyns, A., Riboli, E., and Doombos, G. (1987) Diet and esophageal cancer in Calvadas (France), *Nutr. Cancer*, **9**, 81-92.

Valdez, J., Rachid, M., Bru, E. and Perdigón, G. (1997) The effect of yoghurt on the cytotoxic and phagocytic activity of macrophages in tumour-bearing mice, *Fd. Agricult. Immunol.* **9**, 299-308.

Wattenberg, L. (1992) Inhibition of carcinogenesis by minor dietary constituents, *Cancer Res.*, **52**, 2085 s-2091 s.

Wira, Ch., and Prabhala, R. (1993) Sex hormone, glucorticoid and cytokine regulation of mucosal immunity: hormonal influences on antibody levels and antigen presentation in the female genital tract. In *Immunophysiology of the Gut,* (eds. A. Walker, P. Harmatz and B. Wershil), Academic Press, Inc. **13**, 183-205.

Zheng, W., Blot, W. and Shu, X. (1992) Risk factors for oral and pharyngeal cancer in Shanghai, with emphasis on diet cancer, *Epidemiol. Biomarkers Prov.*, **1**, 441-448.

Ziegler, R., Brinton, L. and Hamman, R. (1990) Diet and risk of invasive cervical cancer among white women in the United States, *Am. J. Epidemiol.* **132**, 432-445.

CHAPTER 7

Modulation of Cytokine Expression by Lactobacilli, and its Possible Therapeutic Use

C B M Maassen, J D Laman, W J A Boersma and E Claassen

7.1 Health stimulating lactobacilli

Lactobacilli have been used for many centuries in the preparation and processing of food and beverages. Currently, lactobacilli are also known for their health-stimulating activities. Such intrinsic properties include: anti-carcinogenic activity, control of intestinal infections, improvement of lactose metabolism, control of serum cholesterol levels, as well as positive effects on allergy and experimental autoimmune diseases (du Toit *et al.*, 1998; Salminen *et al.*, 1996). It should be noted that not all strains from the very large and diverse genus *Lactobacillus* exhibit the same health-stimulating properties and may vary in strength of the effect obtained. Although some of the mentioned positive effects of lactobacilli are mediated by non-immune components such as production, stimulation or reduction of vitamins, enzymes, and antibiotics, immunomodulation by lactobacilli seems to be very important (Rao and Shahani, 1987; Fernandes *et al.*, 1987; Shahani *et al.*, 1977). One of the possible mechanisms for lactobacilli to influence allergy, autoimmunity, infection and carcinogenesis is by affecting cytokine expression in a specific or non-specific manner. Modulation of the local cytokine profile in the gut probably is most effective. Therefore, oral administration of lactobacilli could enhance protection and improve treatment of intestinal infections, food allergy and colon cancer by inducing or reducing level of distinct cytokines. But apparently, oral lactobacilli can also influence distinct disease areas, like autoimmune diseases of the brains and cancer of the pancreas and bladder. Figure 7.1 shows which cytokines positively influence certain disorders when their expression is altered by oral administration of lactobacilli.

R. Fuller and G. Perdigon (eds.), Probiotics 3, 176–192.

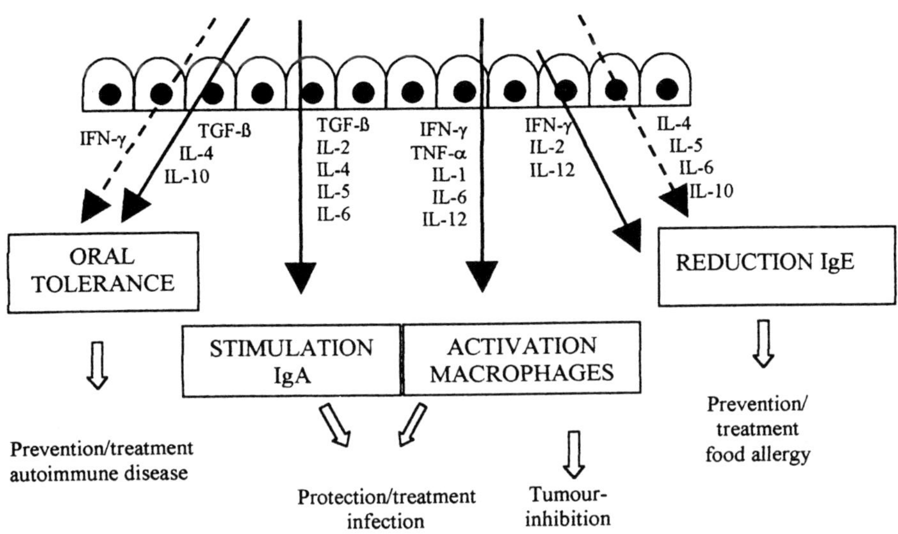

Figure 7.1. Modulation of cytokines by oral administration of lactobacilli can affect disease.

Oral administration of lactobacilli can modulate cytokine expression in the gastrointestinal tract and possibly elsewhere in the body. By inducing (lined arrows) and/or reducing (broken arrows) expression of one or more cytokines positive effects on infection and disease may be achieved. Enhancement of oral tolerance towards orally administered soluble (auto)antigens, even in the periphery, could limit autoimmune disease. Stimulation of IgA production and macrophage activation might improve protection against pathogens that enter *via* the gastrointestinal tract. The cytotoxic action of macrophages can inhibit tumour-growth. Reduction of IgE levels has positive effects on food allergy.

7.2 Defence mechanisms in the gastrointestinal tract

In order to efficiently absorb nutrients from ingested food, the surface of the gastrointestinal tract is very large, over 100 times the area of the skin. As a consequence, a large area of the body may be exposed to many pathogens in the gut. To cope with both pathogens and innocuous substances, the mucosal immune system has generated two major arms of immune reactivity (reviewed by Brandtzaeg, 1995; 1998; Brandtzaeg *et al.*, 1999) : 1) Immune exclusion and elimination. Immune exclusion is a non-inflammatory way of preventing colonization and penetration of harmful foreign material. It results from the physical presence of indigenous bacteria leaving no niche for ingested pathogens, as well as by secretory IgA, which has a higher general cross-reactivity with antigens than has IgG. Immune elimination involves neutralization and removal of foreign material that has penetrated the epithelium by mainly pro-inflammatory, non-specific innate defense mechanisms like complement-activating IgG and IgM and cytokines released from activated T cells and macrophages. 2) Oral tolerance. Oral tolerance is an overall term for immunological mechanisms that may exert suppressive effects on the immune system both locally and in peripheral tissues, mainly against penetrating soluble dietary antigens and the normal microbial gut flora. In addition to anergy and deletion, active cellular suppression is one of the mechanisms of oral tolerance. Active suppression is mediated by the induction of regulatory T cells in the GALT *via* the secretion of suppressive T helper cell 2 (Th2) cytokines such as TGF-ß, IL-4 and IL-10 after antigen-specific triggering (reviewed by Weiner, 1997). Chen *et al.* (1994) have postulated the existence of a Th3 subset of $CD4^+$ T cells, which mainly produces TGF-ß. TGF-ß is thought to be an important factor in down-regulating cell-mediated Th1 as well as humoral Th2-mediated immune responses. These cytokines, TGF-ß, IL-10 and IL-4, are also involved in IgA, IgE and IgG1 isotype switching and proliferation and terminal differentiation of B cells. Local and peripheral T cell tolerance after mucosal administration of the antigen can be regulated by these same cytokines. Consequently, local and peripheral T cell tolerance seems to co-exist with mucosal antibody responses.

7.3 Effect of lactobacilli on cytokine expression

7.3.1 Infection

It has been extensively reported that lactobacilli have probiotic effects which enhance protection against infections (Perdigón et al., 1995; partially reviewed by Salminen *et al.*, 1996). These effects could be due to activation of innate immune defence effector functions (e.g. macrophages) and/or to support of the specific response against infectious agents by upregulation of IgA. These two pathways are discussed below.

The peptidoglycan layer of lactobacilli is thought to be able to activate macrophages (e.g. Schrijver *et al.*, 1999). However, there is some discrepancy between studies as to whether it is the peptidoglycan layer which is responsible for the activation (de Ambrosini *et al.*, 1996); many studies have shown that different strains of lactobacilli are able to activate macrophages under *in vitro* and *in vivo* conditions (Lehman *et al.*, 1988; Nanno *et al.*, 1989; Perdigon *et al.*, 1986; Pool-Zobel *et al.*, 1996; Tomita *et al.*, 1993). *In vitro* upregulation of cytokines produced by macrophages

Table 7.1 a. *Lactobacillus* strains affect cytokine expression *in vitro*

(Possible) effect of lactobacilli	*Lactobacillus* strains	Technique used	Ref
anti-tumour	*L. acodophilu* DDS-1 *L. acidophilus* NRRL 6934 *L. acidophilus* NRRL B4527 *L. acidophilus* NRRL 0734	culture/ ELISA	1
immunomodulation	*L. bulgaricus* Lr 78 *L. bulgaricus* NCK 231	culture/ ELISA	2
prevention IgE-mediated allergy	*L. casei* Shirota	culture/ ELISA	3
influence on vaginal physiology and host defense	*L. crispatus*	culture/ ELISA	4
induction of cardioangitis	*L. casei* (cell wall)	culture/ immunoradiometry (TNF-α) culture/ ELISA (IL-1ß, INF-γ	5
resistance bacterial infections	L. bulgaricus (lysozyme lysate)	thymocyte proliferation/ immuno-fluorescence	6
physiologically functional food	*L. gasseri*	culture/ 50% plaque reduction/ neutralization, rt-PCR	7
physiologically functional foods	*L. acidophilus* (4 strains)	culture/ neutralization	8
prevention/ treatment of food allergy	*L. plantarum* ***L-137***	culture/ ELISA	9
prevention IgE-mediated allergy	*L. casei* Shirota *L. johnsonii* JCM 0212	culture/ ELISA	3
induction of pulpitis	*L. casei* (peptidoglycan)	rt-PCR	10
immunomodulation	*L. bulgaricus*	culture/ immunoradiometry	11
immunomodulation	*L. helveticus* 5089 (medium)	culture/ ELISA	12
immunomodulation	*L. paracasei ssp paracasei* E506 *L. paracasei ssp paracasei* E510 *L. acidophilus* E507 *L. plantarum* E98 *L. rhamnosus* E509 *L. rhamnosus* GG E522 *L. bulgaricus* E585	culture/ ELISA, Northern blot	13, 14
immunomodulation	*L. bulgaricus* Lr 78 *L. bulgaricus* NCK 231	culture/ ELISA	2*

References including remarks: [1]Rangavajhyala et al., 1997 (*L. acidophilus* DDS-1 far best inducer); [2]Marin et al., 1998; [3]Shida et al., 1998; [4]Klebanoff et al., 1999; [5]Tomita et al., 1993; [6]Popova et al., 1993; [7]Kitazawa et al., 1994; [8]Kitazawa et al., 1992;

Table 7. 1 b. *Lactobacillus* strains affect cytokine expression *in vitro*

Lactobacillus strains	Analyzed cytokine producing cells	Cytokines analyzed												
		IL-12	IL-1	IL-1V	IL-1ß	TNF-V	INF-V/E	INF-(	IL-2	IL-4	IL-5	IL-6	IL-10	
L. acodophilu DDS-1	macrophage cell line (RAW 264.7)			8		8								1
L. acidophilus NRRL 6934				8		8								
L. acidophilus NRRL B4527				8		8								
L. acidophilus NRRL 0734				8		8								
L. bulgaricus Lr 78	macrophage cell line (RAW 264.7)					8						8		2
L. bulgaricus NCK 231						8						8		
L. casei Shirota	macrophage cells J774.1	8												3
L. crispatus	macrophage cell line (THP-1)				8	8								4
L. casei (cell wall)	human blood monocytes				8	8		-						5
L. bulgaricus (lysozyme lysate)	human blood monocytes		8			8								6
L. gasseri	spleen macrophages						8	-						7
	PP adherent cells						8	-						
L. acidophilus (4 strains)	peritoneal macrophages						8							8
L. plantarum L-137	peritoneal macroph.	8												9
	splenocytes	8						8						
L. casei Shirota	splenocytes	8						8		9	9			3
L. johnsonii JCM 0212		-						-		-	-			
L. casei (peptidoglycan)	dental pulp cells											8		10
L. bulgaricus	human PBMC				8	8		8						11
L. helveticus 5089 (medium)	human PBMC							8	9					12
L. paracasei ssp *parac.*E506	human PBMC					8						-		13, 14
L. paracasei ssp *parac.*E510						-						-		
L. acidophilus E507						8						-		
L. plantarum E98						8						8		
L. rhamnosus E509		8			8	8	8			-		8	8	
L. rhamnosus GG E522		8			8	8	8			-		8	8	
L. bulgaricus E585		-			8	8	-			-		8	8	
L. bulgaricus Lr 78	T-helper cell line (EL4.IL-2)								8		8			2*
L. bulgaricus NCK 231									8		8			

[9]Murosaki et al., 1998; [10]Matsushima et al., 1998; [11]Solis-Pereyra et al., 1997; [12]Laffineur et al., 1996 (in 2 out of 4 strains); [13]Miettinen et al., 1998; [14]Miettinen et al., 1996 (fixed bacteria: no cytokine induction, IL-18 induced by *L. rahmnosus* and *L. bulgaricus*, other strains not tested) * only with co-stimulation by phorbol 12-myristate-13-acetate.

Tables 7.1a and 7.1b show an overview of studies on the *in vitro* effects of *Lactobacillus* strains on cytokine expression. From top to bottom the analyzed cytokine producing cells are divided in macrophages, mixed cell populations and T-cells. All experiments were performed with material from mice or humans. The experiments using human material are indicated in the column with cytokine producing cells. Northern blotting and rt-PCR were used to determine mRNA levels of cytokine genes. The cytokines analysed are indicated by 8 (induction), 9 (inhibition) or – (no effect).

TNF-α, IL-1, IL-6, IL-12 and/or IFN-α/β was found in different studies with macrophage cell lines, human blood monocytes, spleen macrophages, Peyer's patch (PP) adherent cells or peritoneal macrophages (Table 7.1)(Kitazawa *et al.*, 1992; 1994; Klebanoff *et al.*, 1999; Marin *et al.*, 1998; Murosaki *et al.*, 1998; Popova *et al.*, 1993; Shida *et al.*, 1998; Tomita *et al.*, 1993). Since IFN-γ is the major macrophage activating cytokine, induction of this cytokine by lactobacilli provides indirect evidence of macrophage activating properties of lactobacilli (Laffineur *et al.*, 1996; Murosaki *et al.*, 1998; Shida *et al.*, 1998; Solis-Pereyra *et al.*, 1997). Intraperitoneal administration of *Lactobacillus casei* cell wall, leading to macrophage activation, is now being used as a model for Kawasaki disease (cardiac arteritis) (Okitsu-Negishi *et al.*, 1996; Tomita *et al.*, 1993; Lehman *et al.*, 1988). When lactobacilli were added to *in vitro* cultures of mixed cell populations like splenocytes or human PBMC, upregulation or no effect on expression of IL-12, IL-1, IL-6, IFN-α/β, IFNγ and TNF-α was found (Laffineur *et al.*, 1996; Matsushima *et al.*, 1998; Miettinen *et al.*, 1996; 1998; Murosaki *et al.*, 1998; Shida *et al.*, 1998; Solis-Pereyra *et al.*, 1997). This could reflect activation of the monocyte lineage, but may be partially due to modulation of lymphocytes. *In vivo* administration of lactobacilli can also result in activation of macrophages. In different studies one or more of the cytokines IL-12, IL-1, TNF-α and IL-6 were upregulated by peritoneal macrophages after oral, intramuscular or intraperitoneal administration of the lactobacilli (Table 7.2) (Murosaki *et al.*, 1998; Okitsu-Negishi *et al.*, 1996; Popova *et al.*, 1993; Saito *et al.*, 1987). Although almost all *Lactobacillus* strains could activate macrophages, the extent of cytokine induction differed between strains. TNF-α was also induced in the gut after oral administration of different *Lactobacillus* strains (Maassen *et al.*, 1999b). Increased numbers of TNF-α producing cells in the gut villi and in the submucosa were demonstrated by immunohistochemistry after feeding BALB/c mice with *L. reuteri* (Fig. 7.2).

Lactobacilli can affect infection by macrophage activation (immune elimination), but also by stimulating IgA production (immune exclusion). It has been shown previously that lactobacilli are able to upregulate IgA, locally as well as systemically (Perdigon *et al.*, 1991; Link-Amster *et al.*, 1994; Kaila *et al.*, 1995; Majamaa *et al.*, 1995). This is probably linked to upregulation of one or more cytokines. For instance, TGF-ß is necessary for the isotype switch to IgA (reviewed in Brandtzaeg, 1995). Terminal differentiation of B cells into plasma cells in the secretory tissues involves cytokines such as IL-5, IL-6 and IL-10 and possibly IFN-γ. These cytokines can all be produced by mucosal T-cells (Nilsen *et al.*, 1995). Not much is known about the cytokine profile or other micro-environmental requirements for the enhancement of J chain production by mucosal B cells, a necessary component of secretory IgA and IgM. Probably IL-2, IL-5 and may be IL-6 are involved in its upregulation, whereas IL-4 may have a the opposite effect (Brandtzaeg, 1994). In a T cell line the expression of cytokines IL-2 and IL-5 was enhanced, possibly correlating with the upregulation of J-chain expression (Table 7.1)(Marin *et al.*, 1998). In other cultures no effect or increased expression of IFN-γ, IL-2, IL-4, IL-6 and IL-10 was measured (Table 7.1). It is noteworthy that IL-4 levels remained either unaffected or were down regulated. This is consistent with the results found *in vivo* when, after intraperitoneal or oral application of lactobacilli, IL-4 levels were down-regulated (Table 7.2) (Kato *et al.*, 1998; Maassen *et al.*, 1999b; Matsuzaki *et al.*, 1998; Murosaki *et al.*, 1998). By modulation of cytokine expression lactobacilli may reduce infection.

7.3.2 Tumour growth

Lactobacilli show anti-tumour effects not only in rodents, but also in humans. In particular, intralesional injection of lactobacilli effectively inhibits tumour growth (lung carcinoma) (Masuno *et al.*, 1991), but also oral application of lactobacilli can prevent tumours (colon/bladder cancer) (Aso *et al.*, 1995). IL-1 and TNF-α secreted by macrophages exhibit cytostatic and cytocidal effects on several tumour cell lines *in vitro* (Onozaki *et al.*, 1985; Urban *et al.*, 1986). It is thought that the tumour-suppressive activity of lactobacilli is dependent on the activation of macrophages producing IL-1 and TNF-α (Table 7.1 and 7.2) (Davidkova *et al.*, 1992; Matsuzaki *et al.*, 1996; 1998; Rangavajhyala *et al.*, 1997). IFN-γ not only activates macrophages but also natural killer cells, which can nonspecifically kill tumour cells. Therefore, induction of IFN-γ by lactobacilli could positively affect anti-tumour activity as well.

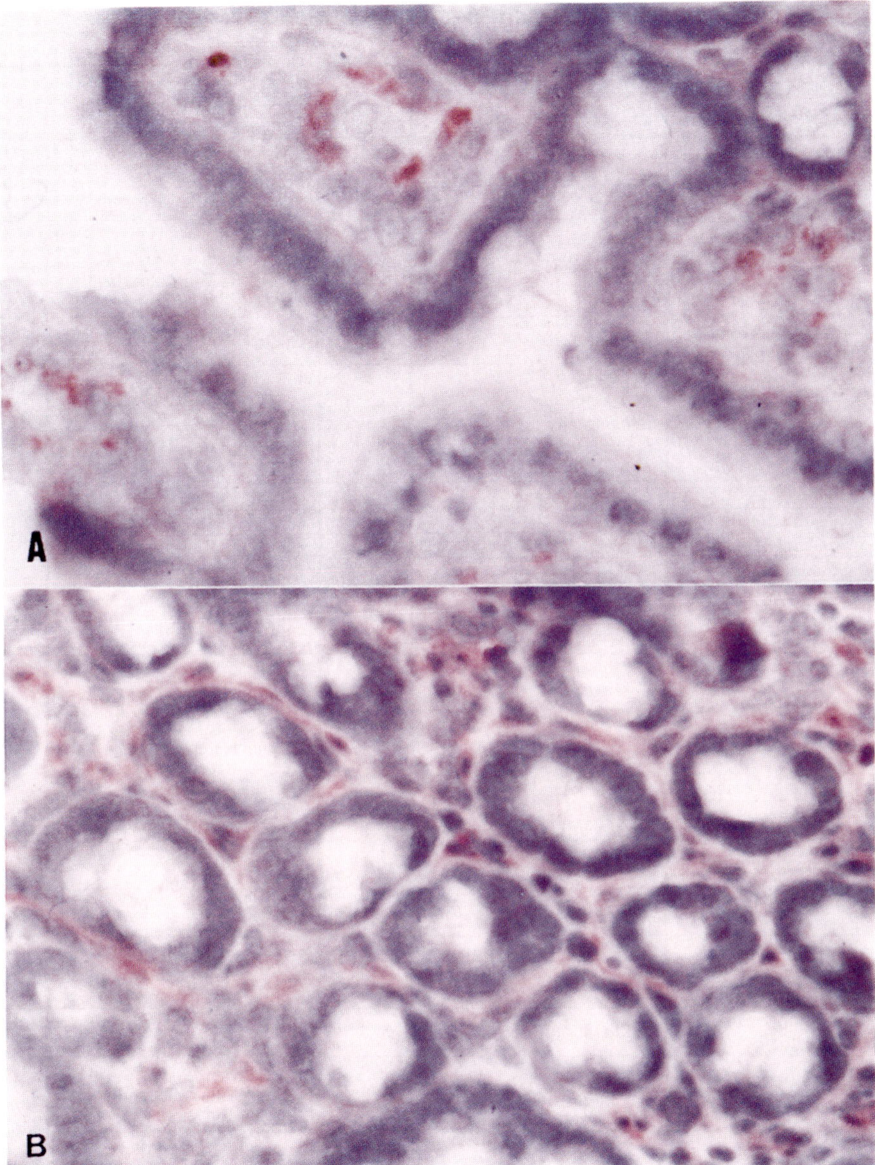

Figure 7.2. Induction of TNF-α producing cells in the gut after oral administration of *L. reuteri*.

Top: TNF-α producing cells in the lamina propria of a mouse fed L. reuteri and immunised with Chikungunya virus. Bottom: Localisation of TNF-α positive cells in submucosa of a mouse fed *L. reuteri* and immunised with Chikungunya virus. BALB/c mice were fed *Lactobacillus reuteri* on days 0, 2, 4 and 6. On day 0 the mice were also immunized i.p. with 25µg UV-inactivated Chikungunya virus in PBS. One day after the last feeding the mice were euthanized. In frozen sections of the first 10 cm of the small intestine containing the Peyer's patches TNF-α positive cells were detected using anti-TNF-α antibodies (bright red precipitate). The slides were counterstained with hematoxylin. Very few TNF-α positive cells were detected in mice immunized with Chikungunya virus fed buffer only.

Table 7. 2 a. *Lactobacillus* strains affect cytokine expression *in vivo*

Possible effect of lactobacilli	*Lactobacillus* strains	Route	Technique used	Ref
resistance bacterial infections	*L. bulgaricus* (lysozyme lysate)	po	thymocyte proliferation/ immunofluorescence	1
anti-infection	L. casei YIT9018	im	^{3}H thymidine incorporation	2
induction of cardioangitis	*L. casei* (cell wall)	ip	culture/ ELISA (TNF-∀), proliferation of B3B1 cells (IL-6), Northern blot (IL-1ß, TNF-∀)	3
prevention/ treatment of food allergy	*L. plantarum* L-137	ip	culture/ ELISA	4
probiotic	*L. casei* *L. acidophilus* *L. helveticus* *L. gasseri* *L. reuteri*	po v	culture/ ELISA	5
reduction CIA	*L. casei* Shirota	po v	culture/ ELISA	6
prevention IDDM	*L. casei*	po nv	culture/ ELISA	7
treatment NIDDM	*L. casei*	po nv	culture/ ELISA	8
inhibition of IgE production	*L. casei* Shirota	po nv	culture/ ELISA	9
anti-tumour	*L. casei* Shirota	ipl	culture/ ELISA, rt-PCR	10, 11
immunomodulation	*L. reuteri* *L. brevis* *L. gasseri* *L. murinus* *L. plantarum* NCIB *L. plantarum* 14917 *L. casei* *L. fermentum*	po v	immunohistochemistry	12
immunomodulation	*L. brevis* ssp. *coagulans*	po v po nv	2'-5' A synthetase	13
treatment neoplastic disease	*L. bulgaricus* (lysozyme lysate)	po	ELISA	14
food processing	*L. bulgaricus*	ip	ELISA	15
anti-Trichinella spiralis infection	*L. casei*	ip v	ELISA	16
prevention/ treatment of food allergy	*L. plantarum* L-137	ip	ELISA	4
anti-tumour	*L. casei* YIT9018	il	^{3}H thymidine incorporation (IL-1, IL-2), ELISA (IFN-(), cytostasis (TNF-∀)	10, 17

Tables 7.2a and 7. 2b show an overview of studies on the *in vivo* effects of *Lactobacillus* strains on cytokine expression. From top to bottom the analyzed cytokine producing cells are divided in macrophages, mixed cell populations, T-cells and soluble components. All experiments were performed in mice or humans. The experiments in humans are indicated in the column with cytokine producing cells. The route of administration is indicated as follows; orally (po), intramuscular (im), intraperitoneally (ip), intrapleural (ipl), intralesional in the lung of tumour-bearing *L. casei* primed mice (il). Where known it was indicated whether viable (v) or non-viable (nv) lactobacilli were used. Experiments which demonstrated that lactobacilli had no effect on cytokine expression are not included in this table. Experiments are also excluded with mixed bacterial cultures where the effect of lactobacilli could not be positively identified. ^{3}H-thymidine incorporation in cells dependent for their growth on the cytokine of interest, was used as a measure for specific cytokine production of the effector cells. Northerm blotting and

Table 7. 2b. ***Lactobacillus*** **strains affect cytokine expression** ***in vivo***

Lactobacillus strains	Analyzed cytokine producing cells	Cytokines analyzed												
		IL-12	IL-1	IL-1A	IL-1ß	TNF-A	INF-A/E	INF-(	IL-2	IL-4	IL-5	IL-6	IL-10	
L. bulgaricus (lysozyme lysate)	peritoneal macrophages		8											1
L. casei YIT9018	peritoneal macrophages		8											2
L. casei (cell wall)	peritoneal macrophages				8	8						8		3
L. plantarum L-137	peritoneal macrophages splenocytes	8						- 		9				4
L. casei	peritoneal leukocytes	8				-		-				8		5
L. acidophilus		8				-		8				8		
L. helveticus		-				-		9				9		
L. gasseri		-				-		9				9		
L. reuteri		-				-		9				9		
L. casei Shirota	splenocytes							9		-				6
L. casei	splenocytes							9	8				8	7
L. casei	splenocytes							9	9					8
L. casei Shirota	splenocytes	8						8	8	9	9	9	9	9
L. casei Shirota	thoracic exudated cells	8			8	8		8				8		10, 11
L. reuteri	gutvilli			-	8	8		-	8	-			-	12
L. brevis				-	-	8		-	8	-			-	
L. gasseri				-	-	8		-	-	-			-	
L. murines				-	-	8		-	-	-			-	
L. plantarum NCIB				-	-	8		-	-	-			-	
L. plantarum 14917				-	-	8		-	-	-			-	
L. casei				-	-	8		-	-	-			-	
L. fermentum				-	-	-		-	-	-			-	
L. brevis ssp. (v)	human PBMC			8										13
coagulans (nv)				-										
L. bulgaricus (lysozyme lysate)	serum					8								14
L. bulgaricus	serum					8	8							15
L. casei	serum							8						16
L. plantarum L-137	serum	8												4
L. casei YIT9018	peritoneal exudate				8	8		8	8					10, 17

were used to determine mRNA levels of cytokine genes. The cytokines analysed are indicated by 8 (induction), 9 (inhibition) or – (no effect). References including remarks: [1]Popova *et al.*, 1993; [2]Saito *et al.*, 1987 (only with infection); [3]Okitsu-Negishi *et al.*, 1996 (depicted results obtained from experiments done in BALB/c, in C3H/HeJ mice no cytokine induction); [4]Murosaki *et al.*, 1998; [5]Tejada-Simon et al., 1999 (no effects detected in splenocytes and Peyer's patches); [6]Kato *et al.*, 1998 (only after collagen immunization); [7]Matsuzaki et al., 1997a; [8]Matsuzaki *et al.*, 1997b; [9]Matsuzaki *et al.*, 1998a; [10]Matsuzaki, 1998b; [11]Matsuzaki *et al.*, 1996; [12]Maassen *et al.*, 1999b; [13]Kishi et al., 1996; [14]Davidkova *et al.*, 1992; [15]Pereyra *et al.*, 1991; [16]Bautista-Garfias *et al.*, 1999; [17]Matsuzaki *et al.*, 1990.

7.3.3 *Autoimmunity*

Many of the autoimmune diseases are chronic inflammatory disorders mediated by Th1 cytokines, such as IFN-γ and TNF-α (Liblau *et al.*, 1995; Powrie and Coffman, 1993). Examples of such autoimmune diseases are multiple sclerosis, diabetes and rheumatoid arthritis. In animal models such diseases can be prevented when the peripheral Th1 type of response is turned into a Th2 type of immune response (Liblau *et al.*, 1995; O'Garra, 1998; Powrie and Coffman, 1993; Scott *et al.*, 1994; O'Garra and Murphy, 1993). This skewing of the T helper pathway can also be achieved by oral administration of the autoantigen, because active suppression is one of the mechanisms evoked after oral administration of soluble antigens, thereby inducing regulatory Th2 or Th3 cells (reviewed by Weiner, 1997). Because large amounts of autoantigen are necessary to skew the response towards the non-inflammatory side, a local environment more permissive for this type of response would be desired. Treatment with *Lactobacillus* strains that stimulate production of TGF-ß, IL-10 and IL-4 locally in the gut could enhance tolerance induction against autoantigens. Unfortunately, a *Lactobacillus* strain with these inducing properties has not been found yet. Only *L. casei* tended to enhance expression of both IL-10 and TGF-ß in the gut villi, but these increases were not significant (Maassen *et al.*, 1999b). Down-regulation of the Th1 pathway can also be beneficial. Several reports show that *Lactobacillus* strains can positively affect experimental autoimmune diseases, such as arthritis and diabetes. In all these reports at least IFN-γ was down regulated after oral administration of lactobacilli (Kato *et al.*, 1998; Matsuzaki *et al.*, 1997a; 1997b).

7.3.4 *Food allergy*

Food allergy is thought to be caused by production of IgE against dietary antigen in atopic individuals, due to inappropriate generation and activation of Th2 cells. The Th2-type cytokine IL-4 not only induces switching of B cells to IgE-producing cells, but also inhibits the production of the Th1-type cytokine IFN-γ (Gascan *et al.*, 1991; Peleman *et al.*, 1989; Pene *et al.*, 1988). Conversely, IFN-γ inhibits the proliferation of Th2 cells and suppresses the switching of B cells. IL-12 is known to stimulate Th1 cells to produce IFN-γ, resulting in inhibition of Th2-type of immune responses, but IL-12 is also capable of preventing Th2 responses independently of IFN-γ (Kiniwa *et al.*, 1992). Lactobacilli that induce IL-12 and/or IFN-γ could help to prevent or treat IgE-mediated food allergy. From Table 1 and 2, it is clear that some strains are able to induce IL-12 or IFN-γ sometimes both. When *L. casei* Shirota was administered orally, the Th2 response against OVA, which was injected i.p, was skewed towards a Th1 response, also reducing the OVA specific IgE response (Shida *et al.*, 1998). Even intraperitoneal administration of *L. plantarum* L-137 reduced casein specific IgG1 and IgE antibodies in casein fed mice (Murosaki *et al.*, 1998). This indicates that lactobacilli can have a role in treatment of food allergy (Shida *et al.*, 1998).

7.4 Concluding remarks

Clearly, selected *Lactobacillus* strains are able to modulate immune responses by affecting cytokine expression *in vitro* and *in vivo*, thus having the potential to suppress infection, autoimmunity, cancer and allergy. The most prominent feature of lactobacilli is that most strains can induce TNF-α, probably correlating to activation of macrophages. Although for most tested cytokines either no induction or enhanced expression was found, especially the data for cytokines IL-6 and IFN-γ were conflicting. This is probably due to the use of different mouse strains, routes of administration, dosages, bacterial viability and effector cells in individual studies. For instance, *L. casei* Shirota showed opposite effects in different experimental set-ups (Kato *et al.*, 1998; Matsuzaki *et al.*, 1996; 1998; Matsuzaki, 1998). On the other hand, various *Lactobacillus* strains within the same experiment differentially affected cytokine expression, indicating that the obtained effect also depends on the *Lactobacillus* strain used (Maassen *et al.*, 1999b; Miettinen *et al.*, 1996; 1998; Shida *et al.*, 1998; Tejada-Simon *et al.*, 1999).

The levels of induction/reduction of cytokines vary greatly and are difficult to compare due to different techniques used. Furthermore, it is difficult to estimate the impact of up- or down-regulation of a particular cytokine *in vivo*. This hampers accurate investigation of whether application of lactobacilli can result in (partial) prevention or treatment of disease. Since many pathogens enter the body *via* the gastrointestinal tract, it is likely that the local cytokine profile at those sites is decisive for the kind of response. Already some reports show that cytokine expression induced by a *Lactobacillus* strain is directly correlated with disease inhibition. However, further study is needed to determine the effects of lactobacilli at the effector sites, together with, as complete as possible, a picture of the local cytokine profile. The cytokine profile which a particular *Lactobacillus* strain induces after oral administration may be important in deciding which strains can be used as probiotics, and also for other applications, such as oral vaccination with recombinant *Lactobacillus* strains. In addition to genetically engineered *Lactobacillus* strains which express protein antigens from pathogens for the use as oral vaccines, *Lactobacillus* strains have been transformed to produce myelin antigens for oral therapy in the autoimmune disease multiple sclerosis (Maassen *et al.*, 1999a).

Acknowledgement

The publication cost for the colour figures were met by Yakult Nederland B.V.

References

Aso, Y., Akaza, H., Kotake, T., Tsukamoto, T., Imai, K., and Naito, S. (1995) Preventive effect of a *Lactobacillus casei* preparation on the recurrence of superficial bladder cancer in a double-blind trial. The BLP Study Group, *Eur. Urol.* **27**, 104-109.

Bautista-Garfias, C.R., Ixta, O., Orduna, M., Martinez, F., Aguilar, B., and Cortes, A. (1999) Enhancement of resistance in mice treated with *Lactobacillus casei*: effect on *Trichinella spiralis* infection, *Vet. Parasitol.* **80**, 251-260.

Brandtzaeg, P. (1994) Distribution and characteristics of mucosal immunoglobulin-producing cells. in P.L. Ogra, J. Mestecky, M. Lamm, W. Strobe, J.R. McGhee and J. Bienenstock (eds), *Handbook of Mucosal Immunology*, Academic press, Orlando, Florida, pp. 251-262.

Brandtzaeg, P. (1995) Molecular and cellular aspects of the secretory immunoglobulin system, *APMIS* **103**, 1-19.

Brandtzaeg, P. (1998) Development and basic mechanisms of human gut immunity, *Nutr. Rev.* **56**, S5-18.

Brandtzaeg, P., Baekkevold, E.S., Farstad, I.N., Jahnsen, F.L., Johansen, F.E., Nilsen, E.M., and Yamanaka, T. (1999) Regional specialization in the mucosal immune system: what happens in the microcompartments? *Immunol. Today* **20**, 141-151.

Chen, Y., Kuchroo, V.K., Inobe, J., Hafler, D.A., and Weiner, H.L. (1994) Regulatory T cell clones induced by oral tolerance: suppression of autoimmune encephalomyelitis, *Science* **265**, 1237-1240.

Davidkova, G., Popova, P., Guencheva, G., Bogdanov, A., Pacelli, E., Auteri, A., and Mincheva, V. (1992) Endogenous production of tumor necrosis factor in normal mice orally treated with Deodan--a preparation from *Lactobacillus bulgaricus* "LB51", *Int. J. Immunopharmacol.* **14**, 1355-1362.

de Ambrosini VM, Gonzalez, S., Perdigon, G., de Ruiz Holgado AP, and Oliver, G. (1996) Chemical composition of the cell wall of lactic acid bacteria and related species, *Chem. Pharm. Bull. (Tokyo)* **44**, 2263-2267.

du Toit, M., Franz, C.M., Dicks, L.M., Schillinger, U., Haberer, P., Warlies, B., Ahrens, F., and Holzapfel, W.H. (1998) Characterisation and selection of probiotic lactobacilli for a preliminary minipig feeding trial and their effect on serum cholesterol levels, faeces pH and faeces moisture content, *Int. J. Food Microbiol.* **40**, 93-104.

Fernandes, C.F., Shahani, K.M., and Amer, M.A. (1987) Therapeutic role of dietary lactobacilli and lactobacillic fermented dairy products, *FEMS Microbiol. Rev.* **46**, 343-356.

Gascan, H., Gauchat, J.F., Roncarolo, M.G., Yssel, H., Spits, H., and de Vries J.E. (1991) Human B cell clones can be induced to proliferate and to switch to IgE and IgG4 synthesis by interleukin 4 and a signal provided by activated CD4+ T cell clones, *J. Exp. Med.* **173**, 747-750.

Kaila, M., Isolauri, E., Saxelin, M., Arvilommi, H., and Vesikari, T. (1995) Viable versus inactivated *Lactobacillus* strain GG in acute rotavirus diarrhoea, *Arch. Dis. Child* **72**, 51-53.

Kato, I., Endo-Tanaka, K., and Yokokura, T. (1998) Suppressive effects of the oral administration of *Lactobacillus casei* on type II collagen-induced arthritis in DBA/1 mice, *Life Sci.* **63**, 635-644.

Kiniwa, M., Gately, M., Gubler, U., Chizzonite, R., Fargeas, C., and Delespesse, G. (1992) Recombinant interleukin-12 suppresses the synthesis of immunoglobulin E by interleukin-4 stimulated human lymphocytes, *J. Clin. Invest.* **90**, 262-266.

Kishi, A., Uno, K., Matsubara, Y., Okuda, C., and Kishida, T. (1996) Effect of the oral administration of *Lactobacillus brevis subsp. coagulans* on interferon-alpha producing capacity in humans, *J.Am.Coll.Nutr.* **15**, 408-412.

Kitazawa, H., Matsumura, K., Itoh, T., and Yamaguchi, T. (1992) Interferon induction in murine peritoneal macrophage by stimulation with *Lactobacillus acidophilus*, *Microbiol.,Immunol.* **36**, 311-315.

Kitazawa, H., Tomioka, Y., Matsumura, K., Aso, H., Mizugaki, M., Itoh, T., and Yamaguchi, T. (1994) Expression of mRNA encoding IFN alpha in macrophages stimulated with *Lactobacillus gasseri*, *FEMS Microbiol. Lett.* **120**, 315-321.

Klebanoff, S.J., Watts, D.H., Mehlin, C., and Headley, C.M. (1999) Lactobacilli and vaginal host defense: activation of the human immunodeficiency virus type 1 long terminal repeat, cytokine production, and NF-kappaB, *J. Infect. Dis.* **179**, 653-660.

Laffineur, E., Genetet, N., and Leonil, J. (1996) Immunomodulatory activity of beta-casein permeate medium fermented by lactic acid bacteria, *J. Dairy Sci.* **79**, 2112-2120.

Lehman, T.J., Warren, R., Gietl, D., Mahnovski, V., and Prescott, M. (1988) Variable expression of *Lactobacillus casei* cell wall-induced coronary arteritis: an animal model of Kawasaki's disease in selected inbred mouse strains, *Clin. Immunol. Immunopathol.* **48**, 108-118.

Liblau, R.S., Singer, S.M., and McDevitt, H.O. (1995) Th1 and Th2 CD4+ T cells in the pathogenesis of organ-specific autoimmune diseases, *Immunol. Today* **16**, 34-38.

Link-Amster, H., Rochat, F., Saudan, K.Y., Mignot, O., and Aeschlimann, J.M. (1994) Modulation of a specific humoral immune response and changes in intestinal flora mediated through fermented milk intake, *FEMS Immunol. Med. Microbiol.* **10**, 55-63.

Maassen, C.B.M., Laman, J.D., den Bak-Glashouwer, M.J., Tielen, F.J., van Holten-Neelen, J.C.P.A., Hoogteijling, L., Antonissen, C., Leer, R.J., Pouwels, P.H., Boersma, W.J.A., and Shaw, D.M. (1999a) Instruments for oral disease-intervention strategies: recombinant *Lactobacillus casei* expressing tetanus toxin fragment C for vaccination or myelin proteins for oral tolerance induction in multiple sclerosis, *Vaccine* **17**, 2117-2128.

Maassen, C.B.M., van Holten-Neelen, J.C.P.A., Balk, F., Heijne den Bak-Glashouwer, M.J., Leer, R.J., Laman, J.D., Boersma, W.J.A., and Claassen, E. (1999b) Strain dependent induction of cytokine profiles in the gut by orally administered *Lactobacillus* strains, *Vaccine,* in press.

Majamaa, H., Isolauri, E., Saxelin, M., and Vesikari, T. (1995) Lactic acid bacteria in the treatment of acute rotavirus gastroenteritis, *J. Pediatr. Gastroenterol. Nutr.* **20**, 333-338.

Marin, M.L., Tejada-Simon, M.V., Lee, J.H., Murtha, J., Ustunol, Z., and Pestka, J.J. (1998) Stimulation of cytokine production in clonal macrophage and T-cell models by *Streptococcus thermophilus*: comparison with *Bifidobacterium* sp. and *Lactobacillus bulgaricus*, *J. Food Prot.* **61**, 859-864.

Masuno, T., Kishimoto, S., Ogura, T., Honma, T., Niitani, H., Fukuoka, M., and Ogawa, N. (1991) A comparative trial of LC9018 plus doxorubicin and doxorubicin alone for the treatment of malignant pleural effusion secondary to lung cancer, *Cancer* **68**, 1495-1500.

Matsushima, K., Ohbayashi, E., Takeuchi, H., Hosoya, S., Abiko, Y., and Yamazaki, M. (1998) Stimulation of interleukin-6 production in human dental pulp cells by peptidoglycans from *Lactobacillus casei*, *J. Endod.* **24**, 252-255.

Matsuzaki, T. (1998) Immunomodulation by treatment with *Lactobacillus casei strain Shirota*, *Int. J. Food Microbiol.* **41**, 133-140.

Matsuzaki, T., Hashimoto, S., and Yokokura, T. (1996) Effects on antitumor activity and cytokine production in the thoracic cavity by intrapleural administration of *Lactobacillus casei* in tumor- bearing mice, *Med. Microbiol. Immunol.(Berl.)* **185**, 157-161.

Matsuzaki, T., Nagata, Y., Kado, S., Uchida, K., Kato, I., Hashimoto, S., and Yokokura, T. (1997a) Prevention of onset in an insulin-dependent diabetes mellitus model, NOD mice, by oral feeding of *Lactobacillus casei*, *APMIS* **105**, 643-649.

Matsuzaki, T., Shimizu, Y., and Yokokura, T. (1990) Augmentation of antimetastatic effect on Lewis lung carcinoma (3LL) in C57BL/6 mice by priming with *Lactobacillus casei*, *Med. Microbiol. Immunol.(Berl.)* **179**, 161-168.

Matsuzaki, T., Yamazaki, R., Hashimoto, S., and Yokokura, T. (1997b) Antidiabetic effects of an oral administration of *Lactobacillus casei* in a non-insulin-dependent diabetes mellitus (NIDDM) model using KK-Ay mice, *Endocr. J.* **44**, 357-365.

Matsuzaki, T., Yamazaki, R., Hashimoto, S., and Yokokura, T. (1998) The effect of oral feeding of *Lactobacillus casei* strain Shirota on immunoglobulin E production in mice, *J. Dairy Sci.* **81**, 48-53.

Miettinen, M., Matikainen, S., Vuopio-Varkila, J., Pirhonen, J., Varkila, K., Kurimoto, M., and Julkunen, I. (1998) Lactobacilli and streptococci induce interleukin-12 (IL-12), IL-18, and gamma interferon production in human peripheral blood mononuclear cells, *Infect. Immun.* **66**, 6058-6062.

Miettinen, M., Vuopio-Varkila, J., and Varkila, K. (1996) Production of human tumor necrosis factor alpha, interleukin-6, and interleukin-10 is induced by lactic acid bacteria, *Infect. Immun.* **64**, 5403-5405.

Murosaki, S., Yamamoto, Y., Ito, K., Inokuchi, T., Kusaka, H., Ikeda, H., and Yoshikai, Y. (1998) Heat-killed *Lactobacillus plantarum L-137* suppresses naturally fed antigen-specific IgE production by stimulation of IL-12 production in mice, *J. Allergy Clin. Immunol.* **102**, 57-64.

Nanno, M., Shimizu-Takeda, T., Mike, A., Ohwaki, M., Togashi, Y., Suzuki, R., Kumagai, K., and Mutai, M. (1989) Increased production of cytotoxic macrophage progenitors by *Lactobacillus casei* in mice, *J. Leukoc. Biol.* **46**, 89-95.

Nilsen, E.M., Lundin, K.E., Krajci, P., Scott, H., Sollid, L.M., and Brandtzaeg, P. (1995) Gluten specific, HLA-DQ restricted T cells from coeliac mucosa produce cytokines with Th1 or Th0 profile dominated by interferon gamma, *Gut* **37**, 766-776.

O'Garra, A. (1998) Cytokines induce the development of functionally heterogeneous T helper cell subsets, *Immunity* **8**, 275-283.

O'Garra, A. and Murphy, K. (1993) T-cell subsets in autoimmunity, *Curr. Opin. Immunol.* **5**, 880-886.

Okitsu-Negishi, S., Nakano, I., Suzuki, K., Hashira, S., Abe, T., and Yoshino, K. (1996) The induction of cardioangitis by *Lactobacillus casei* cell wall in mice. I. The cytokine production from murine macrophages by *Lactobacillus casei* cell wall extract, *Clin. Immunol. Immunopathol.* **78**, 30-40.

Onozaki, K., Matsushima, K., Aggarwal, B.B., and Oppenheim, J.J. (1985) Human interleukin 1 is a cytocidal factor for several tumor cell lines, *J. Immunol.* **135**, 3962-3968.

Peleman, R., Wu, J., Fargeas, C., and Delespesse, G. (1989) Recombinant interleukin 4 suppresses the production of interferon gamma by human mononuclear cells, *J. Exp. Med.* **170**, 1751-1756.

Pene, J., Rousset, F., Briere, F., Chretien, I., Bonnefoy, J.Y., Spits, H., Yokota, T., Arai, N., Arai, K., and Banchereau, J. (1988) IgE production by normal human lymphocytes is induced by interleukin 4 and suppressed by interferons gamma and alpha and prostaglandin E2, *Proc. Natl. Acad. Sci. USA* **85**, 6880-6884.

Perdigon, G., Alvarez, S., and Pesce de Ruiz Holgado A.A. (1991) Immunoadjuvant activity of oral *Lactobacillus casei*: influence of dose on the secretory immune response and protective capacity in intestinal infections, *J. Dairy Res.* **58**, 485-496.

Perdigon, G., Alvarez, S., Rachid, M., Aguero, G., and Gobbato, N. (1995) Immune system stimulation by probiotics, *J. Dairy Sci.* **78**, 1597-1606.

Perdigon, G., de Macias, M.E., Alvarez, S., Oliver, G., and Pesce de Ruiz Holgado, A.A. (1986) Effect of perorally administered lactobacilli on macrophage activation in mice, *Infect. Immun.* **53**, 404-410.

Pereyra, B.S., Falcoff, R., Falcoff, E., and Lemonnier, D. (1991) Interferon induction by *Lactobacillus bulgaricus* and *Streptococcus thermophilus* in mice, *Eur. Cytokine Netw.* **2**, 299-303.

Pool-Zobel, B.L., Neudecker, C., Domizlaff, I., Ji, S., Schillinger, U., Rumney, C., Moretti, M., Vilarini, I., Scassellati-Sforzolini, R., and Rowland, I. (1996) *Lactobacillus*- and bifidobacterium-mediated antigenotoxicity in the colon of rats, *Nutr. Cancer* **26**, 365-380.

Popova, P., Guencheva, G., Davidkova, G., Bogdanov, A., Pacelli, E., Opalchenova, G., Kutzarova, T., and Koychev, C. (1993) Stimulating effect of DEODAN (an oral preparation from *Lactobacillus bulgaricus* "LB51") on monocytes/macrophages and host resistance to experimental infections, *Int. J. Immunopharmacol.* **15**, 25-37.

Powrie, F. and Coffman, R.L. (1993) Cytokine regulation of T-cell function: potential for therapeutic intervention, *Immunol. Today* **14**, 270-274.

Rangavajhyala, N., Shahani, K.M., Sridevi, G., and Srikumaran, S. (1997) Nonlipopolysaccharide component(s) of *Lactobacillus acidophilus* stimulate(s) the production of interleukin-1 alpha and tumor necrosis factor-alpha by murine macrophages, *Nutr. Cancer* **28**, 130-134.

Rao, D.R. and Shahani, K.M. (1987) Vitamin content of cultured dairy products, *Cult. Dairy Prod. J.* **22**, 6-10.

Saito, H., Tomioka, H., and Nagashima, K. (1987) Protective and therapeutic efficacy of *Lactobacillus casei* against experimental murine infections due to Mycobacterium fortuitum complex, *J. Gen. Microbiol.* **133**, 2843-2851.

Salminen, S., Isolauri, E., and Salminen, E. (1996) Clinical uses of probiotics for stabilizing the gut mucosal barrier: successful strains and future challenges, *Antonie Van Leeuwenhoek* **70**, 347-358.

Schrijver, I.A., Melief, M.J., Eulderink, F., Hazenberg, M.P., and Laman, J.D. (1999) Bacterial peptidoglycan polysaccharides in sterile human spleen induce proinflammatory cytokine production by human blood cells, *J. Infect. Dis.* **179**, 1459-1468.

Scott, B., Liblau, R., Degermann, S., Marconi, L.A., Ogata, L., Caton, A.J., McDevitt, H.O., and Lo, D. (1994) A role for non-MHC genetic polymorphism in susceptibility to spontaneous autoimmunity, *Immunity* **1**, 73-83.

Shahani, K.M., Vakil, J.R., and Kilara, A. (1977) Natural antibiotic activity of *L. acidophilus* and *bulgaricus*. II. isolation of acidophilin from *L. acidophilus*, *Cult. Dairy Prod. J.* **12**, 8-11.

Shida, K., Makino, K., Morishita, A., Takamizawa, K., Hachimura, S., Ametani, A., Sato, T., Kumagai, Y., Habu, S., and Kaminogawa, S. (1998) *Lactobacillus casei* inhibits antigen-induced IgE secretion through regulation of cytokine production in murine splenocyte cultures, *Int. Arch. Allergy Immunol.* **115**, 278-287.

Solis-Pereyra, B., Aattouri, N., and Lemonnier, D. (1997) Role of food in the stimulation of cytokine production, *Am. J. Clin. Nutr.* **66**, 521S-525S.

Tejada-Simon, M.V., Ustunol, Z., and Pestka, J.J. (1999) Ex vivo effects of lactobacilli, streptococci, and bifidobacteria ingestion on cytokine and nitric oxide production in a murine model, *J. Food Prot.* **62**, 162-169.

Tomita, S., Myones, B.L., and Shulman, S.T. (1993) In vitro correlates of the *L. casei* animal model of Kawasaki disease, *J. Rheumatol.* **20**, 362-367.

Urban, J.L., Shepard, H.M., Rothstein, J.L., Sugarman, B.J., and Schreiber, H. (1986) Tumor necrosis factor: a potent effector molecule for tumor cell killing by activated macrophages, *Proc. Natl. Acad. Sci. USA* **83**, 5233-5237.

Weiner, H.L. (1997) Oral tolerance: immune mechanisms and treatment of autoimmune diseases, *Immunol. Today* **18**, 335-343.

CHAPTER 8

Bioactive Peptides from Fermented Foods: Their Role in the Immune System

C Matar, J Goulet, R L Bernier and E Brochu

8.1 Introduction

Fermented foods can be described as products whose physical, chemical and biological characteristics have been modified by the activity of microorganisms. They are known to contain specific microbial metabolites such as alcohol, lactic acid, propionic acid, acetic acid, carbon dioxide and exopolysaccharides, as well as bioprocessed molecules derived from the original food material. These derived products, which could be named "tertiary metabolites", can play a significant role in the biological activities of fermented products. The fermentation of milk by lactic acid bacteria (LAB) is a good illustration of this phenomenon. We have suggested, about ten years ago (Goulet *et al.*,1989), that part of the beneficial effect of probiotics might be related to their ability to release bioactive molecules from the substrates on which they are cultivated. Since then, the occurrence of biologically potent molecules derived from the proteolytic attack of milk caseins and whey proteins has been clearly demonstrated and this will be reviewed in this chapter.

Dietary proteins are certainly among the most potent sources of physiologically active molecules in food. Their breakdown by proteolytic enzymes during the digestion process is known to release short or medium size peptides whose structures may be identical or very close to that of animal or human hormones. Because some of these peptides can get across the intestinal mucosa (Gardner, 1987) or interact with biological receptors at this level (Meisel *et al.*, 1989), it is obvious that they may induce or amplify some biological responses. Several bioactive peptidic fractions derived from milk proteins through enzymatic proteolysis have been isolated and characterized. These physiologically active peptides include opiates (Brantl *et al.*, 1979), angiotensin converting enzyme inhibitors (Maruyama *et al.*, 1987), platelet aggregation inhibitors (Jollès *et al.*, 1986), antibacterials (Lahov *et al.*, 1996), digestive system regulators (Yvon *et al.*, 1994) and immunodulators (Parker *et al.*, 1984).

The identification of several bioactive sequences in dietary proteins highlights the major role that these molecules could play as precursors of

R. Fuller and G. Perdigon (eds.), Probiotics 3, 193–212.

bioregulating peptides. These, "formones" (Meisel *et al.*, 1989), could be considered as very potent biological messengers (Goulet and Matar, 1993). Two important observations reported by Ariyoshi (1993) support this hypothesis: the multifunctionality of the active sequences found in milk proteins and their distribution among a large number of mammalian species. Surprisingly, the bioactive peptides are located almost in the same protein regions in all mammalian milk tested. These regions, also called "strategic zones" (Migliore-Samour *et al.*, 1989), are endowed with multiple physiological activities (morphino-mimetic and immuno-modulating) in the β-casomorphin fragments. The antihypertensive peptides from C-terminal α_{s1} casein and the peptide 177-183 from β-casein may also exhibit an immunostimulation activity (Maruyama *et al.*, 1987; Migliore-Sammour *et al.*, 1989). This later peptide is found in the β-casein structure of different species (human, cow, sheep, rat and mouse) reflecting the presence of homologous regions in the sequence of this milk protein fraction (Ariyoshi, 1993). The multifunctionality of physiologically active peptides derived from milk and their wide distribution among mammals could confer on them a role of messenger molecules. Their contribution to the health of the newborn would be three-fold: an easily assimilated source of organic nitrogen, a good source of essential amino acids and a potential source of bioactive molecules.

There is more and more scientific evidence suggesting links between the health benefits of fermented dairy products, specific enzymatic activities of LAB and several components of milk. The microbial acidification process, as well as the proteolytic activities of the LAB, significantly alter the complex structure of the casein molecules. It is obvious that the protein hydrolysates resulting from the action of mammal digestive enzymes will differ in their peptide profile if the native structure of the protein molecule has been previously modified by environmental conditions such as a significant drop in pH and the presence of microbial proteases. Bioactive peptides might then be released prior to, during or after the attack of the milk proteins by pepsin, trypsin and other digestive enzymes. The physiological activities of these peptides could be at least as important as many other primary or secondary bacterial metabolites.

LAB might be indirectly involved in the modulation of the immune response of the host by contributing, during the fermentation process, to the release of peptides bearing hormone-like activities. The mechanism responsible for the health benefits of LAB is probably multifactorial and would result from complex interactions between milk proteins, LAB and the intestinal mucosa (Matar, 1996).

8.2 The proteolytic activities of LAB

Even if most LAB are not highly proteolytic, they rely essentially on proteins or peptides to fulfill their nitrogen needs for growth. The degree of proteolysis during the commercial fermentation of most dairy products is around 2% (Prichard and Goolbear, 1993). Apart from the readily available proteose peptone fraction, the main protein substrate for LAB during milk fermentation is the caseins. Because of their porous structure and poor solubility, differing markedly from that of whey proteins, casein micelles allow bacterial proteolytic enzymes to attack their peptide bonds. This relatively easy access of the proteolytic enzymes to the complex molecular structure of casein is well illustrated by the action of the rennet enzymes. The addition of a relatively low concentration of these proteolytic enzymes (from animal or microbial origin) induces a rapid and spectacular destabilization of the casein micellar structure through very specific attacks of the Phe-Met peptide bonds of κ-casein (Visser, 1993).

During the fermentation of milk by LAB, caseins undergo a slight proteolysis capable of generating potentially bioactive peptides (Matar *et al.*, 1996). *Lactobacillus helveticus* for example is known for its very efficient proteinase and peptidase activities towards milk proteins. The peptides released by the action of LAB proteases on milk proteins often contain several hydrophobic residues such as proline showing good resistance to further hydrolysis. This might be interpreted as an interesting mechanism of protection for a molecule whose primary structure could bear hormone-like messages. Each probiotic organism possesses a unique profile of proteolytic enzymes whose specific activities may contribute to the release of a wide variety of potentially bioactive peptides. Enzymograms of LAB differ from one species to another as well as from one strain to another within the same species; there is thus a very large diversity of peptides that can be released from the proteins of fermented foods.

Cell wall proteases catalyze the first phase of protein hydrolysis, and this activity is often encoded in a plasmid (Kok, 1990). There are two types of cell wall proteases (PI and PIII) that have been isolated from *Lactococci* and classified according to their specificity toward α_{s1} or β-caseins (Visser *et al.*, 1986). A slow proteolytic variant was isolated by (Morelli *et al.*, 1986) from a culture of *L. helveticus* in milk. The analysis of the plasmidic profile of this variant has shown a good correlation between its proteolytic activity and the presence of a 3.5 MDa plasmid.

Figure 8.1. Schematic representation of the proteolytic system of lactic acid bacteria (adapted from Desmazeaud et al., 1983)

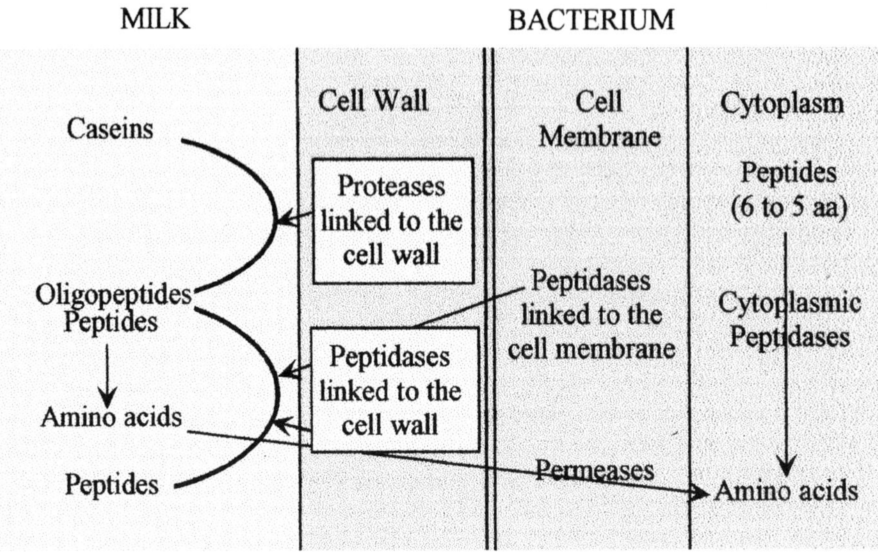

The specificity of proteinases may also differ markedly between strains of the same species of LAB. The hydrolytic activity of two cell wall proteases isolated from *L. helveticus* L89 (Martin-Hernandez *et al.*, 1994) and *L. helveticus* CNRZ 303 (Zevaco and Gripon, 1988) were shown to give very distinct peptide profiles.

Proteinase enzymes can act either individually or in combination with endopeptidases or exopeptidases. Oligopeptides released by the cell wall proteinases are further degraded into smaller peptides by various peptidases (Fig.8.1). According to Tan *et al.* (1993), peptides with molecular weights exceeding 2000 Da would be too large to be attacked by an aminopeptidase isolated from *L. lactis* subsp. *cremoris*. On the other hand, aminopeptidases and dipeptidases isolated from various LAB have been extensively studied (Prichard and Goolbear, 1993), and their hydrolytic activities have been linked to the appearance of bitter peptides during cheese aging. Peptidases are key enzymes for the metabolic activities and growth performance of LAB and the absence of a highly specific aminopeptidase such as prolyl dipeptidyl aminopeptidase, strongly affects the growth kinetics of LAB in milk (Nardi *et al.*, 1991; Matar *et al.*, 1996).

The capacity of LAB proteolytic enzymes to release biologically active peptides from dietary proteins relies on their specificity toward given peptide bonds and their specific activities. Some of these bonds in milk proteins are more readily attacked by specific microbial proteinase and peptidase enzymes than by digestive enzymes. It has been shown indeed that native milk proteins degraded by lactobacillus enzymes instead of trypsin and pepsin, may generate tolerogenic peptides (Sütas *et al.*, 1996a). This reflects a difference in the mechanisms by which the primary structure of the proteins is attacked.

In fermented dairy products, the combined action of LAB proteinases and peptidases yields numerous peptides from unselective casein cleavage sites. Under such conditions, the production of hydrophobic peptides is favoured and these are cleaved at sites different from those usually observed with pepsin or trypsin only. Bioactive peptides such as VPP and IPP (Nakamura *et al.*, 1995) are produced during the fermentation, but are not released by an isolated proteinase of *L. helveticus*. The proposed mechanism suggests a sequential action of proteinases followed by peptidases.

8.3 The release of biologically active peptides in fermented foods

Among dietary proteins, milk proteins are likely to contain a large amount of information due to their molecular complexity and their role in fulfilling the physiological needs of the newborn. The release of information from the milk protein molecule can be accomplished by the "unfolding" of the molecule through external factors such as alterations in pH, ionic strength, or surface tension. This "unfolding" may also be accomplished by the mild action of certain microbial enzymes (Goulet and Matar, 1993).

Matar and Goulet (1996) demonstrated that bioactive peptides (β-casomorphins) can be released during the fermentation of milk by *L. helveticus* (Fig. 8.2). Whey fractions of milk fermented by *L. helveticus* or *L. delbrueckii* subsp. *bulgaricus* were also shown by Yamamoto *et al.* (1994) to give higher Angiotensin I-Converting Enzyme (ACE) inhibitory activities than milk fermented by other LAB species. Those species had stronger enzyme activities than lactoccocci. Moreover, their proteolytic activity could be correlated with the peptide concentration of the fermented milks. Proteinase specificity, which differs markedly among species of LAB, may also have a major impact on the peptide pattern produced during the food fermentation process. In addition the extent of proteolysis may be determined by the fermentation conditions (Fig. 8.3), and consequently may have an affect the bioactivity of the released peptides.

Figure 8.2. HPLC elution profiles after extraction of peptides by charcoal adsorption/desorption with methanol/chloroform

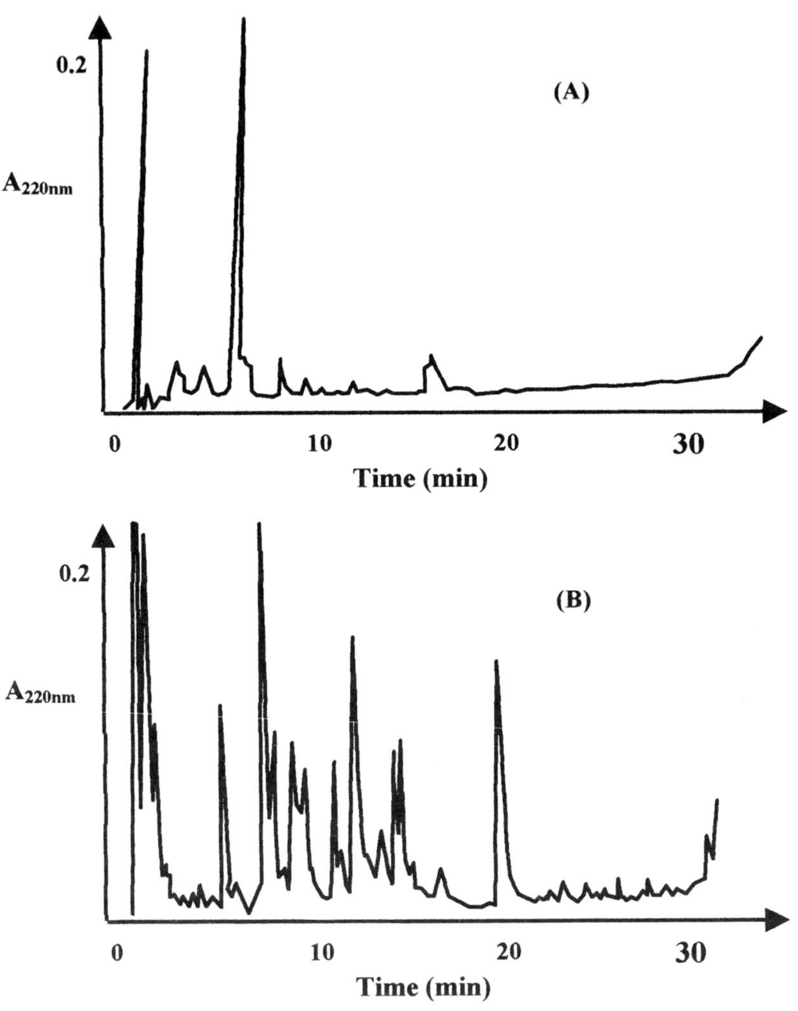

(A) from unfermented milk; (B) from fermented milk with *Lactobacillus helveticus* (X-PDAP-deficient mutant strain) under pH control at 24 h. (β-casomorphin-4 elutes after 20 (min)

A slight or moderate degree of protein hydrolysis may sometimes markedly enhance the release of bioactive peptides. As demonstrated *in vitro* by Matar *et al.* (1996), a significant release of peptides from milk proteins was noticed in the first minutes of hydrolysis under mild digestion conditions. Similar observations were made by Mullally *et al.* (1997), with whey protein concentrate (WPC) hydrolysates giving a significant inhibition of ACE. These ACE inhibitory peptides were released during the first 20 min of hydrolysis, and further digestion up to a degree of hydrolysis value of approximately 8% did not result in an increased development of inhibitory activity. The authors also concluded that it is the specificity of the enzyme(s) and not the final degree of hydrolysis, that determines the development of the ACE inhibitory peptides.

The bioactivity of whole casein is known to be much less important than its hydrolysates. The effect of a caseinomacropeptide hydrolysate on the stimulation of cholecystokinin release was much higher than that of whole casein (Beucher *et al.*, 1994; Cuber *et al.*,1990). It is obvious that the peptide bond(s) being attacked during the enzymatic hydrolysis are likely to have a determining effect on the bioactivity and the potency of the released peptides. The high specificity of chymosin for the Phe-Met bond of β-casein is a good illustration of how a limited proteinase action can have a spectacular impact on very complex protein structures.

Apart from milk caseins, whey-soluble proteins might also favour the release of potentially bioactive peptides when they are submitted to the fermentative action of *Kluyveromyces marxianus var. marxianus* (Bellem*et al.*, 1999).

Among other bioactivities related to milk fermented by *L. helveticus* and somewhat correlated to the degree of protein hydrolysis, is the protective effect on mice against infection with *Klebsiella pneumoniae* resulting from administration of the fermented milk for a 8 days (Moineau and Goulet, 1991); the antimutagenic activity, against 4-nitroquinoline-N'-oxide (4NQO) of a similar fermented milk was also reported by Matar *et al.* (1997). The fermentation of milk by a yoghurt culture was correlated with an increased level of a hormone component, cyclo (His-Pro)-, that elicits activities related to the central nervous system (Prasad *et al.*, 1995). Such a measurable increase could very likely be attributed to the proteases and peptidases of the yoghurt culture.

Figure 8. 3. Electrophoretogramm (SDS-PAGE) of milk proteins following fermentation of skim milk by *Lactobacillus helveticus* at 37°C

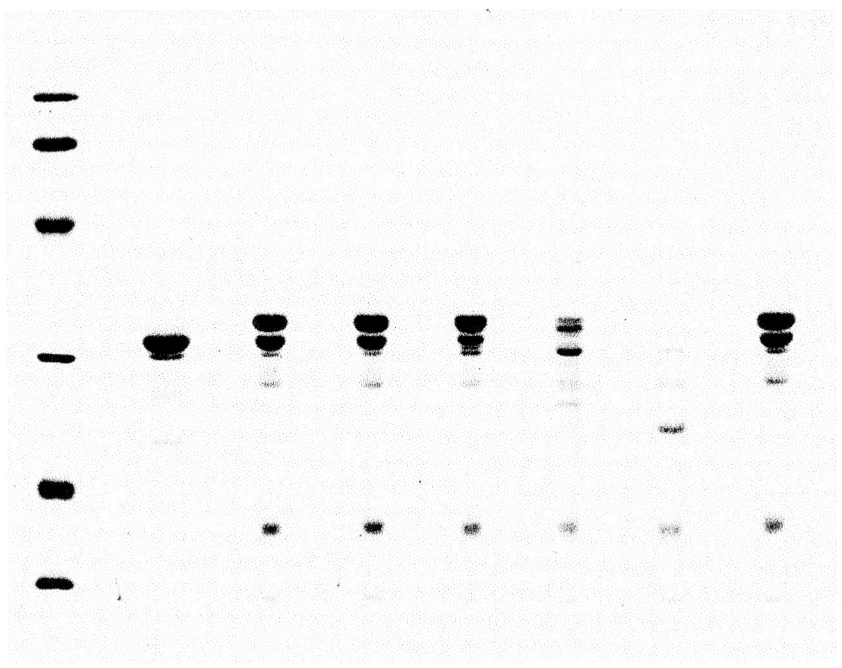

Lane 1, Molecular size markers (Top to bottom: phosphorylase b, (97.4 KDa), BSA (66.2 KDa), ovalbumin (45 KDa), Carbonic anhydrase (31 KDa), Soybean Trypsin inhibitor (21 KDa), and lysozyme (14.4 KDa); Lane 2, purified β-casein; Lane 3 to 7, fermented milk at 0, 6, 9, 12 and 24 hours; lane 8 uninoculated skim milk (24 h at 37°C)

8.4 The release of biologically active peptides derived from fermented milk in the GI tract

It is obviously much more difficult to demonstrate the release of bioactive peptides *in vivo* than *in vitro*. That is why very little evidence is found in the literature on the biological activity of dietary protein derived peptides in the gastrointestinal tract. Matar *et al.*(1996) demonstrated, using a digestion cell roughly simulating the *in vivo* protein hydrolysis process, that the fermentation of milk with a proteolytic strain of LAB can favour the release of novel peptides as compared to a non-fermented milk. The hydrolytic pattern of the proteins as measured by HPLC fractionation was strongly influenced by the fermentative activity of the LAB which favoured the release of larger concentrations of peptides of different hydrophobicities. The HPLC profile of the peptides released after LAB fermentation and gastrointestinal enzymatic digestion differs markedly if the ingested milk has been fermented, suggesting a higher probability of obtaining bioactive peptides.

The contribution of bacterial activity to the release of potentially bioactive peptides during the *in vivo* digestion process of fermented milk is subordinate to the activity of pepsin and trypsin. This was corroborated recently by an *in vivo* study with healthy human subjects (Chabance *et al.*, 1998). It was shown, by an HPLC analysis of the gastric digest of these persons, that the release of peptides is greater after ingestion of yoghurt than non-fermented milk. It was reported in the same study that an the C-terminal end of an immunostimulating peptide (residue 63-68 of β-casein) was released 4 h after the ingestion of milk.

8.5 Biologically active peptides from plant and animal proteins

Many sequences corresponding to those of biologically active peptides have been localized in the primary structure of plant and animal proteins. Some of those sequences could be released either during the chemical processing of these food products, or following the activity of bacterial enzymes as *Streptococcus thermophilus* proteinases (Dziuba *et al.*,1995). The localization of potentially bioactive peptide sequences in the primary structure of plant seed proteins with advanced computer programs have led to the identification of many potentially active peptides, in oats, rice, sorghum, soybean, pumpkin and sunflower. The major identified peptides would be antihypertensive.

Peptides EAE and LLY which can elicit an immunodulatory response were shown to be present in the amino acid sequences of pumpkin and sunflower seed storage proteins (Dziuba *et al.*,1995). The EAE peptide is also known to stimulate the secretion of lymphokines such as α-and γ-interferons, T-cell growth factor and migration inhibiting factor (Mokotoff *et al.*, 1990).

Short chain peptides derived from sardines have been reported to show a potent angiotensin I converting enzyme (ACE) inhibitory activity (Seki *et al.*, 1995). Moreover, an immunostimulating peptide oryzatensin has been isolated from the tryptic digest of the rice albumin (Takahashi *et al.*, 1996). This peptide which is involved in the contraction of longitudinal muscle strips of guinea pig ileum, also stimulates human polymorphonuclear leukocytes and acts as a complement C3a receptor agonist (Table 8.1).

Table 8.1. Immunostimulating peptides from vegetable protein sources

Source	Peptides	Activity	References
δ-chain pumpkin	EAE (42-44)		Dziuba *et al*., (1 995)
Acidic chain sunflower	LLY (71-73)		Dziuba *et al*., (1 995)
Pepsin digest of soybean	AEINMPDY IEEGN SGFAP	Blastoid formation against The splenocytes of mice	Chen *et al*., (1995)
Rice albumin	GYPMYPLPR	Stimulates human polymorphonuclear leukocytes (PMN)	Takahashi *et al*., (1996)

Three immunostimulating peptides have been isolated from pepsin digests of soybeans (Chen *et al.,* 1995). They were shown to activate blastoid formation against the splenocytes of mice. The active fractions have a molecular weight ranging from 300-5000. Many traditional soybean fermented foods are prepared by using bacteria or bacteria-yeast mixed cultures such as Kimena (Himalaya), Dawadawa (West Africa) and Natto (Japan) (Tamang, 1998). These products are all derived from the fermentation of soybeans by highly proteolytic strains of *Bacillus subtilis*, whose fermentative activity might certainly release potentially bioactive peptides from soy proteins. Other fermented foods such as Miso, Shoyu and Tauco, which use blends of proteinaceous plant material, might also be interesting sources of biologically active peptides. The antitumorigenic activities of soy sauce (Benjamin *et al.,* 1991) and miso (Watanabe *et al.,* 1991), have indeed been reported.

8.6 Biologically active-milk derived peptides and the immune system

Several casein-derived peptides may play a significant role in the stimulation of the immune system. The structure of these immunopeptides has been characterized and they have been found to exert a protective effect against microbial infections and to enhance some functions of the immune system (Migliore-Sammour *et al.,* 1989). Immunostimulating peptides were isolated from a tryptic-chymotryptic digest of human caseins (Parker *et al.,*1984). Hydrolysates of α_{s1}- and β-caseins from tryptic and chymotryptic digests of caseins were shown to stimulate the *in vitro* phagocytosis of sheep red blood cells (SRBC) by murine peritoneal macrophages and to protect mice against *K. pneumoniae* infection. After many screening steps, the active peptides were sequenced as VEPIPY (from human casein) and PGPIPD (from bovine casein). Berthou *et al.*

(1987) isolated two immunostimulating tripeptides: one from bovine β-casein (LLY) and the other (GLF) from human lactalbumin. LLY was shown to enhance *in vitro* phagocytosis but did not protect mice against *K. pneumoniae* infection. GLF stimulates macrophage activity against *K. pneumonia*. This tripeptide has been reported to interact with human phagocyte cells through specific binding with a complement component (Jarizi *et al.*, 1992). Costé *et al.* (1992) have obtained the evidence that peptide 193-209 from bovine β-casein can enhance lymphocyte proliferation (Table 8.2). The mechanism by which the LAB and fermented milk products stimulate the immune system is not yet completely elucidated but part of the answer may lie in the complex interactions between the probiotics and their culture medium.

Table 8.2. Immunodulating peptides derived from milk proteins

Source	Peptides	Activity	Reference
Human β-casein Human α-lactalbumin	VEPIPY (54-59) GLF (51-53)	Activate phagocytosis of sheep red blood cells by mice peritoneal macrophages; *in vivo* protection against *K. pneumonia*.	Parker *et al.* (1984)
Bovine β-casein	PGPIPN (63-68) LLY (191-193) C-terminal peptide (192-209)	Stimulate *in vitro* phagocytosis. Enhances proliferation of rat lymphocytes.	Migliore-Samour *et al.* (1989) Costé *et al.* (1992)
Bovine α_{s1}-casein	TTMPLW (194-199)	Protection against infection.	Parker *et al.*, (1984)
Bovine α-lactalbumin	YGG (1 8-20) YG (18-20,50-51)	Modulate proliferation of human peripheral blood lymphocytes.	Mullally *et al.*(1996)
Bovine κ-casein	YG (38-39) CMP(106-169)	Inhibition of the proliferation of B lymphocytes.	Kayser *et al.* (1996) Otani *et al.* (1993)

Much evidence now exists that fermented milks are more efficient at stimulating the immune response than are non-fermented milks. However, many reports suggest that the fermentation process necessary by itself is the maintaince of a biological response of the immune system and a better immunostimulation response; a fermented mixture of LAB was more effective than the non-fermented ones on the potentiation of the immune response and the inhibition of tumours (Perdigón *et al.,* 1993). Fermented milks seem to give a better immunostimulation than bacterial suspensions (Goulet *et al.,* 1989). Hence, Perdigón *et al.* (1995) attributed the increase of the anti-SRBC in yoghurt stored for 20 days to the stimulation of the lymphoid cells associated with the intestinal mucosa by the peptides released during the storage period. When compared with other food microorganisms, fermentation products by *L. helveticus* have shown to clearly exhibit a mitogenic activity (Fujiwara *et al.*, 1990) and an immunodulatory effect (Laffineur *et al.*, 1996).

Tomioka and Saito, (1992) fed mice infected with *Escherichia coli* with different species of lactobacilli. The survival rate was variable depending on the species of lactobacilli used. The protective activity of lactobacilli was related to the activation of the host macrophage and the mobilisation of blood monocytes to the site of infection. The authors postulated that cell wall components or casein peptides are produced during milk fermentation and may have an enhancing effect on the immune response.

Miyauchi *et al.* (1997) found that a pepsin-generated hydrolysates of lactoferrin display an immunostimulant activity more potent than those of undigested lactoferrin. They also demonstrated that the stimulatory effect of the lactoferrin hydrolysate on the proliferation of splenocytes is not dependent on enhanced release of cytokines from macrophage-like cells. They concluded that the hydrolysate of lactoferrin contains some immunostimulating peptides, which can enhance the proliferation of spleen cells. Kayser and Meisel (1996) have demonstrated the *in vitro* modulation of the proliferation of human peripheral blood lymphocytes by the peptides Tyr-Gly and Tyr-Gly-Gly. They reported on the possible function of peptides derived from milk proteins as orally bioavailable immunopotentiatory compounds. Those peptides Tyr-Gly and Tyr-Gly-Gly were also potentially used for immunotherapy of persons infected with the human immunodefienciency virus (Hadden, 1991). Casein-derived peptides could act as cytokine signal inducers necessary for host response to infection by means of a regulatory system and the action of casein kinase which stimulates interleukin (IL-2) cytokine production in lymphocytes (Ole-Moi Yoi and Brown, 1993). Compounds released during the fermentation of β-casein enriched medium by *L. helveticus* have increased the IFN-γ production acting thus on the cytokine network (Laffineur *et al.*, 1996). Interferon-γ also enhanced the expression of immunoglobulin Fc receptors on macrophages (Keller *et al.*, 1994). The interaction with these receptors might be modulated by the immunodulatory peptides released from milk proteins (Gattegno *et al.*, 1988).

An indirect immunostimulation may result from Angiotensin I converting enzyme (Kininase II; EC 3.4.15.1) (ACE) inhibitory peptides, or antihypertensive peptides. ACE inhibitory peptides as β-casokinin-10, a non-opioid peptide fragment, might act as immunodulators since they stimulate the activity of bradikinin (Meisel and Schilimme, 1994). Bradikinin is a vasodilating nonapeptide that may mediate increased immunostimulatory and neurotransmitter activity. The bradikinin is able to stimulate macrophages, to enhance lymphocyte migration, and to increase secretion of lymphokines. The presence of arginine as C-terminal residue in those peptides is a common feature for ACE-inhibitory peptides and immunodulatory peptides.

Goulet *et al.* (1989) reported a correlation between the stimulation of the non-specific immune response in mice fed with fermented milks and the extent of proteolysis of fermented milk. Feeding mice with milk fermented by *B. longum, Lactobacillus casei or Lactobacillus helveticus* has shown a significant stimulation of phagocytosis by pulmonary macrophages (Moineau and Goulet, 1991). The macrophage activity was more important when *L. helveticus* is administered. It has already demonstrated that an immunological communication exists between intestinal and pulmonary mucous tissues including lung, uterus and mammalian membranes (Lamn et *al.*, 1995). Perdigón *et al.* (1998) suggest that the increased numbers of cells secreting IgA (but not IgG) in the large intestine of mice given yoghurt could contribute to limit the inflammatory immune response. Since IgA is considered to be an immune barrier in colonic neoplasia. The modulation of mucosal inflammation by IgA is important to prevent the tissue damaging consequences of a permanent inflammatory response, which occurs during the development of tumours and neoplasia. An increase of the IgA will induce a major protection at any level of mucosal immunity that can stimulate the immune system cells of bronchus-associated lymphoid tissue (BALT) and might have an immunoenhancing activity at this level. Thus, these observations support the hypothesis that peptides released from milk proteins might induce an increase of the IgA response at the intestinal and pulmonary levels without inflammation. This suggests that the mechanisms by which yoghurt inhibits tumour development could be through the decrease of the inflammatory response. Since the increase of the IgA response might be related to the proteolytic activity of *L. helveticus*, we are currently investigating the role of individual peptides on the immunostimulation and the regression of mucosal tumours.

8.7 Biologically active peptides and cancer prevention

There are evidences that consumption of fermented milk products may help prevent mucosal cancers. A large number of reports stating that fermented milks and yoghurt have successfully prevented, inhibited or cured cancer tumours in experimental animals have been published in the scientific literature (Matzuzaki *et al.*, 1996; Perdigón *et al.*, 1998). However, the nature of the milk components involved in cancer prevention remains to be identified. Recent studies have shown that the inhibition of an intestinal tumour induced chemically with 1,2-

dimethylhydrazine (DMH) and a protective effect against entero-pathogenic infections was related to the enhancement in the number of IgA-producing cells in the lamina propria of the large intestine (Valdez *et al.*, 1997). In addition, it has been suggested that many peptides are likely to interact with cellular DNA. According to MacDonald *et al.*, (1994), peptides may reduce the risk of colon cancer by altering the intestinal kinetics. The anticarcinogenicity of hydrophobic peptide fractions isolated from cheese slurries was reported by Kim *et al.* (1995).

Proteins have already been shown to exhibit antimutagenic (Van Boekel, 1993) and anticarcinogenic activities (Bounous *et al.*, 1991; Mclntosh *et al.*,1995). The antimutagenicity, against MNNG, of sodium caseinate, soy and ovalbumin increased after enzymatic digestion (Vis *et al.*, 1998). In addition, a pepsin-generated peptide of lactoferrin was shown to inhibit tumour metastasis produced by highly metastatic murine tumour cells (Yoo *et al.*, 1997); since this effect could not be related to the iron-binding function of lactoferrin, it can be presented as another example of bioactive peptide derived from dietary proteins. These studies confirmed that the antimutagenic and anticarcinogenic activities were greater in fermented milk and casein hydrolysates than in unfermented milk and native casein. This might be considered as more indirect evidence that peptides resulting from the proteolytic action of LAB on milk proteins may act in a prophylactic manner. The limited proteolysis of milk proteins by lactic acid bacteria may also produce substances with antimutagenic activity. *In vitro* studies by Matar *et al.* (1997) demonstrated that antimutagenic activities are related to a limited proteolysis of milk proteins by LAB. Bioactive peptides produced during bacterial fermentation may alter the risk of colon cancer *via* modification of cell proliferation in the colon (Ganjam *et al.*, 1997).

8.8 Bioactivity of the released peptides

The biological activity of the peptides is closely related to their amino acids sequence. The presence of some amino acids such as proline, arginine or the branched amino acids strongly affects the relation between structure and activity of the peptide. The proline-rich immunostimulating peptides such as the heptapeptide (PGPIPN) and its homologue from the human casein are able to resist hydrolysis of gastric and pancreatic enzymes; their action is thus prolonged. However, enzymes, such as dipeptidyl peptidase, present at the brush border could easily attack the proline bonds. The presence of proline also enhances the hydrophobicity of the peptide and it was thought that by this mechanism the peptide could cross the biological barrier. Many proline residues in the same peptide might also open the structure and favour the accessibility of enzymes. The existence of proline residues in the peptide (YPLPR) derived from rice albumin hydrolysis could maintain the three dimensional structure of the peptide and enhance its interaction with the C3a receptor (Takahashi *et al.*, 1996). An active site within an immunostimulating peptide could consist of proline and branch-chain amino acids (leucine, isoleucine, and valine) (Suetsuna *et al.*, 1991). Arginine present on the C-terminal residue of many antihypertensive peptides and some immunodulatory peptides contributes to the bioactivity of the peptides since the positively charged arginine enhances the interaction with the different receptors (Meisel., 1993). Demin *et al.* (1994) assumed that the highly basic side groups in bioactive peptides, such as tuftsin, might ensure the selective interaction of these peptides with the cell surface receptors, which, contain carboxyl groups of glutamic, aspartic and sialic acids. They estimated also that peptides possessing an increased content of amino acids with basic side groups might be able to interact with T-lymphocyte membranes and exhibit immunodulating activities.

Biologically active peptides could reach their receptors at the intestinal level or at the peripheral sites after being absorbed. Peptides such as casomorphins, immunodulating and antihypertensive peptides, may produce local effects on the gastrointestinal tract and stimulate the immunocompetent cells before mucosal absorption. Meisel *et al.* (1989) reported that casomorphins could act not only as modulators of the postprandial hormone release but also as immunodulating agents. The possible immunostimulating effect of opioid peptides, such as β-casomorphins, derived from casein could be attributed to its relation with the a ligand of μ-type opioid receptors that have also been found on the surface of human T-lymphocytes and on human phagocytic leucocytes.

The structure of the proteins has also an effect on the biological activity. The exposure of the inner protein groups after enzymatic digestion increases the antimutagenic capacity of caseins (Vis *et al.*, 1998). The protein chain folding facilitates the accessibility of peptides for enzymes. Casein had little organised structure, which allows it to maintain the bioactivity even after heating. However, whey proteins undergo denaturation after heating, and some authors attributed the differences in immunoreactivity of different whey preparations to the extent of denaturation by heat (Bounous *et al.*, 1991).

8.9 Conclusion

Fermented food products have been consumed through many centuries by millions of human beings long before the existence of microorganisms was scientifically demonstrated. Their nutritive value and therapeutic properties have been and still are widely recognized in all parts of the world and allow them to be classified as nutraceuticals. Not too long ago, the probiotic properties of LAB were thought to be almost exclusively limited to their cellular constituents and enzymatic activities and to their secondary metabolites. More and more evidence is now suggesting that substrate derived molecules may play a significant role in the reported beneficial effects of some of these products. Several peptides derived from milk proteins, mainly caseins and whey proteins, have already found interesting applications in pharmaceutical preparations or dietary supplements. Bioactive peptides, isolated from fermented dairy products mainly, have strengthened the evidence that "tertiary metabolites" resulting from the enzymatic alterations of native or denatured proteins, might be responsible for many of the so called probiotic effects of traditional and newly developed fermented food products.

One might foresee very promising applications in the field of functional foods and nutraceuticals particularly with regard to the prevention or attenuation of several symptoms related to physiological or infectious diseases. The synbiotic approach combining fermented products with prebiotic constituents such as fructo-oligosaccharides can offer a very efficient way of maximizing the probiotic effect of LAB. These combinations of special strains of bacteria, specific substrates and optimal fermentation/growth conditions are likely to yield synergies that would not be observed in conventional fermented products or in freeze-dried concentrates of pure bacterial strains. Some of these synergies might be very helpful for people experiencing sudden or gradual loss of their physiological and immunological abilities.

There are many aspects of prebiotics, probiotics and synbiotics still remaining to be explored and investigated. More and more clinical research should be conducted with humans consuming fermented food products. Probiotics are not drugs: most of the bacterial and yeast strains used for such purposes are on the GRAS (Generally Recognized As Safe) list in America. Since they have been consumed as foods for such a long period of human history, their safety is well established. They should be the subject of further clinical research work.

Most surprising is the immense research interest that dietary protein derived peptides are currently generating. Molecular biology, bio-chemistry, microbiology, chemistry and many other fields of knowledge will certainly contribute to a better understanding of what can be considered as a new level of interaction between foods, microorganisms and the digestive system of most animal species including man. As human beings who try to communicate with the rest of the universe using pictograms and other universal signs launched from our planet, microbial cells might have been successful in establishing new lines of communication with humans and most animals. To decipher such a new reservoir of biological messages that is well encrypted in our food is quite a challenge. Fortunately we can count on probiotics to help us better understand this new language and continue to improve our quality of life.

References

Ariyoshi, Y. (1993) Angiotensin-converting enzyme inhibitors derived from food proteins, *Trends Food Sci. Tech.* **4,** 139-144.

Benjamin, H., Storkson, J., Krewson, J., Sheng, K., Liu, W. and Pariza, M.W. (1991) Inhibition of benzo(a)pyrene-induced mouse forestomach neoplasia by dietary soy sauce, *Cancer Research.* **51,** 2940-2942.

Bellem, M.A.F., Gibbs, B.F. and Lee, B.H. (1999) Proposing sequences for peptides derived from whey fermentation with potential bioactive sites, *J. Dairy Sci.* **82,** 486-493.

Berthou, J., Migliore-Samour, D., Lifehitz, A., Delettré, J., Floc'h, F. and Jollès, P. (1987) Immunostimulating properties and three-dimensional structure of two tripeptides from human and cow caseins, *Fed. Euro. Biochem. Soc. Lett.* **218,** 55.

Beucher, S., Levenez, F., Yvon, M. and Corring, T. (1994) Effet du caséinomacropeptide sur la libération de cholecystokinine chez le rat, *Reprod. Nutr. Dev.* **34,** 613-614.

Bounous, G., Papenberg, R., Kongshavn, P.A.L., Gold, P. and Fleiszerzer, D. (1988) Dietary whey protein inhibits the development of dimethylhydrazine induced malignancy, *Clin. Invest. Med.* **11,** 213-217.

Bounous, G., Batist, G. and Gold, P. (1991) Whey proteins in cancer prevention, *Cancer Lett.* **57,** 91-94.

Brantl, V., Teschemacher, H., Bläsig, J., Henschen, A. and Lottspeich, F. (1982) Opioid activities of β-casomorphin, *Life Science* **28,** 1903-1909.

Chabance, B., Marteau, P., Rambaud, J.C. Migliore-Samour, D., Boynard, M., Perrotin, P., Guillet, R., Jollès, P. and Fiat, A. M. (1998) Casein peptide release and passage to the blood in humans during digestion of milk or yogurt, *Biochimie* **80,** 155-165.

Chen, J.R., Suetsuna, K. and Yamauchi, F. (1995) Isolation and characterisation of immunostimulative peptides from soybean, *J. Nutr. Biochem.* **6,** 310-313.

Costé, M., Rochet, V., Léonil, J., Mollé, D., Bouhallab, S. and Tomé, D. (1992) Identification of C-terminal peptides of bovine β-casein that enhance proliferation of rat lymphocytes, *Immunol. Let.* **33,** 41-46.

Cuber, J. C., Bernard, G., Fukiki, T., Bemard, C., Yamanishi, R., Sugimoto, E. and Chayvialle, J. A. (1990) Luminal CCK-releasing factors in the isolated vasculary perfused rat duodenojejunum, *Am. J. Physiol.* **259,** G191-197.

Demin, A. A., Malinin, V.V. Shataeva, L. K. and Chernova, I. A. (1994) Chromatographic methods for isolation of immunostimulating peptides of milk whey. *Appl. Biochem. Microbiol.* **30,** *255-259.*

Desmazeaud, M. (1983) L'état des connaissances en matière de nutrition des bactéries lactiques, *Lait* **63,** 276-274.

Dziuba, J., Minkiewicz, P., Puszka, K. and Dabrowski, S. (1995) Plant seed storage proteins as potential precursors of bioactive peptides, *Polish J. Food Nutri. Sci.* 4/45, **8,** 31-42.

Fujiwara, S., Kadooka, Y, Hirita, T and Nakazato, H. (1990) Screening for mitogenic activity of food microorganisms and their skim milk culture supernatants. *J. Jpn. Soc. Nutr. Food Sci.* **43,** 203.

Jarizi, M., Migliore-Samour, D., Casabianca-Pignède, M., Kedad, K., Morgat, J. L. Jollès, P. (1992) Specific binding sites on human phagocytic blood cells for Gly-Leu-Phe and Val-Glu-Pro-Ile-Pro-Tyr- immunostimulating peptides from human milk proteins, *Biochem. Biophys. Acta* I **160,** 251-261.

Jollès, P., Levy-Toldano, S., Fiat, A.M., Soria, C., Gillessen, D., Thamaidis, A., Dunn, F. W. and Caen, J.P. (1986) Analogy between fibrinogen and casein. Effect of an undecapeptide isolated from β-casein on platelet function, *Euro. J. Biochem.* **158,** 379-382.

Hadden, J. W. (1991) *Trends Pharmaceut. Sci.* **12,** 107-111.

Ganjam, L.S., Thornton, W.H. Marshall, R.T. and Macdonald, R.S. (1997) Antiproliferative effects of yogurt fractions obtained by membrane dialysis on cultured mammalian intestinal cells. *J. Dairy Sci.,* **80,** 2325-2329.

Gardner, M. (1987) Passage of intact peptides across the intestine, *Advances in the Biosciences* **65,** 99-106.

Gattegno, L., Migliore-Sammour, D, Saffar, L and Jollès, P. (1988) Enhancement of phagocytic activity of human monocytic-macrophagic cells by immunostimulating peptides from human casein. *Immunol. Lett.* **18**, 27.

Goulet, J., Saucier, L. and Moineau, S. (1989) *Yoghurt-Nutritional and health properties,* Chandan RC (eds), USA.

Goulet, J. and Matar, C. (1993) *Yogurt: myth versus reality conference*, Curtis *Communication and Research* (Ed).

Kayser, H. and Meisel, H. (1996) Stimulation of human peripheral blood lymphocytes by bioactive peptides derived from bovine milk proteins. *FEBS letters,* **383,** 18-20.

Keller, R., Keist, R. and Joller, P. W. (1994) Macrophage response to bacteria and bacterial products: modulation of Fcγ receptors and secretory and cellular activities, *Immunology* **81**, 161.

Kim, H.D., Lee, H.J., Shin, Z.I. Nam, H. S. and Woo, H. J. (1995) Anticancer effects of hydrophobic peptides derived from cheese slurry, *Food. Biotech.* **4,** 268-272.

Kok, J. (1990). Genetics of the proteolytic system of lactic acid bacteria, *FEMS MicrobioL Rev.* **87**,15-24.

Laffineur, E., Genetet, N. and Léonil, J. (1996) Immunodulatory activity of β-casein permeate medium fermented by lactic acid bacteria, *J. Dairy Sci.* **79**, 2112-2120.

Lamn, M., Mazanca, M., Nedrud, J. and Kaetzel, C. (1995) *Advances in Mucosal Immunology,* J. Mestecky *et al.,* (eds), Plenum Press, New York.

Lahov, E. and Regelson, W. (1996) Antibacterial and immunostimulating casein-derived substances from milk: casecidin, isracidin peptides, *Food Chem. Toxicol.* **34** (1), 131-145.

MacDonald, R.S., Thornton, W.H. & Marshall, R.T. (1994) A cell culture model to identify biologically active peptides generated by bacterial hydrolysis of casein, J. *Dairy Sci.* **77,** 1167-1175.

Martin-Hernandez, C., Alting, A.C. and Exterkate F.A. (1994) Purification and characterisation of the mature membrane-associated-cell-envelope proteinase of *Lactobacillus helveticus L89, Appl. Microbiol. Biotechnol.* **40,** 828-834.

Maruyama, S., Mitachi, H., Awaja, J., Kurono, M., Tomizaka, N. and Suzuki, H. (1987) Angiotensin 1-converting enzyme inhibitory activity of C-terminal hexapeptide of α_{s1}-casein, *Agri. Biol. Chem.* **51,** 2557-2561.

Matar, C. (1996) Effet de la fermentation du lait par *Lactobacillus helveticus* sur la liberation de peptides potentiellement bioactifs . Ph. D. thesis. Université Laval, Canada.

Matar, C., Amiot, J., Savoie, L. and Goulet, J. (1996) The effect of milk fermentation by *Lactobacillus helveticus* on the release of peptides during *in vitro* digestion, *J. Dairy Sci.* **79,** 971-979.

Matar, C. and Goulet, J. (1996) β-casomorphin-4 from milk fermented by a mutant of *Lactobacillus helveticus, Int. Dairy J.* **6,** 383-397.

Matar, C., Nadathur, S., Bakalinsky, A. and Goulet, J. (1997) Antimutagenic effects of milk fermented by *Lactobacillus helveticus* L89 and a protease-deficient derivative, *J. Dairy Sci.* **80,** 1965-70

Matsuzaki, T., Hashimoto, S. and Yokokura, T. (1996) effects on antitumor activity and cytokine production in the thoracic cavity by intrapleural administration of *Lactobacillus casei* in tumor-bearing mice, *Med. Microbiol. Immunol.* **185**: 157-161.

McIntosh, G.H., Regester, G.0., Leu, R.K.L., Royle, P.J. and Smithers, G.W. (1995) Dairy products protect against dimethylhydrazine-induced intestinal cancer in rats. *J. Nutr.* **125,** 809-816.

Meisel, H., Frister, H. and Schlimme, E. (1989) Biologically active peptides in milk proteins, *Z. Ernährungswiss* **28,** 267-278.

Meisel, H. (1993) *New Perspectives in Infant Nutrition.* G. Sawazki and B. Renner, Stuttgart.

Meisel, H. and Schlimme, E. (1994) *β-Casomorphins and Related Peptides: recent developments,* Brantl, V. and Teschemacher, H. (eds), VCH-Weinhein.

Migliore-Samour, D., Floc'h, F. and Jollès, P. (1989) Biologically active peptides implicated in immunodulation, *J. Dairy Res.* **56:** 357.

Miyauchi, H., Kaino, A., Schinoda, I., Fukuwatari, Y. and Hayasawa, H. (1997) Immunodulating effect of bovine lactoferrin pepsin hydrolysate on murine splenocytes and Peyer's patch cells. *J. Dairy Sci.* **80**, 2330-2339.

Moineau, S. and Goulet, J. (1991) Effect of feeding fermented milks on the pulmonary macrophage activity in mice, *Milchwissenschaft* **46,** 551-554.

Mokotoff, M., Zhao, H., Roth, S.M., Shelly, J.A., Slavoski, J.N. and Koutlab, N.M. (1990) Thymosin like peptides as potential immunostimulants. Synthesis via the polymeric reagent method, *J. Med. Chem.* **33,** 354-360.

Morelli, L., Vesco, M. Coaonelli, P. S. and Botazi, V. (1986) Fast and slow milk coagulating variants of *Lactobacillus helveticus* HLM1. *Can J. Microbiol.* **32**, 758.

Mullally, M., Meisel, M. and Fitzgerald, R. (1997) Angiotensin-I-converting enzyme inhibitory activities of gastric and pancreatic proteinase digests of whey proteins, *Int. Dairy J.* **7**, 299-303.

Nakamura, Y., Yamamoto, N., Kakai, A., Okubo, S., Yamazaki, S. and Takano, T. (1995) Purification and characterisation of angiotensin I-converting enzyme inhibitors from sour milk, *J. Dairy Sci.* **78,** 777-783.

Nardi, M., Chopin, M.C., Chopin, A., Cals, M.M. and Gripon, J.C. (1991) Cloning and DNA sequence analysis of X-prolyl-dipeptidyl aminopeptidse from *Lactococcus lactis* subsp. *lactis NCD0763, Appl. Environ. Microbiol.* **57**, 45-50.

Ole-Moi Yoi, O. K. and Brown, W. C. (1993) Evidence for the induction of casein kinase II in bovine lymphocytes transformed by the intracellular protozoan parasite *Theileria parva. EMBA J.* **12**, 1621-1631.

Otani, H. and Monnai, M. (1993) Inhibition of proliferative responses of mouse spleen lymphocytes by bovine κ-casein digests, *Food Agri. Immunol.* **5,** 219-229.

Parker, F., Migliore-Samour, D., Floc'h, F., Zerial, A., Werner, G. H. Jollès, J., Casaretto, M., Zahn, H. and Jollès, P. (1984) Immunostimulating hexapeptide from human casein: amino acid sequence, synthesis and biological properties. *Euro. J. Biochem.* **145,** 677-682.

Perdigon, G., De Jorrat, M. E., De Petrino, S. F. & Rachid, M. (1993) Antitumor activity of orally administered *Lactobacillus casei*: significance of its dose in the inhibition of a fibrosarcoma in mice, *Food Agri. Immun.* **5**, 39-49.

Perdigon, G., Alvarez, S., Medici, M., Vintini, E., De Giori, G., De Kairuz, M. and Holgado de Ruiz, A. P. (1995) Effect of yogurt with different storage period on the immune system in mice, *Milchwissenschaft* **50**(7), 367-371.

Perdigon, G., Valdez, J. C. and Rachid, M. (1998) Antitumor activity of yogurt: study of possible immune mechanisms, *J. Dairy Res.* **65,** 129-138.

Prasad, C., Kumar, S., Adkinson, W and McGregor, J. (1995) Hormones in foods: abundance of authentic cyclo(His-Pro)-like immunoreactivity in milk and yogurt, *Nutr. Res.* **15,**1623-1635.

Prichard, G.G. and Goolbear, T. (1993) The physiology and biochemistry of the proteolytic system in lactic acid bacteria, *FEMS Microbiol. Rev.* **12,** 179-206.

Seki, E., Katsuhiro, 0., Matsufuji, H., Matsui, T. and Osajima, Y. (1995) *Nippon Nögeikagaku Kaishi,* **69,**1171-1174.

Suetsuna, K., Chen, J.R. and Yamauchi, F. (1991) Immunostimulating peptides derived from sardine muscle and soybean protein; amino acid sequence, synthesis and biological properties, *Clin. Rep.* **25** (15), 75-86.

Sütas, Y., Soppi, E., Korhonen, H., Syvdoja, E.L., Saxelin, M. and Rokka, T. (1996a) Suppression of lymphocyte proliferation *in vitro* by bovine caseins hydrolysed with *Lactobacillus casei* GG-derived enzymes, *J. Allergy Clin. Immunol.* **98,** 216-224.

Sütas, Y., Hume, M. and Isolauri, E. (1996b) Downregulation of anti CD3 antibody-induced II-4 production by bovine caseins hydrolysed with *Lactobacillus* GG-derived enzymes, *Scand. J. Immunol.* **43,** 687-689.

Takahashi, M., Moriguchi., S., lkeno, M., Kono, S., Ohata, K., Usui, H., Kurahashi, K., Sasaki, R. and Yoshikawa, M. (1996) Studies on the ileum-contracting mechanisms and identification as a complement C3a receptor agonist of oryzatensin, a bioactive peptide derived from rice albumin, *Peptides* **17,** 5-12

Tamang, J. P. (1998) Role of microorganisms in traditional fermented foods, *Indian Food Industry,* **17**(3), 162-167.

Tan, P.S., Van Kessel, T A., Veerdonk, F.M. Zurendock, P.F. Buins, A.P. and Konnings, W.N. (1993) Degradation and debittering of a tryptic digest from β-casein by arninopeptidase N from *Lactococcus lactis* subsp. *cremoris WG2. Appl. Environ. Microbiol.* **59,** 1430-1436.

Tomioka, H. and Saito, R. (1992) Lactic Acid Bacteria, *Elsevier Applied Science,* London.

Van Boekel, M.A J.S., Weerens, C.N.J.M., Holstra, A., Scheidtweiler, C.E. and Alink, G.M. (1993) Antimutagenic effects of casein and its digestion products, *Food Chem. Toxicol.* **31** (10),731-737.

Valdez, J. C., Rachid, M., Bru, E. and Perdigon, G. (1997) The effect of yoghurt on the cytotoxic and phagocytic activity of macrophages in tumor-bearing mice, *Food. Agri. Immunol.* 9, 299-308.

Vis, E., Plinck, A., Alink, G. and Van Boekel, M.A.J.S. (1998) Antimutagenicity of heat-denatured ovalbumin, before and after digestion as compared to caseinate, BSA, and soy proteins, *J. Agric. Food. Chem.* **46,** 3713-3718.

Visser, S., Exterkate, F.A., Slangen, C.J. and de Veer, G.J.C.M. (1986) Comparative study of action of cell wall proteinases from various strains of *Streptococcus cremoris* on bovine (α_{s1}-, β- and κ-casein, *Appl. Environ. Microbiol.* **52,** 1162-1166.

Visser, S. (1993) Proteolytic enzymes and their relation to cheese ripening and flavor: an overview. *J. Dairy Sci.* **76**, 329-350.

Watanabe, H., Takahashi, T., Ishimoto, T. and Ito, A. (1991) The effect of miso diet on small intestinal damage in mice irradiated by X-ray. *Sci. Technol. Miso.* **39,** 29-32.

Yamamoto, N., Akino, A. and Takano, T. (1994) Antihypertensive effects of the peptides derived from casein by an extracellular proteinase from *Lactobacillus helveticus* CP790, *J. Dairy Sci.* **77,** 917-922.

Yvon, M., Beucher, S., Guilloteau, P., Le Hueron-Luron, I. and Corring, T. (1994) Effects of caseinomacropeptide (CMP) on digestion regulation, *Reprod, Nutr. Dev.* **34,** 527-537.

Yoo, Y.C., Watanabe, S., Watanabe, R., Hata, K., Shimazaki, K. and Azuma, I. (1997). Bovine lactoferrin and lactoferricin, a peptide derived from bovine lactoferrin, inhibit tumor metastasis in mice, *Jpn. J. Cancer Res.* **88,** 189-190.

Zevaco, C. and Gripon, J.C. (1988) Properties and specificity of the cell-wall proteinase from *Lactobacillus helveticus, Lait* **68,** 393-408.

CHAPTER 9

Mechanisms Involved in the Immunostimulation by Lactic Acid Bacteria

G Perdigón and A Pesce de Ruiz Holgado

9.1 Introduction

The beneficial role played by lactic acid bacteria (LAB) on the host has been extensively reported. Numerous studies have demonstrated (Kato et al., 1981; 1985; Matsuzaki et al., 1985) the antitumour properties of these microorganisms as pure cultures or as fermented milks such as yoghurt. This last aspect will be developed in an other part of this book. The enhancement by LAB of antitumour capacity and resistance to pathogens are undoubtedly associated with an activation of the immune system of the host. LAB or their wall components act by activating the cells involved in the immune response. So it has been demonstrated that certain lactobacilli can induce an increase in the cellular or humoral systemic immune response (Bloksma et al., 1979; Perdigón et al., 1988; Saito et al., 1983) and can also influence the cells such as macrophage involved in the inflammatory immune response (Kato et al., 1983; Perdigón et al., 1986 a; b; 1987; Kato et al., 1984) . There are also reports about the effect of LAB or yoghurt as immunostimulator and as inducer of cytokine release (De Simone et al., 1986; 1993; Link-Amster et al.,1994; Pereira and Lemonnier, 1993; Schiffrin et al., 1995).

However, reports suggest that LAB do not always produce beneficial effects on the host. Some species and strains of lactobacilli are associated with harmful effects such as endocarditis and abscesses which favour tumour growth (Sharpe *et al*., 1973; Iwasaki *et al*., 1983; Davies *et al*., 1986; Maskell and Pead, 1992; Harty *et al.*, 1994). This fact shows the importance of the elucidation of the mechanisms by which the different lactic acid bacteria or at least of those included in food are able to stimulate the immune system to avoid undesireable effects and to make possible their use for therapeutic purposes. Since lactic acid bacteria are usually ingested as part of the normal daily diet it is more important to understand, how they interact or how they influence the behaviour of the immune cells associated with the secretory or mucosal immune system.

R. Fuller and G. Perdigon (eds.), Probiotics 3, 213–233.

Bacterial or viral intestinal infections produce diarrhoea, which is one of the major causes of infant mortality in developing countries and it constitues a risk for travellers from developed countries.There are numerous host mechanisms for the defence against mucosal bacterial infection as well as that afforded by the autochthonous flora. The physical barrier of epithelial cells and their mucous coat, the physical removal by cilia, the peristalsis in the intestinal tract, the pH of the mucosal environment and bile salts or metabolites of the normal indigenous flora are other mechanisms employed by the host to avoid intestinal infections.

Protection against some enteropathogens could be obtained by vaccination , but at present there are no effective oral vaccines to protect against diarrhoeas with different etiologies. LAB have also been used to protect against enteropathogenic agents (Perdigón *et al.*, 1990 a; b; Isolauri *et al.*, 1991; Corthier, 1997; Perdigón and Alvarez, 1992).These microorganisms could inhibit pathogenic bacteria by bacteriocin production, competition for nutrients competition for attachment sites on epithelial cells, or by immunomodulatory mechanisms. However, there is a strong possibility that viral infection may be prevented by the immunomodulatory effect excerted by LAB. This last topic will be discussed elsewhere in this book. The major immunological barrier against enteropathogens is secretory IgA, therefore it is important to know if the LAB are able to increase the number of the IgA secreting cells. It has already been reported that oral administration of lactobacilli or bifidobacteria increased intestinal IgA production during diarrhoea in infants (Yasui *et al.*, 1992; Kaila *et al.*, 1992; Oliver and Gonzalez, 1992; Gonzalez *et al.*,1990). However, the complex interactions among enteropathogens, microflora, host and microbial oral adjuvants, makes it difficult to predict the effect induced by LAB on the intestinal microenvironment, and its influence on the immune response. These observations open up the field for extensive research on the mechanisms involved in immunostimulation by LAB.

9.2 Adjuvanticity of lactobacilli on gut associated immune cells

The major component of bacterial cell walls of Gram-positive microorganisms is muramyldipeptide (MDP) which has adjuvant properties (Allison, 1998). MDP stimulates resistance to bacterial infection but it is also pyrogenic and can induce harmful effects in the host. The immunomodulatory effects of bacterial constituents will be discussed in other part of this book. A great number of MDP analogues have been synthesized which differ in their biological properties. *In vitro* studies have shown that MDP stimulates the release of IL1, IL6 and TNF (Le Contel *et al.*, 1993). The different biological activities of MDP analogues could be related to their profile of induction of cytokine release, which is a limitation for their therapeutic use even when they retain adjuvant activity and are not pyrogenic.

An immunological adjuvant can be defined as any substance which when incorporated directly to the host or *via* vaccine formulation acts generally to accelerate, prolong or enhance the quality of immune response. In the selection of a substance as adjuvant we must know its mechanisms of action. The mechanism of action may vary according to the route of administration chosen and the immune response desired. In mucosal adjuvants it is important to know which kind of immune cells are stimulated and so that we can predict the behaviour. Adjuvants that enhance Th1 immune response induce the release of proinflammatory cytokines such as IFNγ, delayed type hypersensitivity (DTH) and also elicit the production of IgG. These would not be suitable as mucosal adjuvant however, they are important when administered by the systemic route because IgG is able to fix complement and mediate effector mechanisms (Allison and Byars, 1991; Phillips and Emili, 1992). Adjuvants, which preferentially drive Th2 responses, have been shown to enhance IgA and IgE (Xu-Amano *et al.*, 1993; Lindsay *et al.*, 1994) antibody production. This kind of adjuvant could enhance protection against mucosal infections through augmentation of IgA concentration. It is important to select adjuvants which enhance immunogenicity but do not induce adverse reactions. Local adverse reaction includes increase of the inflammatory immune response. In oral bacterial adjuvant is also important to ensure that the effect on the microflora remains unaltered. Adjuvant safety must be evaluated before use for humans. This evaluation (Phase I clinical testing) should be conducted in animals in which the adjuvant has an effect, using the same route anticipated for use in humans. Although not all the results can be extrapolated to humans, these studies must be performed. It is especialy important when developing new products for humans to have available knowledge of the basic immunology such as antigen presentation, or modulation of immune response by cytokines and the requirements needed to reach a protective immunity against infections.

For mucosal adjuvanticity there are many proposed adjuvants (Nardelli *et al.*, 1994; Eldridge *et al.*, 1991; O'Hagan *et al.*, 1993), most of them are lipid-in water systems which can transport antigen to lymphoid tissues; most antigens are ineffective when they are orally administered. Systemic immunization with pilus-associated adhesins have also been reported to protect against mucosal infections (Pere *et al.*, 1987; Hultgren *et al.*, 1993). Non-toxic mutant *E. coli* was also proposed to protect against oral and vaginal infections (Spangler, 1992; Douce *et al*, 1995).

In this chapter we will evaluate the adjuvant capacity of a strain of *Lactobacillus casei* and will demonstrate its use as oral adjuvant or as an oral vaccine vector We studied: 1) evaluation of the safety of the proposed adjuvant, 2) action on the gut associated immune cells and its protective effect against *Sal. typhimurium* infection, establishing the optimal conditions to achieve this protective property, 3) the behaviour of other LAB commonly used in the dairy industry on the mucosal immune system. Elucidating the mechanisms of interaction at the gut level and factors used to predict their effects as adjuvant on the mucosal immune mechanisms.

9.2.1 *Determination of side effect induced by oral administration of Lactobacillus casei*

The importance of the secretory IgA (S-IgA) production in protection of the mucosal surface against enteric infection is well established. We evaluated the effect of the *L. casei* CRL 431 as oral adjuvant on the protection against *Salmonella typhimurium* and *E. coli* infection and the capacity to induce specific anti-pathogen S-IgA (Perdigón *et al.*, 1991 a). We determined the effect of feeding of *L. casei* administered 2, 5 and 7 consecutive days (daily dose 1.2 x 10^9 CFU) on the protection against enteropathogens and on the concentration of specific S-IgA. We observed the importance of the dose required to prevent infection. We obtained total protection with 2 days of feeding of *L. casei*, no protection with 5 days and partial protection with 7 days. We also saw that low doses were better in the production of specific S-IgA production (See Table 9.1).

Table 9.1. Effect of different oral doses of *L. casei* on protection against enteropathogen and on stimulation of specific S-IgA

	Log_{10} CFU/ liver		# S-IgA	
Days of *L. casei*	*Sal. typhimurium* challenged	*E. coli* challenged	*Sal. typhimurium* challenged	*E. coli* challenged
2	0	0	2.5±0.03*	1.6±0.04*
5	4.2±0.5	4.7±0.02	1.0±0.05	0.87±0.1
7	1.2±0.8	ND	2.0±0.07*	ND

Values are mean n = 6 ± S.D., they were determined on 7th day after challenge with *Salmonella typhimurium* and on 4th day after *E. coli* challenge. Control values expressed in log_{10} CFU/organ of *Sal. typhimurium* control (untreated mice) = 4.5 ± 0.9, *E. coli* control= 4 ± 0.5. O.D. 493 nm S-IgA *Sal. typhimurium* control = 1 ± 0.05, *E. coli* control = 0.9 ± 0.08 * Significant by different P < 0.01 compared with control values. # : OD = 493 nm.

According to these results, previous feeding with *L. casei* was only effective for 2 days, because five days did not increase the local immune response and was ineffective in controlling infection with the enteropathogens tested. This behaviour could be due to an acute inflammatory response produced with a dose of 5 days, which disrupted the protective barrier favouring the invasion by the pathogen through the intestine. So we performed studies to determine the level of β-glucuronidase enzyme in the intestinal fluid as a measure of the inflammatory response. We also analysed histological slices of small intestine to observe alteration in the villus structure as a consequence of intestinal inflammation.

We demonstrated that 5 days of *L. casei* induced a high increase in the levels of β-glucuronidase enzyme (Table 9.2). Histological studies revealed increased infiltration of lymphoid cells in the lamina propria of the small intestine as compared with non-fed animals. We also observed alteration in the villus structure with oedema.

Table 9. 2. Levels of β-glucuronidase enzyme from intestinal fluid of *L. casei* treated mice

L. casei administration	β-glucuronidase (nmol/h/ml)
0	200±50
2	250±20
5	400±50*
7	280±30

Values are mean of n = 4 ± S.D. β-glucuronidase activity was determined after each feeding period. 0 = untreated control. * significant by different $P < 0.05$.

In the light of the evidence presented, we cannot ignore the importance of the inflammatory effect that this or other lactobacilli, could provoke in the host which makes them unsuitable for protection against pathogens when they are used in the wrong dose.

Since *L. casei* administered in the wrong dose can induce an inflammatory response when it is used in the prevention of *Sal. typhimurium* infection, we analyzed the importance of this *Lactobacillus* during the infection against this pathogen. We demonstrated (Perdigón *et al.*, 1993) the uneffectiveness of its use as a therapeutic agent or when it was administered immediately after challenge. Only the repeated stimulation on the 6th day after challenge proved to be effective in 50% of the treated animals. Nor we did obtain an increase in the levels of specific S-IgA. In spite of the desire to find a natural therapy to avoid the undesirable effects induced by antibiotics, LAB treatment should be checked to find the optimal dose. We also studied other side effects such as hepatomegaly and splenomegaly which are common in the bacterial immunomodulators (Warren *et al.*, 1986), levels of inflammatory enzymes in the serum and on the haematological and haematopoietic values. We found (Perdigón *et al.* 1991 b) that a long period of *L. casei* administration of 10 days (1.2 x 10^9 daily dose) did not induce hepato or splenomegaly but, we observed small histological changes in the liver of the mice treated for 10 days. Glutamic pyruvic transaminase (GPT) levels were increased in the animals treated with *L. casei* after 5 days of administration. The number of leukocytes was increased for 7 days but we did not have an alteration in the haematopoietic response as judged by the percentage of cells from bone marrow (Table 9.3).

Table 9.3. Effect of different doses of *L. casei* on various biological functions of the host

Days of *L.casei* administration	Spleen weight (g)	Liver weight (g)	GPT levels (IU/ml)	Leukocytes (mm^3)
2	0.11±0.01	1.23±0.05	4±1.1	6,200±500
5	0.10±0.01	1.20±0.09	1.0±1*	6,500±620
7	0.095±0.05	0.95±0.05	2.6±1.5*	8,900±340**
10	0.090±0.01	1.0±0.02	1.1±1.5*	5,850±328
Untreated control	0.090±0.015	1.05±0.05	4.0±0.4	5,000±100

Values are mean of n = 10 ± S.D. Significant by different from control values * P <0.01 and ** P < 0.05.

9.2.2 Determination of the optimal conditions to induce good intestinal mucosal immunostimulation by lactobacilli

The knowledge of the kind of immune cells associated with the intestinal mucosa that must be stimulated by the adjuvants to achieve a good secretory immune response is very important; we focused our study on those cells associated with the lamina propria of small intestine. We performed experiments to find out whether or not *L. casei* might be considered as a possible oral adjuvant. For this purpose we determined: a) how long the immunostimulation lasted after *L. casei* administration in optimal dose? The protective effect of *L. casei* against *Sal. typhimurium* infection was compared with that obtained with another adjuvant substance such as lipopolysaccharide (LPS), b) number of boosting treatments, their frequency and duration of the booster stimulation (Perdigón *et al.*, 1995; Alvarez *et al.*, 1998), c) the number of $CD4^+$, $CD8^+$ T cells, IgA^+, IgM^+ B lymphocytes, the immune cells involved in the inflammatory immune response and the importance of this population in maintaining good stimulation of the mucosal immune system which was able to protect against infection without inducing side effects.

We measured the protective effect of *L. casei* immunostimulation against *Salmonella typhimurium* infection by liver colonization assays and specific S-IgA production. We observed that the protective effect of optimal dose was maintained for only 5 days after feeding. For this period, we did not have total protection, although we had a small liver colonization. The levels of specific S-IgA were slightly increased but they were not enough to stop the infection. These previous results led us to study whether a mixture with LPS (constituent of enterobacterial cell wall) would increase the duration of the stimulation and the resistance to infection. We demonstrated that the mixture of *L. casei* plus LPS was able to induce a total protective effect with high levels of S-IgA, while LPS alone showed a small liver colonization. In the determination of the preventive effect of the above mixture we saw that the effect was maintained until 7 days post-treatment with an increase in S-IgA levels (Table 9.4).

Table 9.4. Duration of the preventive effect of LPS and *L. casei* plus LPS against *Sal. typhimurium* infection.

	Log_{10} CFU/liver			# S-IgA		
Challenge on different days post-treat.	*L.casei*	LPS	*L.c* + LPS	*L.casei*	LPS	*L.c.* +LPS
1	0	$1.5^{*}\pm0.2$	0	$2.5^{*}\pm0.03$	$2.1^{*}\pm0.02$	$2.4^{*}\pm0.02$
3	$1^{*}\pm0.2$	2.1 ± 0.1	0	$1.8^{*}\pm0.02$	1.6 ± 0.01	$2.2^{*}\pm0.03$
5	2.5 ± 0.1	3.5 ± 0.5	$1.1^{*}\pm0.2$	1.5 ± 0.01	1.0 ± 0.04	$2.0^{*}\pm0.01$
7	3.8 ± 0.4	ND	$1.3^{*}\pm0.1$	1.1 ± 0.02	ND	$2.1^{*}\pm0.02$
10	ND	ND	$2.5^{*}\pm0.1$	ND	ND	$1.8^{*}\pm0.03$

Results are the values of $n = 5 \pm$ S.D. obtained on 7th day post-challenge. Colonization control values expressed as $\log_{10}$. number bacteria/organ = 4.5 ± 0.9. O.D. 493 nm of control animals = 1 ± 0.05. Days post-treatment mean after optimal administration (2 days). * Significant values $P < 0.01$ compared with the respective untreated controls. # OD 493 nm.

The protective capacity of *L. casei* and *L. casei* associated with LPS was shown to be due to the stimulation of the local synthesis of IgA secreted into the intestinal fluid and the effect lasted for 7 days.

In order to improve the protective effect of *L. casei* and the mixture of *L. casei* plus LPS against infection we boosted on the 15th and 30th day post-priming with the optimal dose. In these studies we determined secretory IgM to indicate if the booster induced a primary immune response.

We showed that both boosting systems were effective through an increase in the IgA synthesis, the effect being more marked on 15th day post-priming and for *L. casei* alone,. Although the IgA values found for the mixture were significantly higher than the control, we observed an enhancement of IgM values after boosting with *L. casei*/LPS mixture the on 15th and 30th day.

This might indicate an increase of the primary immune response rather than a major induction of the immunological memory. We also saw that high levels of IgA might not be beneficial; excessive synthesis of IgA could bind more antigen favouring an increase in intestinal permeability as was described in coeliac disease (Brandtzaeg *et al.*, 1993).

We demonstrated that *L. casei* alone has good adjuvant activity at the mucosal level. This capacity was higher than that shown by LPS alone. The response to boosting with *L. casei* on 15th and 30th day, only lasted 4 days.

Some treatments were ineffective in the protection against *Sal. typhimurium*, even when we found, high levels of S-IgA were present. We examined the immune cells associated with the gut mucosa. We determined IgA secreting cells, $CD4^+$ and $CD8^+$ T cells by immunofluorescence test. The number of neutrophils and macrophages were studied on histological slices stained with haematoxylin-eosin. We found increased values of IgA^+ cells for *L. casei*/LPS mixture after boosting on 15th day post-priming. The $CD4^+$ population was enhanced for the mixture when boosting was performed on the 30th day. $CD8^+$ was slightly enhanced following boosting on the 15th day. The number of neutrophils was similar to the untreated control and the macrophages increased after boosting on the 30th day (Table 9.5) (Alvarez *et al.*, 1998).

Table 9. 5. Effect of treatments and boosters with *L. casei* and *L. casei*/LPS on the immune cells associated to the gut

	Number of cells/10 villi				
	Immune cells				
	IgA^+	$CD4^+$	$CD8^+$	Neutrophils	Macrophages
Untreated control	70±5	55±4	40±5	15±3	140±10
L.casei 2 d.	100*±10	75*±6	48±4	16±2	140±10
L.c./LPS 2d.	180*±10	90*±5	50±3	13±3	160±8
Booster *L.c.* on 15th d.	150*±15	70*±6	55±4	14±2	160±7
Booster *L.c.* on 30th d.	100*±8	70*±3	40±5	15±1	250*±10
Boost. *L c*/LPS on 15th d	220*±10	75*±5	57±4	13±3	225*±10
Boost.*Lc*/LPS on 30th d	130*±15	85*±4	45±5	14±2	200*±10

Values are mean of n = 4 ± S.D. Boosters with a single dose were performed after 15th or 30th day post-priming with *L. casei* or *L. casei*/LPS for two consecutive days. * $P < 0.05$ related to the control.

We demonstrated that the protective S-IgA induced with viable *L. casei* after priming with a single boosting on the 15th and 30th day post-priming was correlated with an increase in the number of IgA secreting cells present on the gut. The increase in IgA^{+} cells was also correlated with an increase in CD4^{+} population. This may indicate an activation of lymphocytes that would favour the switch of IgM towards IgA production. However, the increase in CD4^{+} cells could be favouring the Th1 population which is involved in delayed hypersensitivity. CD8+ increase might mean an increase in the cytotoxic activity, an undesirable effect at intestinal level. Thus the increase in IgA^{+} or CD4^{+} does not imply a good intestinal mucosal immune response. They can mediate harmful effects on the gut such as inflammatory response through the cytokines released by Th1 population; IFNγ can induce an over expression of class II histocompatibility antigen (Lionetti *et al.*, 1995) with a consequent increase in antigen capture and an overstimulation of the mucosa. In the gut immunological over-stimulation appears to be mediated *via* the lamina propria by CD4^{+} T cells and their cytokines (Brandtzaeg, 1996). It would be advisable to maintain the relationship between CD4^{+} and CD8^{+} T cells in the same proportion as that observed in control animals without treatment to avoid the above mentioned effect.

It is known that the protection against *Salmonella* is mediated in the early phase of infection by macrophages and neutrophils (Akeda *et al.*, 1981). Specific immunity is developed in the late phase of infection. The antibacterial activity of polymorphonuclear and mononuclear cells seems pivotal for the inducement of the host resistance toward invading *Salmonella* because their virulence is related to the ability to survive and multiply within these cells especially in macrophage (Dichelte *et al.*, 1984). The increase in the number of phagocytosing macrophages would be important as a mechanism of controlling *Salmonella* infection. However, the increase in macrophages and neutrophils can induce an inflammatory immune response and affect the mucosal integrity and the intestinal permeability.

Since *Lactobacillus* strains can be used as carriers of antigens (Claasen *et al.*, 1995) it is important to establish the conditions such as priming dose, frequency, number of boosters that stimulate the adequate immune cell population necessary to maintain the equilibrium among them. This is important information which can be used to evaluate the effect of carriers on the mucosal immune system by different LAB which may be used as oral vaccine vectors.

9.3 LAB interaction with the intestine and mucosal stimulation

The intestinal ecosystem represents a complex environment, in which microbial interaction is the main force that contributes to the homeostasis of the bacterial flora. This flora forms an ecosystem with its host and comprises: a) biotic components such as indigenous and transient microbes and gastrointestinal epithelial cells, b) abiotic components of dietary origin and c) endogenous components coming from saliva, gastric secretions or excretions including enzymes, hormones, mucus, bile, immunoglobulins and others. All these components interact and the result of such interactions is compatible with the healthy survival of the host (Raibaud, 1992). Gastrointestinal disorders can destabilize the ecosystem; it is importance to maintain this sensitive equilibrium. Antimicrobial agents can induce disturbances in the microflora, causing bacterial overgrowth increasing the permeability of the intestinal mucosa and permitting the passage of bacteria from the gastrointestinal tract to extraintestinal organs and the bloodstream. This transport of bacteria has been called translocation (Berg, 1992). Bacteria of the indigenous microflora are not normally found in extraintestinal sites such as the mesenteric lymph node (MLN), spleen, liver or blood; the intact mucosal barrier, provides a physical barrier to prevent translocation.

In the integrity of mucosa of the host the immune system plays an important role, where secretory immunity and cell-mediated immunity are important in protecting against bacterial translocation. S-IgA may bind the bacteria avoiding translocation across the mucosal barrier. Serum immunoglobulins could favour the bacterial clearence when they have entered the lamina propria. T cells appear to be particulary important in preventing the spread of translocating bacteria from MLN. Macrophages of MLN and Kupper's cells in the liver would kill the translocated bacteria by phagocytosis. Summarizing the mechanisms which prevent bacterial translocation they are: a) balanced equilibrium in the microflora avoiding overgrowth of some microbial population, b) the active host immune response and c) intact intestinal mucosal barrier. As a rule bacterial translocation is due to an altered permeability of the intestinal epithelium after situations such as stress, sub-clinical infections, tumours or immunosuppression.

Many bacteria such as LAB are ingested with the diet, but they are eliminated rapidly by intestinal peristalsis. Therefore it is possible to make living bacteria pass through the digestive tract, metabolize the substrates and exert their influence on the immune system during their transit, when they come into contact with lymphoid cells of the gut. Dairy foods (e.g. yoghurt) contain viable bacteria and with their consumption LAB are introduced in the digestive tract in large numbers. The effect on the host will depend on whether or not certain food or bacterial species induce bacterial translocation from the gut. It is possible to modify the microbial ecosystem of the digestive tract by ingestion of living microorganisms contained in foods. Very high numbers of living bacteria may induce alterations in the intestinal ecosystem during their transit through the digestive tract and might induce an inflammatory immune response with decrease in the S-IgA levels. However, some lactic acid bacteria such as *L. delbrueckii* ssp. *bulgaricus* are able to inhibit translocation of Gram-negative bacteria (*E. coli*) present in the gut. This may be due to an increase in the host's immunodefences against translocated *E. coli* (De Simone *et al.*, 1992).

In our study on LAB interaction with the intestine we can not ignore the influence of these microorganisms on the gut ecosystem. We must consider not only the consequence of their ingestion on the mucosal immune system but, also, their ability to induce bacterial translocation. Because the LAB are Gram-postive microorganisms with a common antigenic structure (MDP), we studied whether or not the activation of the secretory immune system was similar for all of them. We also analysed if the immune stimulation was characteristic of the genera or species related.

We also studied the different immune responses induced by LAB and the way in which they influence the host. Finally we attempted to understand the mechanisms of the interaction of LAB with the intestine, which would explain the different mucosal immune responses induced.

9.3.1 Translocation studies

We determined the effect of feeding of various doses (2, 5 or 7 consecutive days with 10^9 cells daily) of different LAB on the bacterial translocation to the liver and spleen. We selected the LAB more frequently used in the food industry. We observed positive translocation with some LAB, but this effect was not related with the dose or genus administered. (Table 9.6). We performed some experiments to check if the LAB induced microflora alteration (Perdigón *et al.*, 1997). The changes were not correlated with the translocation observed. These results led us to think that in our study bacterial translocation was more related to an increase in the inflammatory immune response rather than to changes in the normal microflora.

Table 9.6. Translocation assays

Lactic Acid Bacteria	Bacterial translocation Days of feeding		
	2	5	7
L. rhamnosus	+	+	+
L. acidophilus	-	-	+
L. casei	-	+	-
L..delbr. ssp. bulgaricus	+	+	-
L. plantarum	+	+	+
S. thermophilus	+	-	-
Lactococcus lactis	+	+	-

Results expressed as + or – represent colonization found in the liver or spleen either of enterobacteria or strict anaerobes.

9.3.2 Influence of LAB administration on immune cells associated with gut mucosa and on IgA cells associated with bronchus.

Our previous results, showed that, the immune cells were involved in the inflammatory immune response associated with the gut. We also analysed the IgA^+ secreting cells on the gut and bronchus and T $CD4^+$ lymphocytes, by an immunofluorescence test.

The inflammatory immune response is the mechanism by which phagocytic cells such as neutrophils, macrophages, and soluble factors such as antibody and complement, usually in the peripheral blood circulation, can enter into the tissues invaded by foreign antigens and eliminate them favouring the host. However, this protective mechanism can be increased by a strong stimulation producing a harmful effect such as tissue necrosis (Fargeas *et al.*, 1995). This effect can be potentiated by eosinophils, mast cells, $CD8^+$ T cytotoxic cell population and IgG isotype antibody.

The identification of the cells involved in the inflammatory response can be determined by histological slices stained with haeamotoxilin-eosin. We demonstrated that in general macrophages, neutrophils and eosinophils were increased in those cases where LAB dosing, induced bacterial translocation. This last fact might be due to an increase in the inflammatory response. $CD8^+$ T cells and IgG^+ B cells were only increased by 2 days of *Lactobacillus plantarum* administration (Perdigón *et al.*, 1999 b) (Table 9.7).

Table 9.7. Effect of LAB on the immune cells involved with the inflammatory response

	Number cells / 10 villi				
LAB	Macroph.	Neutroph.	Eosinoph.	$CD8^+$ T cells	IgG^+ B cells
L.rhamnosus	160±8(5d)	25*±3(5-7d)	20*±3(5-7d)	57±2	46±3
L.acidophilus	140±10	15 ± 3	50*±2(7d)	62±3	48±2
L.casei	127±8	25*±3(5d)	20*±1(5d)	54±4	45±4
L.plantarum	138±5	35*±2(2-5d)	15±1(2d)	110*±5(2d)	75*±2(2d)
L.delb.ssp.bulg	150±7	25*±2(2-5d)	18*±2(2-5d)	60±2	50±2
Lac. lactis	200*±15(5-7d)	25*±2(5-7d)	30*±4(5-7d)	61±3	58±3(2d)
S.thermoph.	142±8.	27*±3(2-5-7d)	15±1(2-7d)	59±1	47±4
Control	140±10	15±3	10±2	60±3	48±5

The results expressed are only for the periods of LAB administration in which we found slight or significant differences (* $P < 0.05$) compared with the control. d = days of feeding.

We studied the IgA secreting cells and $CD4^+$ T cells in the gut to determine if the LAB were able to increase the specific secretory immune response. IgA^+ cells in the bronchus were measured in order to determine if the LAB gut interaction induced an increase in the number of cells that enter in the IgA cycle repopulating distal tissues from the gut such as bronchus.

The enhancement in the number of IgA^+ cells on lamina propria indicated celullar mobilization. If the LAB interact at Peyer's patches level they would interact with the M cells and IgA^+ cells to migrate together with T cells along a haemolymphatic cycle before colonizing the intestinal mucosa. This aspect is extensively described elsewhere in this book. If the LAB can interact with M cells, T $CD4^+$ population will also increase on lamina propria of intestine. T $CD4^+$ cells favour the switch of immunoglobulin M to IgA. The entrance of lymphocytes into the tissue is regulated by a multistep process, involving different sets of complementary receptors on the surface of lymphocytes and endothelial cells. The role of the cytokines synthesized by epithelial cells is also important for activation of the immune cells associated with the lamina propria. The profile of cytokine released by T cells present in lamina propria is not similar that those produced by $CD4^+$ cells from Peyer's patches (Williams *et al.*, 1997) However, epithelial interaction also could induce the IgA^+ cells to enter the IgA cycle through the mesenteric node according the model proposed by Weiner (1997) . In such a model epithelial interaction could promote only local expansion of the IgA cells.

We found that the LAB assayed increased the IgA secreting cells associated with the gut and with the exception of *L. acidophilus* they enhanced these cells at the bronchus level. The effect observed was dose dependent. $CD4^+$ T cells were increased only for *L. casei* and *L. plantarum* (Perdigón *et al.*, 1999 a; b) (See Table 9.8).

Table 9.8. Effect of LAB on IgA^+ and $CD4^+$ cells associated with the gut and on IgA^+ cells associated with the bronchus

	Number cells/10 villi		
Lactic Acid Bacteria	IgA^+ cells on gut	IgA^+ cells on bronchus	$CD4^+$ T cells on gut
L.rhamnosus	120±10* (7d)	37±2 (7d)	55±5
L.acidophilus	130±10*(5d)	19±1	60±2
L. casei	110±7 (2d)	48±2 (5d)	110±10* (2-5d)
L. plantarum	120±10* (2d)	50±1(2d)	80±5 (2d)
L.delbr. ssp. bulgaricus	120±10*(2-7d)	37*±1(2d)	59±2
Lac. lactis	100±10 (5d)	53±5(5d)	61±1
S.thermophilus	110±5 (2-7d)	55*±5(5-7d)	57±3
Control	90±5	18±4	58±3

Results showed correspond to the doses that induced a significant increase. * $P < 0.05$ compared with the controls. d=days of feeding

We demonstrated that some LAB induced mainly an inflammatory immune response, and others stimulated the response toward protective IgA on gut and bronchus by increasing the IgA cycle. Finding an increase in the IgA number, led to an investigation of the LAB, and which antigens, could induce a specific response against their epitopes. Thus we determined the anti-LAB antibodies present in the intestinal fluid. We found that *L. casei, L. plantarum, L. rhamnosus* and *Streptococcus thermophilus* were able to induce antibody against their own epitopes. These results would mean that those LAB were processed and presented as antigen to the immune cells (Perdigón *et al.*, 1999 b).

The gastrointestinal tract is in continuous and direct contact with environmental antigens *via* the epithelial cell layer. It is known that to induce a secretory response to non-pathogen or food antigen is not always easy. A population of lymphocytes binding to epithelial cells (intra-epithelial lymphocytes IEL) possesses a regulatory function for the maintenance of oral tolerance and also for the IgA response (Fujihashi *et al.*, 1993). Thus two opposite immune reactions simultaneously occur in order to maintain appropiate immunological and physiological homeostasis to orally encountered antigens. Continuous oral administration of particulate antigens can generate an antigen specific S-IgA. This topic is extensively treated in others chapter of this book. The

IEL population protects the epithelial integrity and provides a initially line of defence against pathogens that interact initially with the epithelial surface (Hayday *et al.*, 1993).

The knowledge that certain LAB favoured the inflammatory immune response led us to perform experiments with LAB to demonstrate that the intestinal permeability was increased as a consequence of the inflammatory response.

For this purpose we used the antigen ovoalbumin orally administered at tolerogenic doses. We determined the level of IgM and IgG antibodies to ovoalbumin present in serum, which were generated by ovoalbumin passing from the intestine due to the increased intestinal permeability. We demonstrated that effectively the increase in the immune cells involved in the inflammatory response induced an enhancement in the intestinal permeability. This might be also explain the bacterial translocation observed in previous studies.

9.3.3 Influence of the different immune responses induced by LAB in the protective effect against Salmonella typhimurium

Considering the previous results, the induction of the inflammatory immune response by LAB would be negative in the protection against enteropathogens. Conversely those that favoured the specific immune response would be the appropiate ones for the protective effect. We observed that the LAB able to protect against *Salmonella* were *L. casei*, *L. delbrueckii* ssp. *bulgaricus* and *S. thermophilus* at doses that did not induce an inflammatory immune response and where the bacterial translocation was negative.

The other LAB assayed (*L. acidophilus*, *L. rhamnosus*, *L. plantarum*, *Lac. lactis*), even when they produced an enhancement in the IgA secreting cells, did not protect. This may be due to an increase in the number of the cells involved in inflammation, because this would increase the intestinal permeability favouring translocation of the pathogen.

The host secretory immune system can be activated by lipo-polysaccharice (LPS) or peptidoglican (PG) in an indirect manner. The major component of the bacterial cell wall of LAB is the PG. This component can stimulate the immune cells through an endogenous mediator released by other cells e.g. epithelial cells, which are endowed with biological activity. During recent years enormous progress has been made in understanding how LPS and PG stimulate the immune system (Hamann *et al.*, 1998). Thus today, it is known, that LPS and PG mediate cell stimulation by a receptor-dependent process involving the cell surface antigen CD14 present in immune cells, endothelial and epithelial cells. The CD14 molecule is required for signal transduction. The characterization of such signal transducer molecules is still under investigation. When the cells are activated by these microbial components, they release endogenous mediators such as cytokines. The binding of LPS to CD14 is of high affinity and its action is mediated by a serum protein called LPS binding protein (LBP). PG has also been shown to bind CD14 but in contrast to LPS, this binding is LBP independent. Due to the utilization of the same receptor it is likely that both LPS and PG might activate at least some similar pathways (Hamann *et al.*, 1998). On the other hand, the microorganisms can increase the expression of the glycoprotein receptors on the epithelial cells favouring the adhesion to the cell. However, to induce signals it is necessary that 1) the microorganisms reach a critical density, 2) that LPS or PG can transmit signals by interaction with the receptor CD14 present in the cellular surface. As was mentioned elsewhere in this book, epithelial cells release cytokines by interaction with the antigens. LAB could induce this effect by increasing the cellular aflux and activating the cells to release cytokines, or enhance the IgA cycle.

What are the biological implications of our results? We believe that the different behaviours observed in the gut mucosal response could be due to the different ways of interaction with the gut, even when all of them have PG as common microbial immunomodulator. In the light of our research those bacteria that induce an increase in the IgA^+ cells associated with gut and bronchus, $CD4^+$ cells on the gut and antibody produced against their epitopes, could interact in the intestine at the Peyer's patches level. This kind of interaction is the only one able to induce the migration of T cells and IgA B cells increasing this population in the lamina propria of the intestine and in distant tissues such as bronchus. We think that the LAB that induced only the IgA cycle without an increase in T cells on the intestine, would interact with the epithelial cells which might or might not process and present the LAB as antigen to the immune cells. If the LAB only induce increase in the IgA associated with the intestine with no antibody against the LAB and no increase in the IgA cycle, the interaction would also be with the epithelial cells but, the effect achieved would be restricted to the gut. This was the case seen in our studies with *L. acidophilus* (Perdigón *et al.*, 1999 b).

Another important field to investigate is cytokine release concentrating on those involved in mechanisms of immune down regulation such as IL10, TGFβ. This knowledge would permit a better use of LAB in for example illneses such as autoimmunity or allergy where, the immune down regulation is necessary.

9.4 Conclusions

After *L. casei* administration, we established the importance of the dose, frequency and number of stimuli needed to maintain the different immunological parameters in equilibrium without high exacerbation of activity of the mucosal associated immune cells. This gave good mucosal immunity able to protect against infection. This knowledge would be important especially if the LAB are to be used as a vaccine vector.

Not all the LAB can stimulate the mucosal immune system in the same way. The immunostimulatory capacity was not related to the genus or species but was strain specific. The different immunomodulating activities of the LAB would be related to the mechanisms of interaction of these microorganisms with the intestine (Peyer's patches or epithelial cells) and with the intensity of such interaction that initiates the intercellular signals tranductions which activate the immune system. The importance of the interaction of LAB with Peyer's patches or epithelial cells in this hypothesis remains to be confirmed, as does the finding that the epitopes of the LAB involved in the antibody response are the same in all the LAB that were able to induce antibody for their epitopes.

Acknowledgements

The authors whish to thank Dr. Marta Medici for typing the manuscript, and also the coworkers from the Immunology Department at CERELA and of Immunology Laboratory at Microbiology Institute of Tucuman University. This research was supported by grants from CONICET PIP 5011/97, CIUNT 96/98 and 98/2000.

References

Akeda, H., Mitsuyama, M., Tatsukawa, K., Nomoto, K. and Takeya, K. (1981) The synergistic contribution of macrophages and antibody to protection against *Salmonella typhimurium* during early phase of infection *J.Gen. Microbiol.* **123**, 209-213.

Allison, A. (1998) The mode of action of immunological adjuvants. In *Modulation of the Immune Response to Vaccine Antigens* ((eds. F. Brown, L. Haaheim) Dev. Biol Stand. Basel Karger, **92**, 3-11.

Allison, A., Byars, N. (1991) Immunological adjuvants: Desirable properties and sie-effects. *Molecular Immunology* **28**, 279-284.

Alvarez, S., Gobbato, N., Bru, E., P. de Ruiz Holgado, A. and Perdigón, G. (1998) Specific immunity induction at the mucosal level by viable *Lactobacillus casei*: A perspective for oral vaccine development. *F. Agricul. Immunol.* **10**, 79-87.

Berg, R. (1992) Translocation and the indigenous gut flora. In *Probiotics The Scientific Basis.* (ed. R. Fuller,) Chapman and Hall, London, pp 54-85.

Bloksma, N., de Heer, E., van Dijk, M. and Willers, M. (1979) Adjuvanticity of lactobacilli. I. Differential effect of viable and killed bacteria. *Clin. Exp. Immunol.* **37** 367-375.

Brandtzaeg, P. (1996) Lymphoepithelial interaction in the human mucosal immune system (Abstract) *Mucosal Immunol. Update* **4**, 22-23.

Brandzaeg, P., Halstensen, T., Hvatum, M., Kvale, D. and Scott, H. (1993) The serologic and mucosal immunologic basic of celiac disease. In *Immunophysiology of the Gut* (eds. A. Walker, P. Harmatz and B. Wershill) Academic Press, New York, NY, USA. Vol II, pp 295-.353.

Claasen, E., Van Winsen, R., Posno, M., and Boersma, J. (1995) New and safe oral live vaccines based on Lactobacillus. In *Advances in Mucosal Immunology* (eds. J. Mestecky, *et al.*) Plenum Press, New York, pp. 1553-1558.

Corthier, G. (1997) Antibiotic-associated diarrhoea: treatments by living organisms given by the oral route (probiotics). In *Probiotics 2: Applications and Practical Aspects* (ed. R. Fuller) Chapman and Hall, London. 40-64.

Davies, A., James, P. and Hawkey, P. (1986) *Lactobacillus* endocarditis. *J. Infect.* **12**, 169-174.

De Simone, C., Bianchi Salvadori, B., Negri, R. *et al.* (1986) The adjuvant effect of yogurt on production of gamma-interferon by Con A stimulated human peripheral blood lymphocytes.*Nutr. Reports Int.* **3**, 419-431.

De Simone, C., Bianchi Salvadori, B., Tzantzglou, S., Jirillo, E., Camaschella, P., Cislaghi, S., Ciardi, A. and Vesely, R. (1992) Bacterial translocation and Immunological Responses in Mice Monoassociated or Biassociated with *Lactobacillus bulgaricus* and *Escherichia coli.* In *Dynamic Nutrition Research* (eds. M. Paubert-Braquet, Ch. Dupont, R. Paoletti) Vol. 1, pp 57-65. Karger.

De Simone, C., Vesely, R., Bianchi Salvadori, B. and Jirillo, E. (1993) The role of probiotics in modulation of the immune system in man and in animals. *Int. J. Immunother.* **9**, 23-28.

Dichelte, G., Kaspereit, F. and Sedlaced, H. (1984). Stimulation of cell-mediated immunity by Bestatin correlates with reduction of bacterial persistence in experimental chronic *Salmonella typhimurium* infection. *Infect. Immun.* **44**, 168-172.

Douce, G., Turcotte, C., Cropley, I., Roberts, M., Pizza, M., Domenighini, M., Rappuoli, R., Dougan, G. (1995) Mutants of Escherichia coli heat-labile toxin lacking ADP-ribosyltransferase activity act as non-toxic, mucosal adjuvants. *Proc. Natl. Acad. Sci. USA* **92**, 1644-1648.

Eldridge, J., Staas, J., Meulbroek, J., McGhee, J., Tice, R. and Gilley, R. (1991) Biodegradable microspheres as a vaccine delivery system. *Mol. Immunol.* **28**, 287.

Fargeas, M., Theodorou, V., More, J., Wal, J., Fioramonti, J. and Bueno, L. (1995) Boosted systemic immune and local responsiveness after intestinal inflammation in orally sensitized guinea pigs. *Gastroenterology* **109**, 53-62.

Fujihashi, K., Masafumi, Y., McGhee, J. and Kiyono, H. (1993) Immunoregulatory function and cytokine production by alpha beta TCR+ and gama delta TCR+ T cells for mucosal immune response. In *Mucosal Immunology: Intraepithelial Lymphocytes* (eds. H. Kiyono and J. McGhee) Raven Press, Ltd., New York, 89-114.

Gonzalez, S., Albarracín, G., Locascio de Ruiz Pesce, M., Male, M., Apella, M.C., Pesce de Ruiz Holgado, A. and Oliver, G. (1990) Prevention of infantile diarrhoea by fermented milk, *Microbiol. Alim. Nutr.* **8**, 349-354.

Hamann, L., El-Samalouti, V., Ulmer, A., Hans-Dieter Flad and Rietsche, E. (1998) Components of gut bacteria as immunomodulators. In *International Journal of Food Microbiology* Elsevier Science, pp.141-154.

Harty, D., Oakey, H., Patrikakis, M. et al. (1994) Pathogenic potential of lactobacilli. *Int. J. Food Microbiol.* **24**, 179-189.

Hayday, A., Scott, J. and Dudley, E. (1993) The protection of epithelial integrity by intraepithelial lymphocyte populations: gamma delta T cell receptors constitutively and inducibly associated with epithelia. In *Mucosal Immunology: Intraepithelial Lymphocytes.* (eds. H. Kiyono, J. McGhee) Raven Press, Ltd. New York, 175-183.

Hultgren, S., Abraham, S., Caparon, M., Falk, P., St Geme III, J. and Norwark, S. (1993) Pilus and nonpilus bacterial adhesins: assembly and function in cell recognition. *Cell* **73**, 887-901.

Isolauri, E., Juntunen, M., Rautanen, T. *et al.* (1991) A human *Lactobacillus* strain (*Lactobacillus casei* sp. strain GG) promotes recovery from acute diarrhea in children. *Pediatrics* **88**, 90-97.

Iwasaki, I., Yumoto, N., Iwase, H. and Ide, G. (1983) Potentiation of large intestinal tumorigenicity of cycasin derivative by high fat diet and *Lactobacillus* in germ free mice. *Acta Pathol. Japan.* **33**, 1197-1204.

Kaila, M., Isolauri, E., Soppi, E. et al. (1992) Enhancement of the circulating antibody secreting-cell response on human diarrhea by a human *Lactobacillus* strain. *Pediatric Res.* **32**, 141-144.

Kato, I., Kohayashi, S., Yokokura, T. and Mutai, M. (1981) Antitumor activity of *Lactobacillus casei* in mice. *Gann* **72**, 517-523.

Kato, I., Yokokura, T. and Mutai, M. (1983) Macrophage activation by *Lactobacillus casei* in mice. *Microbiol. Immunol.* **27**, 611-618.

Kato, I., Yokokura, T. and Mutai, M. (1984) Augmentation of mouse natural killer cell activity by *Lactobacillus casei* and its surface antigens. *Microbiol. Immunol.* **28**, 209-217.

Kato, I., Yokokura, T. and Mutai, M. (1985) Induction of tumoricidal peritoneal exudate cells by administration of *L. casei*.*Int. J. Immunopharmacology* 7, 103-109.

Le Contel, C., Temime, N., Charron, D. and Parant, M. (1993) Modulation of LPS-induced cytokine gene expression in mouse bone marrow-derived macrophages by muramyl dipeptide. *J. Immunol.* **150**, 4541-4549.

Lindsay, D., Parton, R. and Wardlaw, A. (1994) Adjuvant effect of pertussis toxin on the production of anti-ovoalbumin IgE in mice and lack of direct correlation between PCA and ELISA. *Int. Arch. Allergy Immunol.* **105**, 281-288.

Link-Amster, H., Rochat, F., Saudan, K. *et al.* (1994) Modulation of a specific humoral immune response and changes in intestinal flora mediated through fermented milk. *FEMS Immunol. Med. Microbiol.* **10**, 55-63.

Lionetti, P., Cheng, S. and McDonald, T. (1995) Relationship between the extent of mucosal T cell and macrophage activation and mucosal damage. In *Mucosal Immunity and the Gut Epithelium: Interactions in Health and Disease. Dynamic Nutrition Research* (eds. S. Auricchio *et al*). Karger, Basel, Vol. 4, pp 84-89.

Maskell, R. and Pead, L. (1992) 4-Fluorochinolones and *Lactobacillus* spp. As emerging pathogens. *Lancet* **339**, 929.

Matsuzaki, T., Yokokura, T. and Azuma, I. (1985) Antitumor activity of *Lactobacillus casei* on Lewis Lung carcinoma and line-10 hepatoma in syngeneic mice and guinea pig. *Cancer Immunol. Immunother.* **20**, 18-22.

Nardelli, B., Haser, P. and Tam, J. (1994) Oral administration of an antigenic synthetic lipopeptide (MAP-P3C) evokes salivary antibodies and systemic humoral and cellular responses. *Vaccine* **12**, 1335.

O'Hagan, D., McGhee, J., Holmgren, J., Mowat, A McI, Donachie, A., Mills, K., Gaisford, W., Rahman, D. and Challacombe, S. (1993) Biodegradable microparticles for oral immunization. *Vaccine* **11,** 149.

Oliver, G. and Gonzalez, S. (1992) Lactobacillus milk for biotherapy of infantile diarrhea, in *Encyclopedia of Fermented Fresh Milk Products (*eds. J. Kurmann , J. Rasic., M. Kroger) pp. 191. An AVI Book, New York.

Perdigón, G. and Alvarez, S. (1992) Probiotics and the immune state. In *Probiotics The Scientific Basis* (ed. R. Fuller,) Chapman and Hall, London. **7,** 146-180.

Perdigón, G., Alvarez, S. and Pesce de Ruiz Holgado, A. (1991 a) Immunoadjuvant activity of oral *Lactobacillus casei*: influence of dose on the secretory immune response and protective capacity in intestinal infections. *J. Dairy Res.* **58**, 485-496.

Perdigón, G., Alvarez, S., Agüero, G., Medici, M. and P. de Ruiz Holgado, A. (1997) Interaction between lactic acid bacteria, intestinal microflora and the immune system.

In. *Progress in Microbial Ecology* .(eds. M. Martins) 311-316. Sociedade Brasileira de Microbiologia. Sao Paulo. Brasil.

Perdigón, G., Alvarez, S., Gobbato, N., V. de Budeguer, M., and P.de Ruiz Holgado, A. (1995) Comparative effect of the adjuvant capacity of *Lactobacillus casei* and lipopolysaccharide on the intestinal secretory antibody response and resistance to *Salmonella* infection in mice. *F. Agricult. Immunol.* **7**, 283-294.

Perdigón, G., Alvarez, S., Medici, M. and P. de Ruiz Holgado, A. (1993) Influence of the use of *Lactobacillus casei* as an oral adjuvant on the levels of secretory immunoglobulin A during an infection with *Salmonella typhimurium*. *F. Agricult. Immunol.* **5**, 27-37.

Perdigón, G., Alvarez, S., Medina, M., Vintiñi, E. and Roux, E. (1999 a) Influence of the oral administration of lactic acid bacteria on IgA producing cells associated to bronchus. *Internat. J. Immunol. .and Pharmacology.* **12**, 97-102.

Perdigón, G., Alvarez, S., Nader de Macías, M.E., *et al.* (1990 a) The oral administration of lactic acid bacteria increases the mucosal intestinal immunity in response to enteropathogens. *J. Food Prot.* **53**, 404-410.

Perdigón, G., Alvarez, S., Nader de Macías, M.E., Margni, R., Oliver, G. and P. de Ruiz Holgado, A. (1986 a) Lactobacilli administered orally induce release of enzymes from peritoneal macrophages in mice. *Milchwiss.* **41**, 344-348.

Perdigón, G., B. de Jorrat, M. E., F. de Petrino, S. and Valverde de Budeguer, M. (1991 b) Effect of oral administration of *Lactobacillus casei* on various biological functions of the host. *Fd. Agricult. Immunol.* **3**, 93-102.

Perdigón, G., Nader de Macías, M.E., Alvarez, S. *et al.* (1987) Enhancement of immune response in mice fed with *Streptococcus thermophilus* and *Lactobacillus acidophilus.J. Dairy Sci..* **70**, 919-926.

Perdigón, G., Nader de Macías, M.E., Alvarez, S. *et al.* (1990 b) Prevention of gastrointestinal infection using immunobiological methods with milk fermented with *Lactobacillus casei* and *Lactobacillus acidophilus*. *J. Dairy Res.* **57**, 255-264.

Perdigón, G., Nader de Macías, M.E., Alvarez, S., Oliver, G. and P.de Ruiz Holgado, A. (1988) Systemic augmentation of the immune response in mice by feeding fermented milks with *Lactobacillus casei* and *Lactobacillus acidophilus*. *Immunology* **63**, 17-23.

Perdigón, G., Nader de Macías, M.E., Alvarez, S., Oliver, G. and P. de Ruiz Holgado, A. (1986 b) Effect of perorally administered lactobacilli on macrophage activation in mice. *Infect. Immun.* **53**, 404-410.

Perdigón, G., Vintiñi, E., Alvarez, S., Medina, M. and Medici, M. (1999 b) Study of the possible mechanisms involved in the mucosal immune system activation by lactic acid bacteria. *J. Dairy Sci.* **82**, 1108-1114.

Pere, A., Nowicki, B., Saxen, H., Siitonen, A. and Korhonen, T. (1987) Expression of P, type-1 and type 1C fimbriae of *Escherichia coli* in the urine of patients with acute urinary tract infection. *J. Infect. Dis.* **156**, 567-574.

Pereyra, B. and Lemonnier, D. (1993) Induction of human cytokines by bacteria used in dairy foods. *Nutr. Res.* **13**, 1127-1140.

Phillips N. and Emili, A. (1992) Enhanced antibody responses to liposome-associated protein antigens: preferential stimulation of IgG2a/b production. *Vaccine* **10**, 151-158.

Raibaud, P. (1992) Bacterial interactions in the gut. In *Probiotics The Scientific Basis* (ed. R. Fuller) Chapman and Hall, London. 2, pp 9-28.

Saito, I., Sato, K., Horikawa, Y. et al. (1983) Enhanced humoral antibody production and delayed type hypersensitivity response in mice by *Lactobacillus casei*. *Hiroshima J. Med. Sci.* **32**, 223-225.

Schiffrin, E., Rochat, F., Link-Amster, H. *et al.* (1995) Immunomodulation of human blood cells following the ingestion of lactic acid bacteria. *J. Dairy Sci.* **78**, 491-497.

Sharpe, M., Hill, R. and Lapage, S. (1973) Pathogenic lactobacilli. *J. Med. Microbiol.* **6**, 281-286.

Spangler, B. (1992) Structure and function of cholera toxin and the related *Escherichia coli* heat-labile enterotoxin. *Microbiol. Rev.* **56**, 622-647.

Warren, H., Vogel, F. and Chedid, L. (1986) Current status of immunological adjuvants. *Ann. Rev. Immunol.* **4**, 369-388.

Weiner, H. (1997) Oral tolerance: immune mechanisms and treatment of autoimmune diseases. *Immunol. Today* **18** 335-343.

Williams, N., Harper, H. and Cochrane, L. (1997). Antigen presenting cells of the small intestinal lamina propria. *Mucosal Immunol. Update*, **5**, 29-32.

Xu-Amano, J., Kiyono, H., Jackson, R., Staats, H., Fujihashi, K., Burrows, P., Elson, C., Pillai, S. and McGhee, J. (1993) Helper T cell subsets for immunoglobulin A responses: oral immunization with tetanus toxoid and cholera toxin as adjuvant selectively induces Th2 cells in mucosa associated tissues. *J. Exp. Med.* **178**, 1309-1320.

Yasui, H., Nagaoka, A. , Mike, A. *et al.* (1992) Deteccion of Bifidobacterium strains that induce large quantities of IgA. *Microbiol. Ecol. Health Dis.* **5**, 155-162.

CHAPTER 10

Probiotic Bacteria as Live Oral Vaccines *Lactobacillus* as the Versatile Delivery Vehicle

W J A Boersma, M Shaw and *E Claassen*

10.1 New Vaccine Strategies

Present vaccines for use in humans for the major part are inactivated and depend upon (new) adjuvants (Claassen and Boersma, 1992; Gupta *et al.*, 1996; Van Regenmortel, 1997). The properties of inactivated vaccines together with the nature of the adjuvants in general led to MHC class II restricted humoral responses which tend to have a bias to immunomodulation supported by T helper 2 type cells, especially in young individuals (Forsthuber et la., 1996; Barrios *et al.*, 1996 a,b; Adkins and Du, 1998). However, protection against a number of diseases, especially viral-induced, offered by these type of vaccines is not sufficient since the activation of cellular immune responses is also required in order to clear the infectious agent and to get rid of infected cells. It has become apparent that the new generation of vaccines which are needed for protection against a number of diseases, but for which still no vaccine exists or for which the present vaccines are not effective, should fulfil several specific requirements (Gupta *et al.*, 1996).

In recent years a plethora of different recDNA model vaccines has been developed such as mutant or marker vaccines, trans-disease vaccines and multi-antigen vaccines. In most cases the principle is similar: a pathogen is transformed to express specific antigens either of homologous of heterologous origin. These live vaccines have the potential to generate both specific humoral and cellular immune responses, as application in veterinary practice often shows. However, their intrinsic pathogenic character requires attenuation, especially for safe application in humans. This attenuation is either based on classical selection methodology or obtained by recDNA techniques which induce mutations or deletions. Pathogens which were successfully applied in vaccines also have been used to generate trans-disease vaccines in which a specific pathogen carries a set of specific protective elements from another pathogen (e.g. Pseudorabies virus which expresses Influenza virus HA or classical swine fever antigens). Nevertheless, here also the character of the carrier pathogen to a large extent determines the safety of these vaccines. In

R. Fuller and G. Perdigon (eds.), Probiotics 3, 234–270.

addition, a specific type of attenuation is presently required to restrict the survival of the transformed micro-organisms, in order to prevent environmental contamination. Attenuation however may lead to insufficient intrinsic adjuvant activity of the vaccine or the vaccine may become deficient in particular in those characteristics for which this category of vaccines was developed, i.e. induction of specific cellular immune responses.

The efficiency of attenuated pathogenic bacteria (*Salmonella typhimurium, Vibrio cholera* and *Listeria monocytogenes*) and viruses (adenovirus, vaccinia) capable of replicating at mucosal surfaces, as putative vaccine carriers for the induction of antigen specific immune responses has been confirmed. However, these pathogen-based vaccines each have their typical limitations (e.g. *Salmonella* derived antigen delivery systems are highly reactogenic), and this induction of *Salmonella*-specific immunity restricts their use in multi-schedule immunisation protocols. An additional limitation encountered with *Salmonella* vectors has been plasmid segregation *in vivo* and consequently loss of antigen production although insertion of the antigen genes into the chromosome can stabilise the presence of the heterologous gene. An alternative to this approach is the construction of translational gene-fusions with the M6 (fibrillar surface protein) gene in the human oral commensal *Streptococcus gordonii* which stabilises the surface-anchored expression of heterologous antigen. However, both strategies restrict gene copy numbers and may limit antigen doses delivered *in vivo*.

In addition to these restrictions, the current vaccine approaches are still constrained by safety and environmental considerations. Over-attenuation or inactivation can have detrimental effects on the immunogenicity of the vectors through a reduction in their invasiveness or colonisation ability, whilst mild attenuation retains the risk of reversion to wild type and therefore virulent forms of the organisms. The risk this poses to a paediatric, geriatric or immuno-compromised recipient is too substantial to enable licensure and regulatory compliance.

Sub-unit vaccines which utilise liposomes, ISCOMS or micro-particles as delivery vehicles may present solutions to some of the safety considerations but observations to date have underlined the superiority of attenuated pathogenic viruses and bacteria over non-replicating antigens for the induction of mucosal immune responses. Sub-unit vaccine approaches based upon peptides or purified recombinant proteins may therefore be deficient in this one important requisite, the induction of protective immunity in the GI-tract or other mucosal tracts

Therefore, for a number of years various groups including those at TNO Prevention and Health have examined the potential to develop vaccines that digress from the Jennerian approaches. These approaches enable the provision of safe, antigen-adaptable vaccines that maintain the capacity to sensitise against pathogen serotypes relevant to particular geographical contexts and immunise by a principle different from that of natural infection. These novel vaccines may provide the rationale for the improvements necessary to facilitate oral vaccination

Here we will discuss various aspects of probiotics such as Lactobacillus (mainly), and as a comparison both Lactococcus lactis and Streptococcus spp will be examined. For these species effective transformation systems have been developed and putative live oral vaccines have been prepared. The promising results obtained with a number of these constructs will be discussed.

10.2 Vaccination of large populations

In vaccination programmes in which large numbers of subjects are involved, the oral route of vaccine administration presents several advantages over the more frequently used parenteral routes, particularly in potentially immuno-compromised and paediatric populations. Many organisations such as the World Health Organisation and the Children's Vaccine Initiative have strongly advocated the development of such vaccines, especially with the potential these vaccines possess to reduce reliance upon medically trained personnel for vaccine administration, to reduced dependence on cold-chains and to increase the likelihood of complete immunisation coverage and enhanced compliance. With projected global cohorts in excess of 125 million children per year, the capacity of new vaccines to impact on the pressures of distribution and administration will represent an important attribute determining acceptance and implementation by national vaccination authorities.

Therefore, a vaccine technology that addresses these demands and facilitates direct vaccination of the mucosal surfaces through which the majority of pathogens gain access to the body, may be a pre-requisite to ensuring the induction of protective immunity in the respiratory, gastro-intestinal and urogenital tracts.

The first line of defence against bacterial, viral or parasitic infection utilises both non-specific (mucus, GI tract peristalsis, gastric acid and enzymes) and immunological protective mechanisms. The immunological mechanisms are adaptive responses which utilise predominantly immunoglobulins secreted across the epithelial cells which line the mucosal surfaces to neutralise, inhibit binding or aggregate infectious micro-organisms. However, antigen-specific cellular components such as cytolytic T-cells are also vital mediators of protection, playing roles both in the prevention of primary infection in addition to the rapid resolution of re-infection.

The route of introduction of the vaccine is decisive in presentation of the antigen and in the localisation of responsiveness. Classical routes of application such as intra-muscular and intra- or sub-cutaneous administration in general lead to systemic immunisation. Most pathogens, however, do enter the body *via* the mucosa of GI-tract, respiratory tract and uro-genital tracts. Protection of the individual against invasion of infectious agents *via* the mucosa therefore should preferably include activation of the mucosal immune system. In the case of parenteral administration of attenuated live vaccines priming is, in general, obtained by a subsequent mucosal booster or challenge. However, effective induction of the mucosal immune system only occurs following an infection *via* the mucosal route (e.g. poliovirus, pseudorabies virus).

In the veterinary practice for poultry, administration *via* aerosols is widely applied and takes care to ensure antigen presentation *via* the nasal mucosa but, following the feather care also *via* the oral route to the gut mucosa. However, inactivated vaccines in general do not induce effective protection after oral application. Therefore, alternative approaches need further investigation.

To date however, for human applications, very few microorganisms which mediate their pathology following infection through the mucosal surfaces can be effectively prevented with currently available vaccines. Polio, cholera, typhoid and more recently the tetravalent rhesus rotavirus vaccine (Rotashield®) which attained FDA licensure at the end of 1998, are the current limited examples of effective disease prevention or reduction following mucosal vaccination. The manipulation of the mucosal immune system in order to facilitate effective immunity induction has been a formidable task. Consequently the majority of vaccines are still administered through invasive puncture procedures and in general are still based around the utilisation of attenuated or killed pathogens as the critical vaccine constituent.

10.3 Assets of probiotics as vaccine candidates

Definitions for probiotic activity like 'general health improvement' in animal science, often have been roughly restricted to enhanced growth, food utilisation and production of milk and eggs (Berg, 1998). Though, in physiological terms, this means a higher level of 'production', the present super-milk-producing cows and super rapid growing chickens show that this is not necessarily a matter of health in terms of well-being of the individual. Use of probiotics for this purpose might lead to ever increasing requirements, which mainly have an economical basis. This might lead to an imbalance of the animal's health since it is driven to the limits of its physiological capacity.

Probiotics according to Fuller (1992) include live microbiological food or feed supplements, such as *Lactobacillus*, *Bifidobacteria*, *Bacillus*, *Streptococcus* and *Enterococcus*, that beneficially affect the host individual by improving its intestinal microbial balance. Tannock (1997) and Tannock *et al.*(1998) also includes yeasts such as *Saccharomyces, Aspergillus* and *Torulopsis*. Applications as probiotics in general terms are mostly found with *Lactobacillus,* and to a lesser extent also with *Bifidobacteria* and *Streptococcus*. *Saccharomyces*, for example *S.boulardi*, may be envisaged as probiotic but its function may be probiotic in an indirect way, through generation of prebiotics for specific microflora species (Tannock, 1997; Tannock *et al.*, 1998).

Consequently, non-pathogenic, food grade or commensal bacterial vectors have received attention for their vaccine potential (Pozzi *et al.*, 1992 a,b; Robinson *et al.*, 1997; Pouwels *et al.*, 1998). *Lactococcus lactis*, a strain used in cheese manufacture does not colonise the GI tract and is not viable following passage through the gastric chamber, thereby limiting its ability to express heterologous genes *in vivo*. *In sensu strictu*, *L. lactis* is not a probiotic micro-organism. However, the molecular genetics of this organism are advanced and notable success in the induction of Tetanus Toxin Fragment C-specific (TTTC-specific) serum IgG has been documented following oral immunisation. Heterologous gene expression systems for the non-pathogenic species of *Staphylococcus carnosus* and *sxylosus* have been developed enabling levels of surface antigen expression which may contribute to the immunogenic potential of the vector. Similarly work with *L. lactis* has indicated that at lower doses of surface exposed antigen is sufficient to induce responses identical to those observed with antigen expressed as an intracellular product.

In our own research probiotic activity has been narrowed down to bacteria with properties which have a direct influence on the animal's health, and from the immunologist's point of view, particularly bacteria which improve the non-specific inflammatory responsiveness and/or the specific immune responses of the recipient. A direct basis for this approach was the demonstration of the adjuvant activity of, for example, lactobacilli. This property made clear that *Lactobacillus* in fact had sufficient potential to fulfil the criteria necessary for modern live oral vaccine carriers, such as: safety, since it is a GRAS organism (Guarner & Schaafsma, 1998), genetic transformability, ease of culture and storage, cheap, entrance to the mucosal immune system and intrinsic adjuvant activity for systemic as well as mucosal responses.

Commensal bacteria and other food derived Gram positives such as *Lactobacillus* can maintain a sophisticated non-invasive ecology with the host and although surveyed by the immune system are not necessarily susceptible to immune clearance from their ecological niches. The predominance of lactobacilli in various regions of the aero-digestive tracts indicates their particular potential as live oral vaccines. Their GRAS status is evident from extensive application as starter or fermentation strains in the food industry. In this context, we consider that lactobacilli, represent a unique opportunity for the delivery of a multitude of serotype-specific candidate antigens to the mucosal immune system whilst limiting risks to the paediatric recipients (Medaglini *et al.*, 1995; Wells *et al.*, 1993, Oggioni *et al.*, 1998). Selected strains, by virtue of being able to colonise mucosal sites, may compete with specific pathogens for representation in the microflora (Blomberg *et al.*, 1993, Coconnier *et al*, 1997, 1998). In addition, the relatively low intrinsic immunogenicity most likely allows repetitive usage of the vectors in vaccination strategies.

The capacity to remain viable following gastric passage enables heterologous gene expression and secretion *in situ.* The opportunity for persistence or colonisation of mucosal surface facilitates the probiotic influences on nutrition and health (Fernandes *et al.*, 1987; Marteau and Rambaud, 1993) that have been documented, for example, during the course of acute rotavirus infection (Kaila *et al.*, 1992 Kaila *et al.*, 1995).

10.4 Immunomodulation by probiotic bacteria

In mice, *in vivo* a-specific polyclonal enhancement of intestinal IgA-secreting cells was observed with indigenous flora components and with selected segmented filamentous bacteria (SFB) (Moreau *et al.*, 1982; Klaassen *et al.*, 1993). In addition, SFB enhanced the ConcanavalinA-induced proliferation of mesenteric lymph node cells (Klaasen *et al.*, 1993). The SFB are mainly localised on the epithelia which cover the Peyer's patches in mice and rats (Klaasen *et al.*, 1991).

Immuno-modulating capacity of probiotic bacteria initially was demonstrated following subcutaneous immunisation of SRBC using live and killed lactobacilli as adjuvants. Responses to these immunogens were unexpectedly high in both plaque forming cell assays (PFC) as well as in DTH. (Bloksma *et al.*, 1979). Feeding of fermented milk containing *L. casei* and of *L.acidophilus* stimulated mouse intra peritoneal macrophages into carbon clearance and led to enhanced PFC responses (Perdigon *et al.*, 1986). From these initial studies there was a follow up in at least three directions: a) analysis of adjuvanticity or enhancement of immune responses, b) induction of cytokines and c) effects on cellular aspects of antigen presentation.

10.4.1 Immuno-adjuvant effect

An intrinsic ability to augment immune responses in either an antigen specific or a-specific manner presents an important criterion governing strain selection. Early work has shown that following parenteral immunisation certain *Lactobacillus* strains were able to confer equivalent levels of adjuvant effect on sub optimal doses of the model antigen Tri Nitro Phenylated-Chicken Gamma Globulin (TNP-CGG) as was observed with a more conventional oil in water emulsion Specol (Fig.10.1). As this adjuvant effect is not equivalent across strains, much work has focused on detailing the basis for the effect (Boersma *et al.*, 1994; Pouwels *et al.*, 1995; Claassen *et al.*, 1994). The capacity to enhance immune responses also has been demonstrated with co-administered DxRRV rhesus-human reassortant oral rotavirus vaccine (Isolauri *et al*, 1995). All these effects are probably attributable to the macrophage-activating and IFN-γ inducing properties of the Gram-positive peptidoglycan and lipoteichoic acid fractions (Cleveland *et al.*, 1996). But these observations underline the unique opportunities *Lactobacillus* presents for oral vaccination. Using *Lactobacillus*, adjuvanticity was demonstrated for humoral immune responses and for DTH reactions in BALB/c mice which are representative of mice which in general tend to respond on a Th2 fashion.

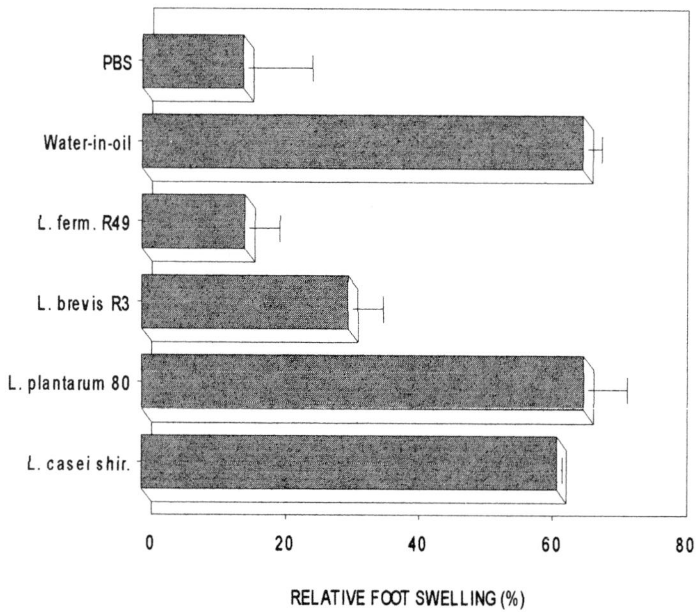

Figure 10.1. Enhancement of DTH responses in mice after immunization with chicken γ globulin conjugated with trinitrophenol (CGG-TNP).
Groups of 5 mice were primed i.p. with a doses of 25 microgram antigen and 10^9 *Lactobacillus fermentum*, *L. brevis*, *L. plantarum* or *L. casei* (Shirota). Differential secondary reactions to the antigen were measured as footswelling in DTH. For comparison control mice were primed with antigen and water in oil adjuvant.

Enhancement of antibody formation by simultaneous oral administration of adjuvant and parenteral immunisation was shown for protein antigens, subunit vaccines (Fig.10.2) and for inactivated virus. The level of enhancement was *Lactobacillus* strain dependent, but for some strains it was as high as was observed with water in oil emulsions (Boersma *et al.*,

1994, Pouwels *et al.*, 1995). *L. casei, L.plantarum, L. acidophilus* and *L. reuteri* demonstrated the highest level of response stimulation. Thus it could be shown that probiotic bacteria had an effect on the GI-tract which led to stimulation of the systemic immune system. In these mouse experiments *L. casei* (type strain), *L. plantarum* and *L. reuteri* were most promising. Both humoral responses and DTH were supported indicating that induction of Th1 biased responses using lactobacilli may be expected (Maassen *et al.*, 1997).

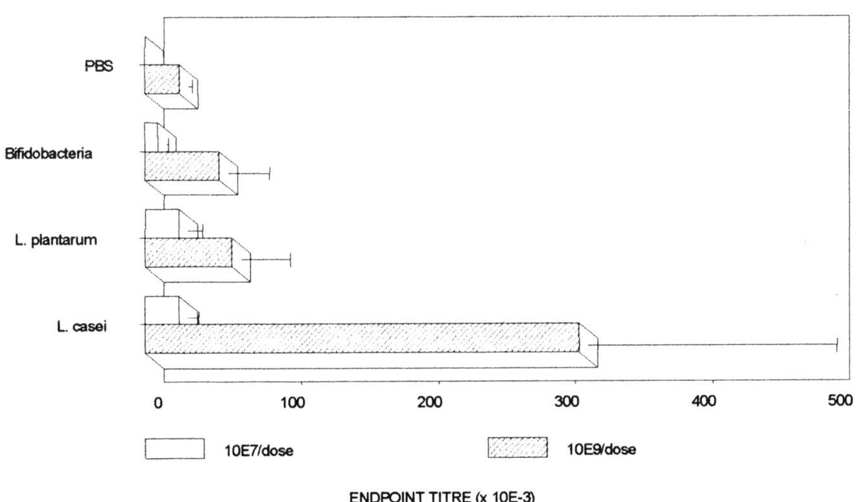

Figure 10.2. Enhancement of secondary response to parenteral immunization.
Groups of six Balb/c mice were immunized s.c. with a suboptimal dose of antigen, 0.5 microgram trivalent heamagglutinin of influenza subunit vaccine, such that no reponse upon priming was observed. *Bifidobacteria, L. plantarum* or *L. casei* were intragastric administered in doses of respectively 10^7 and 10^9 bacteria daily during the experiment. The second immunization was performed four weeks after priming with the same dose of antigen. Seven days after secondary immunization antigen specific IgG was determined in serum. Mean values and SD are shown for end-point titres. Only relatively high doses of *Lactobacilus casei* showed adjuvanticity.

Rook and Stanford (1998) recently hypothesised that aberrant reactivity of the immune system later in life might have its origin earlier during development of the system. In neonates there is a tendency to react to immune stimulation with Th2 biased responses. This effect may be the result of an imprint by the maternal immune system which during pregnancy shows a similar bias (Ragupathy, 1997). It was claimed that, the absence of exposition to environmental pathogens and natural infections and the use of vaccines with adjuvants that direct responses into the Th2 trajectory leads to an increase in prevalence of allergies such as asthma and other Th2 associated deviations of correct responsiveness. To solve this problem they pray 'give us this day our daily germs' or an a-specific adjuvant like micro-organism such as mycobacteria to stimulate the immune system into Th1 type responses (Rook and Stanford, 1998). *Lactobacillus* based live oral vaccine carriers might be applied especially in neonates and young to make use of the intrinsic adjuvanticity. Regular administration of dosages of probiotic bacteria independent on vaccines might already have an adjuvant effect for any infection. This could induce a general skewing of responses and may also be beneficial on concomitant use of non-reproductive or inactivated vaccines used mainly with alum or water in oil adjuvants. We herewith support the view expressed recently by Famularo and De Simone (1998).

10.4.2 Cytokine induction

In situ staining of mucosal tissues obtained following administration of lactobacilli has identified cytokine induction as one mediator of the adjuvant effect. This will be discussed in depth in a separate chapter (Claassen *et al.*). Briefly, in BALB/c mice cells producing cytokines which are active in inflammatory responses were increased in frequency along the GI tract. Interleukin 2 (IL-2), TNF-α and IL-10 levels were all increased in lamina propria cells following oral administration of lactobacilli, but only in response to particular *Lactobacillus* strains. For some strains, the production of IL-2 and interferon γ was also observed. In addition, evidence was found for a polyclonal activation of IgA responses. In SJL mice, which are roughly considered to represent TH1 mice, the results were slightly different indicating that the interaction between host and probiotic will determine to a great extent the response of the immune system.

In pigs, *Streptococcus faecium* (M74) and *Lactobacillus casei* spp. but not *S. thermophilus* and *L. delbrueckii* spp *bulgaricus* were shown to induce Interleukin-2 in illeal tissue, thereby increasing the phagocytic activity of the cells (Tortuero *et al.*, 1995).

PBMC from human volunteers, as well as mouse cells, obtained following consumption of yoghurt show an enhanced production of Interleukin-1- β, Interferon-α and -β and Tumor Necrosis Factor α (TNF-α) (Pereyra and Lemonnier, 1993; Solis-Pereya *et al.*, 1997). Aattouri and Lemonnier (1997) showed that LAB often used in dairy products, such as *Streptococcus lactis*, *Streptococcus thermophilus*, *Lactococcus lactis* and *Lactobacillus acidophilus* spp., were able to enhance *in vitro* production of Interferon-γ and interleukin-6 by PBMC of yoghurt consumers.

Recently it was shown that *in vitro* stimulation of human PBMC was enhanced with live non-pathogenic *L. rhamnosus*, and *L. delbrueckii* spp *bulgaricus*, that are part of the normal microflora or common in dairy food, respectively. These lactobacilli were able to induce PBMC to produce the inflammatory cytokines such as TNF-α, IL-1-β and IL-6 (Miettinen *et al.*, 1996). In addition, the cytokines which are associated with typical TH1 cell profiles such as Interferon-γ, IL-12 and IL-18 were also produced.

L. bulgaricus was deficient in interferon-γ production and this LAB also was relatively low in Interleukin-12 production. Similar experiments with *Streptococcus pyogenes* demonstrated that this pathogenic lactic acid bacterium induced a cytokine profile in PBMC which was very similar (Miettinen *et al.*, 1998). In particular, IL-12 and Interferon γ were produced in concentrations relatively high upon incubation with *S. pyogenes* when compared with the lactobacilli. During an immune response these latter cytokines are initially produced by macrophages. The Interleukin-12 which is produced stimulates the production of Interferon-γ by T cells and NK cells. Interleukin 18 enhances the induction of Interferon-γ. This directs differentiation of naive CD4 positive cells into T-helper 1 cells. In PBMC IL-12 and IL-18 most probably are produced by monocytes. Their synergistic action leads to interferon γ production (D'Andrea *et al.*, 1993; Okamura *et al.*, 1995; Puren *et al.*, 1998).

From this one might expect that lactic acid bacteria may lead to the skewing of T-cell responses toward the T helper 1 type cells. In addition, it suggests, that the cytokine profile induced by harmless bacteria such as the lactobacilli may be as functional in the enhancement of immune responsiveness as the cytokine profiles induced in immune responses toward specific pathogens. However, to moderate the enthusiasm about this finding it must be added that induction of IL-10, though not to high levels, was also observed. Interleukin-4 was not detectable. Interleukin-10 down regulates TH1 responses by modulating the production of the inflammatory cytokines as well as Interferon-γ and Interleukin-12, thereby enhancing the TH2 responses.

Th2 responses are the natural response of the mucosal immune system, since Th2 type cells stimulate IgA production (McGhee and Kiyono, 1993). However, present oral vaccines do not only aim to generate sufficient IgA to exclude pathogens which use the mucosal route as an entry to the body. In addition, these vaccines aim at protective effects at the level of the systemic immune system, first to assure a second line of defence, but more importantly to assure sufficient memory to overcome later challenges.

Interleukin-18 is a cytokine which is thought to have an important role in mucosal immunity (Kohno & Kurimoto, 1998). This makes it likely that the lactobacilli and other lactic acid bacteria have an immunomodulating role in the GI-tract and similarly in other mucosal sites. From these findings Miettinen *et al.* (1998) concluded that the putative cytokine profiles induced with LAB are likely to be beneficial to mucosal immune responses. However, *in vitro* detection of cytokines after stimulation of PBMC is merely an indication of the capacity of cells to produce these specific immuno-modulators but does not prove that *in vivo* the same profile is generated. Moreover the cell distribution in PBMC is quite different from the cells which come into contact with LAB *in situ*, for example enterocytes. These latter cells have been shown to generate the inflammatory cytokines, but thus far Interleukin-12 , IL-18 as well as interferon-γ have not been shown to be produced at mucosal induction sites. However, it cannot be excluded that specialised mucosal antigen presenting cells, such as M-cells, do also respond to LAB with production of these cytokines. An indication for such potential mutual influences is the *in vitro* induction of enterocytes to differentiate into M-cells following stimulation by activated human PBMC (Kerneis *et al.*, 1997).

Recently, pathogens of the GI-tract which in general cannot easily be cleared by their natural hosts, such as *Salmonella* spp. (Chong *et al.*, 1996) and *H.pylori* (Haeberle *et al.*, 1997) were also shown to be able to induce IL-12 and IL-10 respectively. This indicates that the inclusion of co-expressing vectors for various cytokines, as such, does not guarantee the enhancement of protection by LAB based vaccines.

New vaccine vectors are being developed which allow co-expression of cytokines which have been shown to have a beneficial action similar to that of live pathogen based vaccines or infections. However, protection to most pathogens requires that the immune system reacts at different levels. In many infections the reaction of cells and factors of the innate immunity is initially required. Subsequently both humoral and cellular reactions are necessary to overcome disease and infection. As a consequence, for most pathogens the vaccine should be developed such that it assists the host immune system in clearing the pathogen and the infection and therefore both arms of the immune system should be activated. Then induction of cytokines should be such that a balanced response is induced which leads to protection. Skewing of responses to extremes of immune reactivity may lead to unwanted side effects. As far as is presently known lactobacilli may support induction of protective responses beneficially.

10.4.3 Effects on antigen presentation

Whether *Streptococcus gordonii* can be regarded as a probiotic is not clear. However such flora components at least *in vitro* have been shown to have powerful influences on professional APC's. Upregulation of class I and class II MHC antigens was observed on exposure of isolated dendritic cells to transformed *S.gordonii*. Processing and class I antigen presentation of a model antigen ovalbumin expressed on the surface *via* the M6 anchor (see below) was demonstrated (Rescigno *et al.*, 1998).

It is thought that influence of LAB on induction of cytokines in the recipient host will be beneficial. Vaccine trials in which, for example, *L. casei* were used as adjuvants do indeed suggest that such a result may be envisaged (Isolauri *et al.*, 1995). However, for transformed LAB the adjuvant properties should be unaffected by the presence of an expression system for vaccine antigens.

To date most adjuvants which are active at the mucosal surfaces derive from purified or recombinant components of bacterial toxin such as the heat-labile toxin of *E.coli* and both Cholera toxin or its B-subunit. However, safety concerns regarding the application of these adjuvants will obstruct their licensure. To circumvent this, recombinant analogues of these toxins have been investigated and although these preparations deal effectively with the safety considerations they have also resulted in significant decreases in the levels of adjuvant effect. However, the oral administration of *Lactobacillus* spp. Results in the adjuvant effects whilst maintaining, in general, the induction of only low levels of antibody specific for the bacterial carrier itself. Again these observations contrast with those seen with the toxin-derived adjuvants which themselves are intrinsically highly immunogenic, resulting in immense difficulties regarding their application in multi-schedule immunisation.

10.5 Effect on vaccination of specific localisation of *Lactobacillus* in the GI tract

M cell regions overlying the lymphoid follicles mediate the induction and effector phases of mucosal immune responses. Adherence to these epithelial cells lining the mucosa may contribute to localisation and colonisation abilities and therefore present particular advantages from a vaccination perspective. These M cells are specialised epithelial cells. They sample antigen present in the lumen of the GI and nasal tracts and function as a conduit for this antigen, directing its delivery to antigen presenting cells such as the dendritic and macrophage populations present in the dome regions of the Peyer's patch follicle. Adherence to such cells will focus and sustain the antigen stimulus, but adherence to other regions of the GI tract will also afford a competitive advantage over other bacteria present in the tract.

We expect that a relatively short exposure of the mucosal immune system to the vaccine vehicle is an advantage of non-commensal, non-colonising lactobacilli over vectors which lack these properties. In contrast, the prolonged presence or colonisation of vaccine vehicles in the GI-tract such as obtained with *Streptococcus gordonii* may lead to an initial induction of responsiveness. However, upon secondary exposure of the mucosa to repeated vaccination using the same carrier, vaccination will be ineffective due to induced tolerance that developed during the first and relatively long period of contact.

Eleven species of lactobacilli have been detected in either porcine or rodent faecal material with an additional 10 species isolated from either human or other animal sources. This variation between hosts supports the opinion that mucosal adhesion is an important colonisation factor. (Pouwels *et al.*, 1998). However, this colonisation capacity is fragile and *exvivo* manipulation of colonising strains may result in a loss of colonisation capacity. In this respect therefore, the use of *in vitro* techniques to identify appropriate antigen delivery hosts requires a cautious analysis. Adhesion of strains to epithelial cells has been extensively studied using cell lines that are morphologically and phenotypically similar to normal intestinal cells. In this context the Caco-2, HT-29 and HeLa cells have enabled detailed studies to be made on the interactions between the commensal strains and mucosal tissues. The caution required with the *in vitro* techniques is exemplified by the work of Conway and Hendriksson (1993) who demonstrated the inability of a porcine *L. fermentum* strain 104-R to adhere to porcine epithelium *in vitro* but the ability of a human derived strain *L. fermentum* KLD to maintain its adherence characteristics to human tissue whilst demonstrating no specificity to porcine tissue. Therefore *in vitro* analyses are of limited use because they are unable to suitably assess the role of mucus in the adhesion process and more importantly the potential for co-aggregation of *Lactobacillus* species with other resident bacteria.

Polysaccharides and proteins have both been implicated in the mediation of adhesion. *In vitro* work with intestinal epithelial cells correlated adhesion with bacterial hydrophobicity whilst the use of the Caco-2 cells suggested the involvement of both a proteinaceous and a non-proteinaceous factor. A unifying theory centres on lending a lectin function to the proteins with function to cross link the bacterial polysaccharides with the host tissue cell receptors.

Work by Conway and Kjelleberg (1989) identified a surface associated protein that mediated the adherence of the *L. fermentum* 104R strain to porcine mucosa. This 29kDa protein is loosely associated with the cell surface and importantly could bind mucus *in vitro* (Conway and

Kjelleberg, 1989). Sequence analysis has revealed that a structural similarity between this mucus adhesion promoting protein and a virulence factor for *Campylobacter jejuni* and the 85KD A, B and C complex proteins from *Mycobacterium tuberculosis*. The gastric mucosa derived glycoprotein fibronectin and to a lesser extent the collagen, elastin and laminin all components which comprise the extra-cellular matrix demonstrate an affinity to several lactobacilli.

Marteau and Rambaud (1993) established that the *L. plantarum* strain NCIMB 8826 and *L. salivarius* UCC 433118 when administered to humans as a fermented milk product were able to remain viable following passage through the gastric chamber. Importantly, these two strains were able to establish high colony levels in the ileum itself, the section of the GI tract which maintains a high focus of the Peyer's patch lymphoid tissue sites. This *L. plantarum* NCIM 8826 strain, although of human saliva origin was able to transiently implant in the murine vagina for a time period (> 1 week) equivalent to that seen with a murine vaginal isolate *L. paracasei* LbTGS1.4.

In conclusion therefore, the two important considerations for utilising this attribute of lactobacilli for strain selection purposes are, firstly, the host species and tissue origin of candidate strains and secondly the *in vivo* validation of all data collected using the *in vitro* cell line based adhesion assays. In any case it seems inevitable that strain selection will have to be tailored to both the intended host as well as the intended mucosal compartment and that the prospect of a *Lactobacillus* single species with the potential for universal application is remote.

10.6 Construction of putative vaccines

For construction of transformants recDNA technology offers a lot of spare parts such as promoters, genes coding for heterologous proteins, sequences which direct the products of a vector to the right site in the micro-organism. When these assets are put together just as building blocks the result is a vector which in principle has all the necessary technical specifications, but may not be highly effective in generation of the heterologous product required. In general, attempts to transform micro-organisms started with the well known tools developed for *E.coli*. Promoters generally originate from the species actually used for expression. Most effective expression systems have been obtained only after fine tuning to the requirements of the host probiotic.

10.6.1 Streptococcus

Streptococcus lactis also has been used in vaccine development. A structural surface protein from *S.mutans* serotype c was expressed in *S.lactis*. The antigen was not secreted into the supernatant but was found in the cytoplasm of the transformants. Though expression was low oral immunisation led to significant specific IgA in saliva and IgG in serum (Iwaki *et al.*, 1990).

Most *Streptococcus* based vaccines until now are based on *S.gordonii* expressing fusion proteins with the modified M6 surface anchor of the pathogen *Streptococcus pyogenes* (Pozzi *et al.*, 1992a,b; Medaglini *et al.*, 1995). Modification of the M6 was such that the truncated molecule remained effective in support of immune responses, but M6 is sufficiently crippled to silence most of the criticism with respect to pathogenic risks of the M6, which in *S.pyogenes* is an important virulence factor. Chromosomal integration was relatively easily obtained and ensures stable expression (Oggioni & Pozzi., 1996; Pozzi *et al.*, 1992a,b). This highly efficient expression system has led to a considerable number of model vaccines for infectious diseases and model antigens (cf. Fischetti *et al.*, 1996).

S. gordonii expressing M6 fusion proteins with a hornet venom allergen upon oral/nasal administration of a single dose of bacteria led to specific IgA responses in lung washings and saliva as well as specific systemic IgG (Medaglini *et al.*, 1995). In addition, *S.gordonii* expressing human papilloma virus 16 (HPV-16) proteins on the surface easily colonised the mouse vagina and did evoke local IgA immune responses but in addition led to systemic IgG responses (Oggioni *et al.*, 1995; Medaglini *et al.*, 1997). Also intranasal/oral immunisation led to colonisation as well as systemic immune responses. In these experiments it seemed that live and therefore colonising bacteria only were able to evoke immune responses. Killed bacteria were not effective. (Oggioni *et al.*, 1995). This may be an indication that at least for some micro-organisms cohabitation with the host may be a dynamic equilibrium which does not prevent a systemic response (Oggioni *et al.*, 1995; Medaglini *et al.*, 1997). Not only the humoral compartment was activated using *S.gordonii* constructs. Transformants with an HIV-1 gp120 T-cell epitope (human) were able to stimulate T-cells *in vitro* (Pozzi *et al.*, 1994). Both HPV16 and HIV-1 expressing *S.gordonii* have been applied in the vagina in Cynomolgus monkeys. As in mice this resulted in colonisation and local and systemic immune responses (Medaglini *et al.*, 1998; Di Fabio *et al.*, 1998).

Streptococcus vaccines as developed by Pozzi *et al.* (1992a,b) in inactivated form do require a formulation with adjuvants. *S.gordonii*, the strain which was mainly used for vaccine development colonises easily in the mouth and other body cavities. This may be a disadvantage since continuous exposure (> 10 weeks) may harbour the risk of induction of tolerance, though in the present models this has not been observed directly. In contrast, recolonisation with *S.gordonii* in mice ranges from difficult to impossible (Pozzi pers. comm.) and therefore could be indicative of a slowly built up resistance which would make the repetitive use of this vaccine vector impossible.

Since the commensal *S.gordonii* lacks intrinsic adjuvanticity their future application in inactivated form as a loaded vehicle may be restricted to a delivery vector for prebiotics, antigens and pharmaceutical products. Co-expression of cytokines and heterologous antigen may lead to a second chance for *Streptococcus* vaccines.

10.6.2 Lactococcus lactis

Lactic acid bacteria (LAB) have been used for a considerable time in preparation and fermentation of foodstuffs. Bacteriocins from LAB were thought to provide natural substitutes for synthetic preservatives, but apart from nisin not many products have been developed such that their use has become common practice (Lucey and Fitzgerald, 1997). The search for new bacteriocins and expression systems for many enzymes, and the wide use of LAB in industry has led to the investigation of their metabolism and molecular biology. Consequently, when new applications such as the development of vaccine vectors surfaced, most of the tools needed to construct a live vaccine vector were already available.

The T7 polymerase of *E.coli* initially was used to introduce the tetanus toxin fragment C (TTFC) gene into *L.lactis*. The *L.lactis* recombinants obtained were both immunogenic and able to protect mice from lethal challenge (Cherfas, 1993). *Lactococcus lactis* in part is used as a kind of "magic bullet" system (Wells *et al.*, 1993, Norton *et al.*, 1996, 1997). Antigen loaded particles do in fact function as sophisticated alternatives for antigen loaded liposomes. Subsequently, an expression-secretion system was also developed (Wells *et al.*, 1993). Antigen loading which enabled the secretion of the TTFC product by transformed *L.lactis* was slower than the production in the intracellular compartment and as a consequence accumulation of the product occurred (up to 2.9 mg per liter of growth medium).

Pre-treatment of the loaded bacteria with mitomycin-C kills the bacteria and after oral delivery leads to release of its contents in the GI-tract. Constructs which expressed tetanus toxin fragment C in mice have been shown to be very effective in producing responses which were protective to challenge (Robinson *et al.*, 1997). Apart from oral application the intra-nasal administration has also led to protective immune responses (Norton *et al.*, 1997). It is assumed that the protection was supported to a large extent by the systemic responses which were obtained with the *L.lactis* magic bullet system.

In all experiments it has been observed that the immune responses to *L.lactis*, which may become prohibitive in repetitive use of the same vaccine carrier, were relatively low for the vaccine carriers as compared to the wild type *L.lactis* (Norton *et al.*, 1996).

Similar to *Streptococcus*, *L.lactis* lacks intrinsic adjuvanticity. However, Steidler *et al.* (1995, 1998) showed that co-expression of heterologous antigens and secretion of functional cytokines (IL-12 and IL-6) was feasible. However, the mitomycin-C treatment required for intra-gut release of antigen led to a loss of cytokine secretion.

10.6.3 Lactobacillus as an antigen delivery vehicle

The molecular genetics of *Lactobacillus* and consequently their use as antigen delivery vehicles is not at a state of advancement equivalent to that observed with other lactic acid bacteria such as *L. lactis* and *S. gordonii.* The genus is comprised of more than 50 species and this diversity is reflected not only at the level of variety in their industrial applications but also down to the large differences in GC content of their DNA (36% - 50%). The diversity results in an inherently more complex development process as a result, and this review will stress that appropriate strain selection is of equivalent importance to the amenability of the species to genetic modification, in the generation of a potent oral vaccine delivery system. The attributes, which determine the appropriateness of strains, fall into 4 principal categories:

1. Surface structure differences are also prevalent within the genus and this will manifest itself in a variety of capacities of species to adhere to the mucosa and therefore generate some competitive advantage over indigenous species of bacteria.
2. Differences in sugar metabolism dictate that complex media are required to ensure optimum growth of lactobacilli. Therefore, the capacity of certain species of lactobacilli to derive suitable levels of energy from the sugar sources actually available in the intestines will influence their capacity to survive and over express antigens under *in vivo* conditions.
3. Several reports indicate differences in the immunoadjuvant or immunostimulatory effect of *Lactobacillus* spp. and this attribute may have important implications for the potentiation of immune responses to heterologous antigens produced by these vaccine delivery vehicles.
4. The vast diversity of transcriptional and translation controls limits how generally applicable observations of efficient gene expression in one species can be extrapolated to similar organisms.

Therefore, this variety does present an unrivalled diversity of strains that qualify for consideration as antigen delivery vehicles and underlines that strain selection is as important a consideration as is the ability to optimise the gene expression systems that facilitate the vaccine antigen production. This diversity allows for continual improvement in the antigen delivery vehicle; a luxury not afforded to the *Lactococcus* and *Streptococcus* systems which remain extremely limited in availability of strains for analysis.

10.7 Heterologous antigen expression in *Lactobacillus*

The genetic diversity of the genus presents a vast variety of transcription, translation and targeting sequences which are available to implement optimum gene expression. However, in general these gene expression elements maintain considerable species specificity. As a consequence wild type strains selected for use as antigen delivery vehicles do not necessarily have available all the elements necessary for optimum heterologous gene expression. In particular solutions to the problems of the both structural and segregational stabilities of these gene expression elements in a broad range of *Lactobacillus* strains will be critical for identifying host vector combinations which function as effective immunogens.

Lactobacilli did not readily accept ligation mixtures for transformation therefore intact plasmids were required for this procedure. As a consequence relatively large amounts of purified plasmids were needed and these have to be initially isolated from *Lactobacillus casei* which was used as the working organism. Therefore in the process of development of efficient *Lactobacillus* vectors a major drawback was that isolation of plasmid DNA from Gram-positive micro-organisms such as *Lactobacillus* was inefficient because of the resilience of the surface peptidoglycan layer. Mechanical or enzymatic methods to obtain cell lysis were not highly efficient and reproducible and showed large variations between strains of lactobacilli. For cell lysis existing methods (Klaenhammer and Sutherlands, 1980) were optimised by Posno *et al.* (1991a,b) and later by Frere (1994) and by Reinkemeier *et al.* (1996). Maassen (1999) recently described a rapid purification method for the plasmid DNA which proved to be effective for two series of transformed strains based on *Lactobacillus casei* expressing respectively the B subunit of the urease enzyme of *Helicobacter pylori* and *Lactobacillus plantarum* expressing tetanus toxin fragment C (Maassen *et al.*, 1999).

Transformation efficiency is an extremely variable attribute, with numerous strains such as *L. delbrueckii spp bulgaricus* actually refractory to transformation. The majority of gene expression systems for use in lactobacilli have derived from naturally occurring cryptic plasmids, derived from *L. pentosus* and *L. plantarum* strains, with a rolling circle replicative (RCR) mechanism. The cryptic p353-2 plasmid identified by Posno *et al* (1991a,b) has formed the basis for several heterologous gene expression systems. The pLPCR2 plasmid contains the *L. pentosus* xylose operon repressor gene xylR and the xylB.gene terminator. Cloning of the *E. coli* β-galactosidase into the multi-cloning site resulted in the ability to express this protein to levels of 0.2% of total soluble protein. However, fusions of tandem repeats of a foot and mouth disease epitope to the N-terminus of the β-galactosidase resulted in further reductions in the expression levels. Although this low level of expression was solved in *L. pentosus* strains by utilising a bile acid hydrolase gene (cbh) promoter to enable levels of 2%, this solution did not extend to the *L. casei* strains selected for use in vaccination studies.

Mercenier *et al.* (1996) reported the use of replicons obtained from other Gram-positive bacteria in the construction of the pTG2247 plasmid, which combine the (TIR) obtained from *L. plantarum* with the strong P25 promoter of *S. thermophilus* and the replicon of the cryptic lactococcal plasmid pSH71. Expression of fusion proteins comprising the HIV-1 V3 loop epitope (gp41E) and a modified cell wall anchored M6 protein from *S. pyogenes* resulted in expression levels of 0.5% of total soluble protein.

Rush *et al.*, (1995) reported a broad host range vector utilising the *S.aureus* protein A promoter, combined with the TIR and signal sequence to express the variable domain 4 of the chlamydial major outer membrane protein at levels of 10 $mg.l^{-1}$ in numerous *Lactobacillus* strains. The broad host range plasmids are vitally important to vaccine applications and therefore have received considerable attention.

Constitutive expression vectors based upon the Theta Replicating Expression plasmids (pTREX) have been developed to include lactococcal promoters and the bacteriophage T7 gene 10 TIR optimised for complimentarity of the Shine Dalgarno sequence (Wells *et al*, 1996) to the ribosomal 16sRNA of *L. lactis*. This plasmid originally designed for use in *Lactococcus* has now successfully been used to transform *L. paracasei, L. gasseri* and *L. jonsonii* species and enable the expression of the model antigen TTFC (Wells *et al*, 1996).

Though the utilisation of the theta mode plasmid replication has considerable structural stability advantages over the RCR plasmids, the segregational instability is significantly increased in the absence of antibiotic selection markers.

Figure 10. 3. Schematic representation of the pLP401 expression vectors developed by TNO.

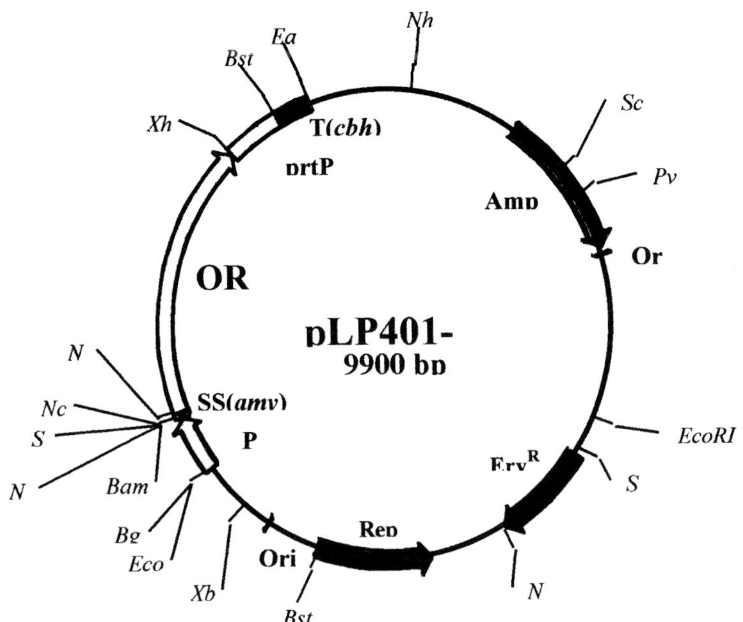

The PCR product coding for bacterial or viral antigens are appropriately digested and ligated into the open reading frames (ORF) of shuttle plasmids (Maasen *et al.*, 1999) prior to *BamHI/Nhe*I subcloning into pLP401T (surface-anchored product) or similarly in the pLP503T (intracellular product) plasmids, respectively. *L. casei* are ultimately transformed with the plasmids detailed, following *NotI* removal of the T*ldh* terminator present in the shuttle vectors. P*ldh* and P*amy* represent the promoters of the L-*ldh* (*lactate dehydrogenase*) gene of *L. casei* and the α-*amy* (α-*amylase*) gene of *L.amylovorus* respectively. T*ldh* and T*cbh* represent transcription terminators of the L-*ldh* (*L. casei*) and *cbh* (conjugated bile acid hydrolase of *L. plantarum*) genes. The anchor *prtP* in the pLP401 plasmid is the sequence from *L. casei* encoding the anchor sequence of the proteinase P gene. SS(amy) refers to the signal sequence of the α-amylase gene, which facilitates transport of the heterologous genes encoded within the ORF through the cell membrane. The determiants encoding for Erythromyocin resistance (Ery), Ampicillin resistance (Amp) and the plasmid origin of replication (Ori+) are also shown.

10.7.1 Development of new Lactobacillus vectors

More recent improvements to the gene expression systems have increased plasmid stability and utilised chromosomal integration systems that can target either specific or random loci. These integrant systems have been based around either non-replicative plasmids or conjugative transposons. The transposon systems enable a rapid testing of antigen expression in numerous host strains, but introduce a substantial risk that (i). integrants will carry an antibiotic resistance marker or (ii). that genes which contribute to the important strain specific attributes of adherence or immunomodulation are corrupted. In this context, the non-replicative plasmid integration system is advantageous in that the $tRNA^{ser}$ locus is utilised for non-disruptive integration. Chromosomal integration in *L. plantarum* has also been achieved with the *L-ldh* locus, which does not

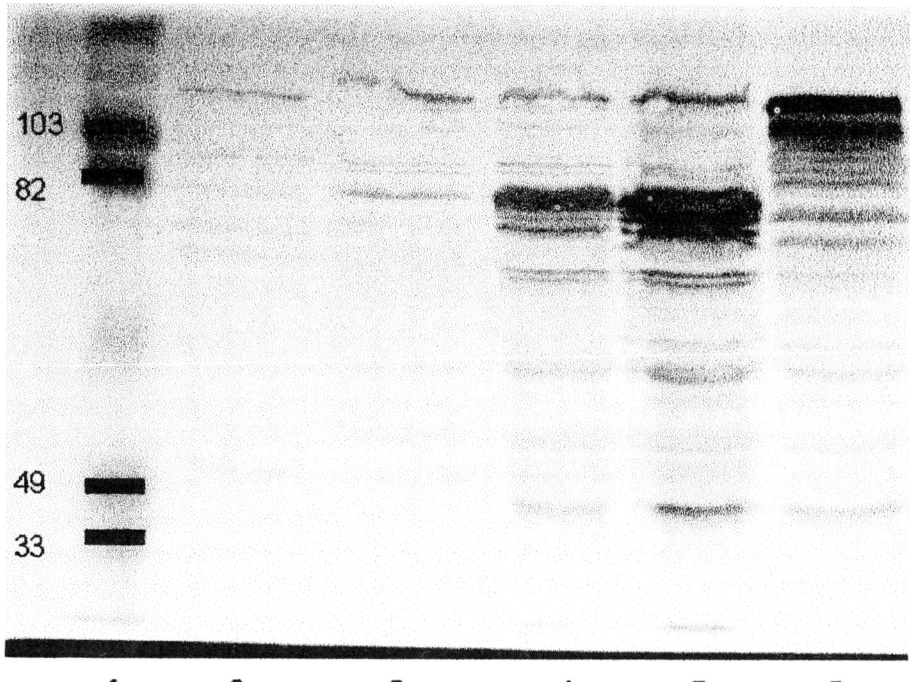

Figure 10.4. Expression of TTFC (approximately 75 kDa) from *L. casei* transformants with plasmids under the transcriptional control of the inducible α-amy promoter derived from *L. amylovorus*.

Cells were transformed with the pLP401-TTFC vectors, that facilitate cell wall anchored expression and were grown in LCM medium + 2% mannitol, supplemented with 5μg/ml erythromycin at 37°C for defined time periods. Cells were analysed following disruption by sonification, separation of proteins on a 10% SDS/polyacrylamide gel and transferred electrophoretically to nitro-cellulose membrane. TTFC was visualised with a polyclonal rabbit anti-TTFC serum. (1.) Bars indicate the migration of molecular weight markers in kDa. TTFC expression is shown following (2.) -two hours, (3.) -four hours, (4.) -six hours, (5.) or 8 hours, after de-repression of the α-amy promoter. (6.) indicates the expression of a TTFC-β glucuronidase fusion protein (approximately 118 kDa) 8 hours following derepression of the α-amy promoter.

compromise growth but does facilitate a second *in vivo* homologous recombination event resulting in the absence of the antibiotic selection marker, by virtue of the antigen coding DNA being carried out as a transcriptional-translational fusion with the *L-ldh* gene. Insertion at the *L-ldh* locus results in higher levels of antigen expression than seen with $tRNA^{ser}$ locus integration, although both systems produce up to five times less antigen than multi-copy plasmid gene expression systems. Researchers at TNO have focused considerable efforts on the generation of structurally and segregationally stable plasmid vectors that maintain sufficiently broad host range to facilitate rational identification of optimum host-vector combinations. However, most vectors were segregationally unstable in *Lactobacillus* in the absence of antibiotic selection with plasmid loss of between 50% -95% within 100 generations (Posno *et al.*, 1991 a,b).

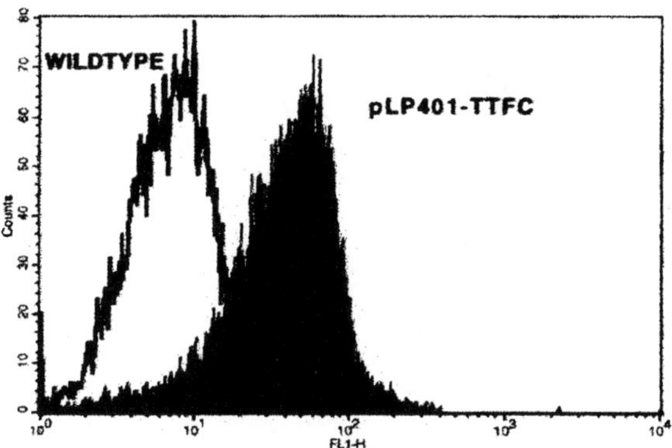

Figure 10.5. Immuno-fluorescence analysis of recombinant *L. casei* (pLP401) expressing TTFC as a surface anchored product.
Lactobacillus cells were gated on the basis of forward and side scatter cytograms and stained with rabbit TTFC-specific antiserum optimally diluted. Bound antibody was detected with optimally diluted FITC-conjugated anti-rabbit antibody and gated cells analysed for fluorescence by FACScan. Peak levels of fluorescence ($FL\text{-}1=10^2$) were demonstrated approximately 8 hours (OD =0.6) following initiation of culture and are shown in histogram form and presented in relation to levels of fluorescence obtained with the non-transformed *L. casei* ($FL\text{-}1 < 10^1$) stained with the TTFC-specific serum diluted 1:500. 10, 000 -20,000 cells were analysed in each experiment.

One important exception was the pLP323 plasmid that we have found to be segregationally stable in many of the *Lactobacillus* strains analysed (Pouwels *et al*, 1996). Using these plasmids expression vectors were developed which allow any antigen of choice to be expressed. Furthermore these vectors allow the expression of antigen at defined cellular locations, namely the intracellular compartment, anchored to the cell wall or secreted. Each of these antigen presentation forms will possess particular advantages or disadvantages for the induction of immunity or tolerance following administration to the GI tract. The pLP323 series of plasmids all utilise *Lactobacillus* derived gene expression elements. Secretion of antigen is directed by the inclusion of the secretion signals and the first few (N terminus) codons of the amylase gene. Cell wall anchored expression of antigen is mediated through the inclusion of the anchor sequence of the proteinase gene of *L. casei.* A variety of antigens was expressed in the cytoplasm at levels of up to 5% of total protein (Fig. 10.3, 10.4) whilst FACS analysis has quantified the levels of antigen accessible on the cell wall at up to 10^4 molecules per cell (Fig. 10.5). In this context the 50 kD ganglioside binding but non-toxic C fragment of tetanus toxin, the A and B subunits of the urease enzyme of *H.pylori* and the VP4, VP6 and VP7 inner and outer capsid proteins derived from rotavirus have all been expressed at levels and efficiencies not previously attainable in *Lactobacillus* (Fig. 10.3, 10.4).

Hols *et al.* (1997) have reported secretion of the M6-gp41E fusion proteins (*S.pyogenes*/HIV-1 gp41) into the culture medium at levels of 13 $mg.l^{-1}$ from *L. para-casei* strain LbTGS1.4. More recently, Maassen *et al.* (1999) described the secretion of encephalitogenic myelin peptides from *L. casei* strains transformed with vectors derived from the pLP323 plasmids, indicating a potential role for these antigen delivery vehicles in the induction of immunological tolerance.

The ability to control expression from these *Lactobacillus* vectors was in general limited due to a lack of regulatable promoters. Constitutive over expression can result in plasmid instability and it has been observed by Leer *et al.* (1992) that this instability extends to segregational instability if certain *E.coli* sequences are inserted. The nisin system developed at NIZO in The Netherlands (Kleerebezen *et al.*, 1997) for use in *L. lactis* was utilised to facilitate *in vitro* analysis of antigen expression. This enabled the expression of genes such as the gp50 glycoprotein of Aujeskys disease virus which had proven impossible in *Lactobacillus* when relying upon constitutive promoters.

However, the elegant nisin system has almost no *in vivo* applicability in the context of vaccine delivery and therefore the group at TNO has utilised the α-amylase promoter obtained from *L. amylovorus* to generate a regulatable expression system under control of catabolite repression (Pouwels *et al.*, 1996). This system has facilitated even the expression of full length rotavirus proteins on the cell wall of several *Lactobacillus* strains at levels equivalent to that documented for the model antigens such as TTFC (Pouwels *et al.*, 1998).

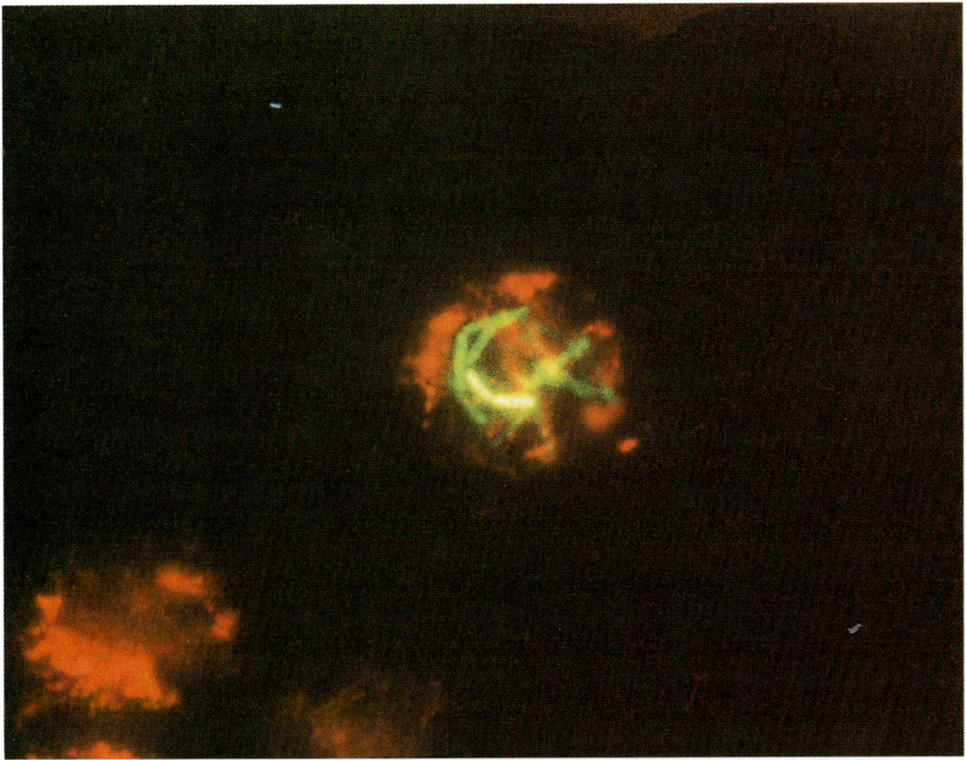

Figure 10. 6. Immuno-fluorescence analysis of phagocytosis of recombinant *L. casei* expressing Green Fluorescent Protein (GFP) by human monocytes. Human PBMC were pulsed for 2 hours with 5 x10^7 *L. casei* transformed with the pLP503-GFP vector which enables intracellular expression of GFP. Following extensive washing monocytes were immuno-stained using a CD68-specific (PE-conjugated) monoclonal antibody and analysed by fluorescence microscopy to identify the macrophage population and GFP-expressing lactobacilli. The figure indicates a single CD68 stained macrophage fluorescing red, with GFP-containing lactobacilli clearly visible within the cell. Approximately 30% of the macrophages in such experiments are doubled stained, indicating substantial uptake of the GFP-expressing lactobacilli. Macrophages that have not taken up the lactobacilli are also visible in the frame.

Apart from cell wall anchored surface expression other alternative ways to express surface antigens have been investigated. Improvements are being evaluated by examining the potential to utilise the surface-layer (S-layer) proteins present on certain *Lactobacillus* strains, including some present in the GI tract (Masuda and Kawata., 1983). The S-layer which envelopes the *Lactobacillus* cells may mediate adhesion to epithelial cells but also presents an opportunity to be utilised in heterologous gene expression. Their periodic structure on the cell wall and their vast numbers that are present per cell ($>3x10^5$) make them ideal for either antigen or antibody expression eg. single chain variable fragment expression. Present research at TNO is aimed at determining which regions within the S-layer protein of *L. acidophilus* may permit the introduction of heterologous antigen or antibody encoding sequences. Recent data indicates that the paracrystalline structure can be maintained when antigen genes are inserted at the N-terminus or at several specified internal locations of the S-protein (Pouwels *et al.*, 1998).

10.7.2 Targetting and uptake of expression vectors

The expression of the Green Fluorescent Protein (GFP) from *Aequorea victoria* by the TNO vectors has enabled the fate to be analysed of the recombinant lactobacilli following intra-gastric delivery. With this system we have been able to establish the uptake of transformed strains in the GI tract. Importantly identification of the GFP-expressing strains in the dome regions of the Peyer's patches has confirmed earlier findings with vital fluorescent staining of non-transformed lactobacilli which were found in the dome of the Peyer's patch. In addition, phagocytosis of GFP transformed *Lactobacillus casei* was shown in human PBMC (Fig.10.5). The utilisation of the GFP vector in a variety of host strains will aid in the *in vivo* determination of preferred host strains, for example those which are seen to adhere either to mucus or epithelial cell surfaces. In particular this facility will enable a direct evaluation of observations such as those of Rojas and Conway (1993) and Stotzer *et al.* (1996) that particular strains such as the *L. fermentum* KLD have a preference for certain sites in the ileum and importantly retain these characteristics following transformation. Similar vectors developed for the *L. plantarum* strain NCIMB 8826 using the nisin system (Mercenier *et al.*, 1999) will enable an evaluation of the survival of transformed strains in the environment to be made.

10.8 Immunological evaluation of mucosal immunisation with *Lactobacillus* spp. expressing antigens

The success seen with the expression of antigens from *Lactobacillus* has provided a solid foundation on which to undertake immunological evaluations of their vaccine potential. Early observations made at TNO demonstrated that lactobacilli were able to provide the T-cell help necessary for the induction of responses specific for haptens (Gerritse *et al.*, 1990). Following oral immunisation with lactobacilli chemically conjugated to TNP serum antibodies specific for TNP were detectable. However, the expression of antigens such as β-galactosidase did not induce either secretory antibody responses in intestinal lavages or in serum. It has been argued that this may have been a consequence of the presence of this antigen in numerous other commensal organisms present in the GI tract (Wells *et al.*, 1996). This possibility is supported by similar observations seen following oral immunisation with strains expressing α-amylase (Claassen *et al.*, 1995).

Both intra-nasal and oral immunisation with the *L. plantarum* TGS1.4 strains expressing the M6-V3 or M6-gp41E fusion proteins has resulted in the induction of M6-specific serum responses when mice received a dose of 10^9 bacteria on two consecutive days (Mercenier *et al.*, 1996). In general, immune responses were only observed after oral administration if booster immunisations are given at designated periods following the priming of mice, suggesting that optimum immunogenicity still had to be attained. In order to allow comparative immunogenicity measurements to be made, several research groups have adopted the model antigen TTFC for analysis.

At TNO *L. casei* and *L. plantarum* strains expressing TTFC as an intracellular product were used to immunise mice both intranasally (i.n.) and orally. In general, the titres of serum IgG specific for TTFC, obtained following sub-cutaneous or intra-peritoneal immunisation are similar to those observed following mucosal vaccination, confirming the potency of this approach. In particular, following intranasal immunisation on days 1-3 both recombinant strains were able to induce serum IgG responses specific for TTFC as early as day 21. Booster immunisations administered i.n. on days 28-30 resulted in rapid and significant boosts to serum IgG levels with end point titres by day 56 in excess of 10^3 (Fig.10.7). Comparative experiments with these strains within the LABVAC network (supported by the fourth framework of the European Commission) has demonstrated that these *Lactobacillus* strains are able to match the immunogenicity levels previously reported for the *L. lactis* system (Mercenier, 1999). Therefore, it is exciting to speculate that they also could also confer the same degree of protection from lethal dose tetanus toxin challenge.

Following nasal or oral immunisation, particulate antigen will be transported to draining lymph nodes by the variety of immune inductor mechanisms already described. Recent results obtained following immunisation of mice with recombinant *L. casei* expressing TTFC has shown *in vitro* that antigen specific T cells can be detected in the cervical lymph nodes that drain the nasal mucosa in addition to lymphoproliferative activity in the spleens of immunised mice. Surprisingly, strains expressing the TTFC as a surface-anchored product were less immunogenic when administered to either BALB/c or C57bl/6 mice by the i.n. route and induced no detectable antibody responses when given orally.

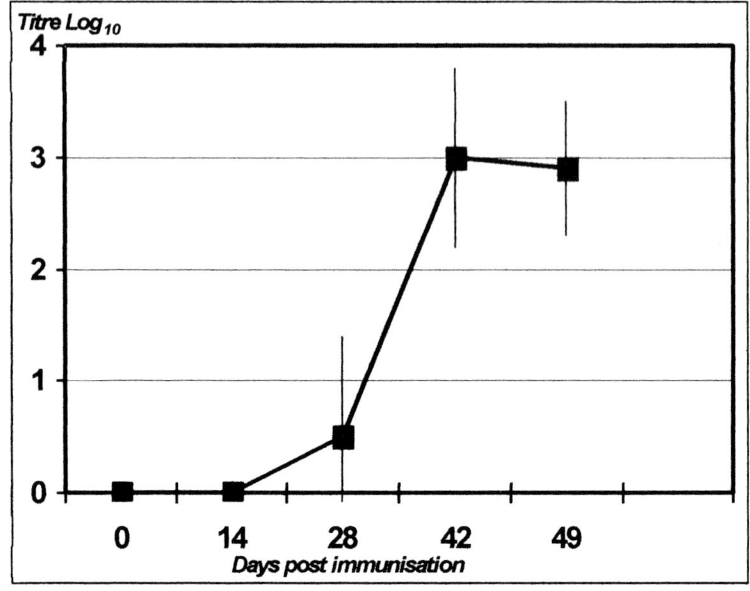

Figure 10.7. TTFC-specific IgG following intranasal immunisation of groups of 3 mice with live recombinant lactobacilli.
Serum was collected from pre-immune mice and at 7 day intervals beginning on day 7. End-point titres of IgG in individual sera were measured by ELISA using microtitre plates (Nunc Maxisorp) coated o/n at 4°C with 5□g/ml of tetanus toxoid in PBS. Bound antibody was detected by the addition of anti-mouse AP conjugate (Nordic, Tilburg) and PNPP substrate. OD_{405nm} values of each well were measured at 90 mins. End-point titres were determined using a cut-off value calculated as the mean OD+ 2 SD's (≈0.2) of pre-immune sera diluted 1:40. Mice vaccinated with irrelevant strains demonstrate no TTFC-specific IgG titres (data not shown). BALB/c mice were immunised intra-nasally with 3 doses of $5x10^9$ *L. casei* pLP503-TTFC [■] in 20□l of PBS on days 1-3. Identical booster immunisations were administered on days 28-30. Data represent the geometric mean of end-point titres of groups of 3 mice ±1 standard deviation.

Boosting vaccinated mice which did not produce TTFC specific antibodies following intranasal administration, with the immunogenic vectors which expressed TTFC as an intracellular product, resulted in rapid high titred serum IgG responses indicating that these mice had been primed by immunisation with the surface-anchored TTFC strains, an observation similar in nature to that reported previously by Mercenier *et al.* (1996). Surface-anchored expression may be particularly susceptible to pH, bile-acid or proteolytic environments encountered following administration. Therefore, attaining high levels of surface anchored antigen may be critical to ensuring sufficient antigen remains accessible to immune-inductive sites. However, the nasal mucosa has proved to be an efficient immune inductive site and this characteristic is well documented, with considerable evidence indicating that the nasal mucosa also possesses the specialised M-like cells also found overlying the Peyer's patches in the gut (Wu *et al.*, 1997). Strain variations in the level of antigen production, as well as the persistence of strains in the GI tract will have pivotal influences on the potency of the recombinant strains. However, the poor intrinsic immunogenicity of specific antigens should not be overlooked. For instance, the failure to induce serum IgG responses failed when the V3 or gp41E peptide of HIV as a component of the M6 fusion protein that was expressed in LbTGS1.4. This was most probably a consequence of both the poor immunogenicity of the peptides but also because the selected mouse strains are poor responders themselves.

The selection of *Lactobacillus* strains that will function as potent carriers in humans is therefore a critical decision for ensuring that all antigens of interest can be presented in an immunogenic form following oral delivery. In addition to the particular strain characteristics already described, the group of Collins, at the University College in Cork, Eire has identified suitable strains that are of human origin. To meet the environmental and safety demands surrounding this technology the modification of such strains to ensure their biological containment is also under progress (Mercenier, 1999).

10.9 Conclusions & future perspectives

This evaluation will be limited to the potential of the probiotic based on *Lactobacillus* spp. For the other vaccine carriers such as *Streptococcus gordonii* and *Lactococcus lactis* molecular biological developments are matter of refinement. The future developments of these vectors will probably aim to design these carriers in order that they, in addition to the heterologous antigens, express properties which are already available naturally in the probiotics.

From this overview it will become apparent that the knowledge with respect to the LAB 'cell factory' and our ability to enable it to work are presently well developed. Nevertheless, for lactobacilli these tools still require further sharpening than that necessary for lactococci and streptococci. This is not because lactobacilli are more refractory to molecular biological modification but rather it is principally due to the fact that they have only recently become the subject of this type of study. In addition, the number of *Lactobacillus* strains over which this interest can be spread are numerous, whereas both for *Lactococcus* and *Streptococcus* the number of potential vaccine hosts is limited. Furthermore, the differences in interesting properties between *Lactobacillus* strains is far greater in every selection criteria for oral vaccine candidates and for molecular biological functioning. However, in reviewing present developments this diversity should be considered more an asset than an obstacle.

Table 10.1. Functional properties of putative oral vaccines

- Support mucosal (IgA) and systemic (IgG) immune responses
- Support cellular immune reactivity
- Immunogenic after repetitive use
- Adjuvant activity
- Cytokine induction
- Skewing to balanced Th1 and Th2 support

The variety in properties allows a selection of those micro-organisms that fit in best for the job intended. The limitations that have been met in *Lactococcus* or *Streptococcus* may be overcome by the wide choice of potentially available *Lactobacillus* strains that may be applied as vector. That means, that for a specific antigen *Lactobacillus* strains can be selected that serve best the production expression with respect to the level and site of expression. *Lactobacillus* ssp. can also be selected to function optimally in the intended host e.g. with respect to localisation or retention. Furthermore, the best combination of antigen, *Lactobacillus* strain and host can be selected in terms of immunogenicity. In this way we can avoid the possibility that antigens which normally are effective immunogens are rendered non-immunogenic when presented in combination with inappropriate expression vehicles. This is a observation that not only arises from work with LAB expression vectors, but rather is actually quite common in the development of combinations of vaccines that are administered simultaneously. It has been observed that certain combinations are detrimental for elicitation of immune responses.

A point which needs still further clarification is the role of intrinsic immunogenicity of the vectors. To direct the response to the heterologous antigens the intrinsic immunogenicity of the vector need not to be beneficial. In this way the complex relationship between vehicle adjuvanticity and immune responsiveness to the expressed antigen starts to emerge. It indeed seems that coexpression of cytokines, that for other vectors may have an important adjuvant effect is effective in live oral vaccines.

Localisation of *Lactobacillus* is a host dependent property. For the purpose of vaccine delivery this is not necessarily detrimental in view of potential tolerance induction, however to date insufficient experimental evidence is available to make proper decisions in this respect. The question remains whether adjuvanticity and immunogenicty of the antigen presented by the vector are mutually influenced. New vectors which are engineered to express both adherence properties and antigens may give some a clues to solve this.

From experiments with *L. lactis* is has become apparent that surface expression is not always beneficial for oral immunisation and subsequent response induction. For some surface expressed antigens there were indications that they might not survive the gastric passage undegraded. However, for live lactobacilli these considerations may be quite different due to the potential for *de-novo* generation in the GI-tract. In addition, expression systems for lactobacilli include both intracellular, surface and excretion of antigens, each of which may have particular applications.

Table 10.2. Selection criteria for *Lactobacillus* oral vaccine candidates

- Expression vectors
- Heterologous gene expression
- Genetic segregation
- Stability of expression
- Level of expression
- Delivery potential
- Homing, localisation capacity
- Adherence to mucosa or mucosal receptors
- Low intrinsic immunogenicity
- Effective heterologous immunogen
- Logistics
- Easy culture
- Stable on freeze/spray drying

At present the selection criteria for *Lactobacillus* vaccine vectors have more or less crystallised. Also the molecular biological tools have been developed such that a rational design of new specific expression vectors can be realised in the specific *Lactobacillus* strains that gives the best opportunity for the results expected.

As the interaction of *Lactobacillus* based oral vaccine vectors and the recipient includes a multifunctional series of events, the complexity probably can best be evaluated in the intact target host. For some species, e.g. humans, this will not be possible for all aspects of interest while for other animals this is rather costly. Therefore, there is certainly a need for new *in vitro* or *ex vivo* methods that allow selection of *Lactobacillus* strains with specific properties such as adherence, induction of cytokines and activation of specific cell types such as Peyer's patch cells and macrophages.

From this it can be concluded that the present vectors or model vaccines available should be considered as a first generation. The new generation of vectors will be tailor made for specific applications with respect to pathogen, host, adherence properties, adjuvanticity and immunogenicity. It is on the basis of the evaluation of these vectors the future of *Lactobacillus* based vaccines will depend.

10.10 Summary

The natural route for the majority of pathogens to enter the body is *via* the mucosa of the gastro-intestinal-, respiratory- and uro-genital tracts. In the development of vaccines, attenuated or genetically modified pathogens have often been applied in order to exploit their natural route of entrance. For pathogens which impose a high risk of unwanted inflammation or for which attenuation led to inactive vaccines, new trans-disease vaccines were developed with pathogens that were used instead as vehicles to the natural site of entry. This made clear that two aspects are of major importance in the development of oral vaccines: to determine the route of entry to the mucosal immune system and to give rise to a level of inflammation sufficient to support induction of local immunity. To facilitate entry to the mucosal system, virus receptors, receptors for toxins and particles of specific size were selected. All provide the correct routing, but they do not necessarily support the induction of immune responsiveness.

Probiotic microorganisms were demonstrated to have an influence on antigen presenting cells and in addition did induce local mucosal immuno-modulating effects as a result of local cytokine production. The enhancement of immune responses by probiotics demonstrated that these immuno-modulating properties could also be applied as local adjuvants. The combination of the particulate aspect and the adjuvant capacity of probiotic bacteria together offer the properties that an oral/mucosal vaccine preferably should possess. This led to investigations of the potential of transformed lactic acid bacteria, such as *Lactobacillus,* as live oral vaccine carriers. These transformants provide adjuvant activity, correct particle size, uptake into the mucosal immune system and - provided proper transformation systems are used- the production of sufficient antigen to elicit specific mucosal responses. Their food grade character makes them a generally regarded as safe (GRAS) tool in a new field of application. In this paper we give an overview of the present status of probiotic lactobacilli as putative oral vaccine carriers.

References

Aattouri N. and Lemonnier D (1997) Production of interferon induced by *Streptococcus thermophilus*: role of CD4 and CD8 lymphocyte. *J.Nutr.Biochem.* **8**, 25-31.

Adkins D. and Du R.Q. (1998) Newborn mice develop balanced Th1/Th2 primary effector responses in vivo but are biased to Th2 secondary responses. *J.Immunol.* **160**, 4217-4224.

Barrios C., Brawand R., Berney M., Brandt C., Lambert P.H. and Siegrist C.A. (1996a) Neonatal and early life immune responses to various forms of vaccine antigens qualitativley differ from adult responses: predominance of a Th2 biased pattern which persists after adult booster. *Eur.J.Immunol.* **26**, 1489-1496.

Barrios C., Brawand R., Berney M., Brandt C., Lambert P.H. and Siegrist C.A. (1996b) Partial correction of the Th1/Th2 imbalance in neonatal murine responses to vaccine antigens through seletive adjuvant effects. *Eur. J.Immunol.* **26,** 2666-2670.

Berg R.D. (1998) Probioitcs, prebioitcs or conbiotics. *Trends in Microbiol.* **6,** 89-92.

Bloksma N., De Heer E., Van Dijk H. and Willers J.M. (1979) Systemic augmentation of the immune response in mice by feeding milks with *Lactobacillus casei* and *Lactobacillus acidophilus. Immunology* **37**, 367-375.

Blomberg L., Hendriksson A. and Conway P.L. (1993) Inhibition of adhesion of *Escherichia coli* K88 to piglet ileal mucus by *Lactobacillus* spp. *Appl. Environm. Microbiol.* **59**, 34-39.

Boersma W.J.A., Zegers N.D., Van Den Bogaerdt A., Leer R.J., Bergmans A., Pouwels P.H., Posno M. and E.Claassen. (1994) Development of safe oral vaccines based on *Lactobacillus* as a vector with adjuvant activity. Proc. ICHEM 2nd. Internatl. Congr. Biotech UK, Brighton: Industrial Immunology pp 43-46.

Cherfas J. (1993) From victuals to vaccines: food organisms burst forth. *Biobulletin* **14**, 8-9.

Chong C., Bost K.L. and Clements J.D. (1996) Differential production of interleukin-12 mRNA by murine macrophages in response to viable or killed *Salmonella. Infect. Immun.* **64**, 1154-1160.

Claassen E. and Boersma W.J.A. (1992) Characteristics and practical use of new-generation adjuvants as an acceptable alternative for Freund's complete adjuvant. 44th Forum in immunology. *Res. Immunol.* **143**, 471-586.

Claassen E., Kottenhage M.J., Pouwels P.H. Posno M., Boersma W.J.A. and Lucas C.J. (1994) The use of *Lactobacillus*, a GRAS (generally regarded as safe) organism as a base for a new generation of 'oral" live vaccines. In:"Recombinant and Synthetic Vaccines". Eds. G.P.Talwar and V.S.R. Kanury. Narosa Publ. New Delhi pp 407-412.

Cleveland M.G., Gorham J.D., Murphy T.L., Tuomanen E. and Murphy K.M. (1996) Lipoteichoic acid preparations of gram positive bacteria induce interleukin-12 through a CD-14 dependent pathway. *Infect.Immun.* **64**, 1906-1912.

Coconnier M.H.;,Lievin V., Bernet-Camard M.F.;,Hudault S. and Servin A.L. Antibacterial effect of the adhering human Lactobacillus acidophilus strain. *Antimicrob-Agents-Chemother.* **41**: 1046-1052

Coconnier M.H. Lievin V., Hemery E. and Servin A.L. (1998) Antagonistic activity against Helicobacter infection *in vitro* and *in vivo* by the human Lactobacillus acidophilus strain LB. *Appl.Environ.Microbiol.* **64**, 4573-4580

Conway P..L. and Kjelleberg S. (1989) Protein mediated adhesion of *Lactobacillus fermentum* strain 737 to mouse stomach squamous epithelium. *J.Gen.Microbiol.* **135**, 1175-1186.

Conway P..L. and Henriksson A. (1993). Strategies for the isolation and characterisation of functional probiotics. In Gibson., (Ed). Human Health: The Contribution of Micro-organisms. Springer. Pp. 75 –93.

D'Andrea A., Aste-Amezaga M., Valiante N.M., Ma X., Kubin M. and Tricheri G. (1993) Interleukin 10 (IL-10) inhibits human lymphocyte interferon γ production by suppressing natural killer cell stimulatory factor IL-12 synthesis in accessory cells. *J.Exp.Med.* **178**, 1041-1048.

Di-Fabio S., Medaglini D., Rush C.M., Corrias F., Panzini G.L., Pace M., Verani P.,

Pozzi G. and Titti F. (1998) Vaginal immunization of Cynomolgus monkeys with Streptococcus gordonii expressing HIV-1 and HPV 16 antigens. *Vaccine* **16**, 485-92.

Famularo G. and De Simone C. (1998) Oral Bacteriotherapy. *Immunol. Today* **19**, 486-87

Fernandes C.F., Shahani K.M. and Amer M.A., (1987) Therapeutic role of dietary lactobacilli and lactobacillic fermented dairy products. *FEMS Microbiol. Revs.* **46**, 343 -356.

Fischetti V.A., Medaglini D. and Pozzi G. (1996) Gram-positive commensal bacteria for mucosal vaccine delivery. *Curr. Opin. Biotechnol.* **7**, 659-66.

Forsthuber T., Yip H.C. and Lehman P.V. (1996) Induction of Th1 and Th2 immunity in neonatal mice. *Science* **271**, 1728-1730.

Frere J. (1994) Simple method for extracting plasmid DNA from lactic acid bacteria. *Lett. Appl. Microbiol.* **4**, 227-9.

Fuller R. (1992) History and development of probiotics. In: *Probiotics: The scientific basis.* (Ed. R Fuller) Chapman and Hall, UK., 1-8.

Gerritse K., Posno M., Schellekens M..M., Boersma W.J.A. and Claassen E. (1990) Oral administration of TNP-*Lactobacillus* conjugates in mice: a model for evaluation of mucosal and systemic immune responses and memory formation elicited by transformed lactobacilli. *Res. Microbiol.* **141**, 955-962.

Guarner F. and Schaafsma G.J. (1998) Probiotics. *Int. J. Food Microbiol.* **39**, 237-238.

Gupta R.K., Griffin P., Chang A.C., Rivera R., Anderson R., Rost B., Cecchini D., Nicholson M. and Siber G.R. (1996) The role of adjuvants and delivery systems inmodualtion of immune response to vaccines. In: Cohen S. and Shafferman A. (eds) Novel strategies in design and production of vaccines. Plenum Press, New York 1996, pp 105-113.

Haeberle H.A., Kubin M., Basmford K.B., Garofalo R., Graham D.Y., El Zaatari F., Karttunen R., Crowe S.E., Reyes V.E. and Ernst P.B. (1997) Differential stimulation of interleukin 12 (IL-12) and IL10 by live and killed *Helicobacter pylori in vitro* and association of IL-12 production with gamma-interferon producing T-cells in the human gastric mucosa. *Infect.Immun.* **65**, 4229-4235.

Hols P., Slos P., Dutot, P., Reymund, J., Charbot, P., Delplace, B. Delcour, J. and Mercenier, A. 1997. Efficient secretion of the model antigen M6-gp41E in *Lactobacillus* plantarum NCIMB 8826. *Microbiol.* **143**, 2733 –2741.

Iwaki M., Okahashi N., Takahashi I., Kanamoto T, Sugita-Konishi Y Aibara K. and Koga T. (1990) Oral immunisation with recombinant *Streptococcus lactis* carrying the *Streptococcus mutans* surface protein antigen gene. *Infect. Immun.* **58**, 2929-2934.

Isolauri E., Joensuu J., Suoalainen H., Luomala M. and Vesikari T. (1995) Improved immunogenicity of oral DxRRV reassortant rotavirus vaccine by *Lactobacillus casei* GG. *Vaccine* **13**, 310-312.

Kaila M., Isolauri E., Soppi E., Virtanen E., Laine S. and Arvilommi H. (1992) Enhancement of the circulating antibody secreting cell response in human diarrhea by a human *Lactobacillus* strain. *Pediatr.Res.* **32**, 141-144.

Kaila M., Isolauri E., Saxelin M., Arvilommi H. and Vesikari T. (1995) Viable versus inactivated lactobacillus strain GG in acute rotavirus diarrhoea. *Arch. Dis.Childh.* **72**, 51-53.

Klaasen H.L.B.M., Koopman J.P., Poelma F.G.J. and Beynen A.C. (1991) Intestinal segmented filamentous bacteria. *FEMS Microbiol. Rev.* **88**, 165-180.

Klaasen H.L.B.M., Van der Heijden P.J, Stok W., Poelma F.G.J, Koopman J.P, Van den Brink M.E., Bakker M.H., Eling W.M.C. and Beynen A.C. (1993) Apathogenic intestinal segmented filamentous bacteria stimulate the mucosal immune system of mice. *Infect. Immun.* **61**, 303-306.

Kerneis S., Bogdanova A., Kraehenbuhl J.-P. and Pringault E. (1997) Conversion by Peyer's patch lymphocytes of human enterocytes into M cells that transport bacteria. *Science* **277**, 949-953.

Klaenhammer T.R. and Sutherlands S.M. (1980) Detection of plasmid deoxyribonucleic acid in an isolate of *Lactobacillus acidophilus*. *Appl. Environ. Microbiol.* **39**, 671-674.

Kleerenbezem M., Beerthuyzen M.M., Vaughan E.E., de Vos W.M.and Kuipers O.P. (1997) Controlled gene expression systems for lactic acid bacteria: Transferable nisin-inducible expression cassettes for *Lactococcus*, *Leuconostoc* and *Lactobacillus* spp. *Appl. Environ. Microbiol.* **63**, 4581-4584.

Kohno K. and Kurimoto M. (1998) Interleukin 18, a cytokine which resembles IL-1 structurally and IL-12 functionally but exerts its effect independently of both. *Clin.Immunol.Immunopathol. J.* **86**: 11-15.

Leer, R.J., Van Luijik, N., Posno, M. and Pouwels, P.H. 1992. Structural and functional analysis of two cryptic plasmids from *Lactobacillus pentosus* MD353 and *Lactobacillus* planatraum ATCC 8014. *Mol. Gen. Genet.* **234**, 265 –274.

Lucey M., and Fitzgerald G. (1997) The biotechnology of lactic acid bacteria. *Food Science Technol. Today* **11**, 230-233.

Maassen C.B.M., Gerritse K., Leer R.J., Heemskerk D., Boersma W.J.A. and Claassen E. (1997) Lactobacillus as a vector for oral delivery of antigens, the role of intrinsic adjuvanticity in modulation of the immune response. 9th Int. Congress Mucosal Immunology, Sydney Australia In: Mucosal Solutions, (Eds. A.J.Husband, K.W. Beagley, A.W. Collins, R.L.Clancy, A.W. Cripps, D.L Emery). *Advances in Mucosal Immunology*, **2**, 235-247.

Maassen, C.B.M., Laman J.D., Heijne den Bak-Glashouwer M.J., Tielen F.J., Van Holten-Neelen J.C.P.A., Hoogteijling L., Antonissen C., Leer R.J.,. Pouwels P.H, Boersma W.J.A. and Shaw D.M. (1999). *Vaccine (in press)*.

Marteau P. and Rambaud J.C. (1993) Potential of using lactic acid bacteria for therapy and immunomodulation in man. *FEMS Microbiol. Rev.* **12**, 207-220.

Masuda, K. and Kawata, T. (1983). Distribution and chemical characterisation of regular arrays in the cell walls of strains of the genius *Lactobacillus*. *FEMS. Microbiol. Lett.* **20**, 145 –150.

McGhee J.R. and Kiyono H. (1993) New perspectives in vaccien development: mucosal immunity to infections. *Infect. Agents Dis.* **2**, 55-73.

Medaglini D., Pozzi G., King T.P. and Fischetti V.A. (1995) Mucosal and systemic immune responses to a recombinant protein expressed on the surface of the oral commensal bacterium *Streptococcus gordonii* after oral colonization. *Proc.Natl.Acad.Sci. USA*. **92**, 6868-6872.

Medaglini D., Rush C.M., Sestini P. and Pozzi G. (1997) Commensal bacteria as vectors for mucosal vaccines against sexually transmitted diseases: vaginal colonization with recombinant streptococci induces local and systemic antibodies in mice. *Vaccine* **15**, 1330-1337.

Medaglini D., Oggioni M.R. and Pozzi G. (1998) Vaginal immunization with recombinant Gram-positive bacteria. *Am. J. Reprod. Immunol.* **39**, 199-208.

Mercenier, A. (1999) Lactic Acid Bacteria as Live Vaccine. In: *Probiotics: A Critical Review*. (Ed. G.W. Tennock) Horizon Scientific Press U.K., pp 113-128.

Mercenier A., Dutot P., Kleinpeter P., Aguirre M., Paris P., Reymaund J. and Slos, P. (1996). Development of lactic acid bacteria as live vectors for oral or lacal vaccines. *Adv. Food. Science* **18**, 73-77.

Miettinen M., Matikainen S., Vuopio-Varkila J. and Varkila K. (1996) Production of tumor necrosis factor α, interleukin 6 and interleukin 10 is induced by lactic acid bacteria. *Infect. Immun.* **64**, 5403-5405.

Miettinen M., Matikainen S., Vuopio-Varkila J., Pirhonen J., Varkila K., Korimoto M. and Julkunen I. (1998) lactobacilli and streptococci induce intereukin 12 (IL-12), IL-18 and gamma interferon prodcution in human peripheral blood mononuclear cells. *Infect. Immun.* **66**, 6058-6062.

Moreau M.C., Raibaud P. and Muller C. (1982) Relation entre developpement du systeme immunitaire intestinal a IgA et l'etablissement de la flora microbienne dans le tube digestif du souriceau holoxenique. *Ann Immunol. (Pasteur)* **133D**, 29-39.

Norton P.M., Brown H.W., Wells J.M., Macpherson A.M., Wilson P.W. and Le-Page R.W. (1996) Factors affecting the immunogenicity of tetanus toxin fragment C expressed in *Lactococcus lactis*. *FEMS Immuno. Med. Microbiol.* **14**, 167-177.

Norton P.M., Wells J.M., Brown H.W., Macpherson A.M. and Le-Page R.W. (1997) Protection against tetanus toxin in mice nasally immunised with recombinant *Lactococcus lactis* expressing tetanus toxin fragment C. *Vaccine* **15**, 616-619.

Oggioni M.R, Manganelli R., Contorni M., TommasinoM.and Pozzi G. (1995) Immunization of mice by oral colonization with live recombinant commensal streptococci. *Vaccine* **13**, 775-779.

Oggioni M.R. and Pozzi G. (1996) A host vector system for heterologous gene expression in *Streptococcus gordonii*. *Gene* **169**: 85-90.

Oggioni M.R., Pozzi G., Valensin P.E., Galieni P. and Bigazzi C. (1998) Recurrent septicemia in an immunocompromised patient due to probiotic strains of *Bacillus subtilis*. *J.Clin. Microbiol.* **36**, 325-326.

Okamura H. Tsutsui H., Komatsu T., Yutsudo M., Hakura A., Tanimoto T., Torigoe K., Okura T., Nukada Y., Hattori K., Akita K., Namba M., Tanabe F., Konishi K., Fukuda S. and Kurimoto M. (1995) Cloning of a new cytokine that induces interferon gamma production by T-cells. *Nature* **378**, 88-91.

Perdigon G., De Macias M.E.N., Alvarez S., Oliver G. and Pesce De Ruiz Helgado A.A.P. (1986) Effect of perorally administered lactobacilli on macrophage activation in mice. *Infect. Immun.* **53**, 404-410.

Pereyra B. and Lemonnier D. (1993) Induction of human cytokines by bacteria used in dairy foods. *Nutr. Res.* **113**, 1127-1140.

Posno, M., Heuvelmans, P.T.M.H., van Giezen, M.J.F. Leer, R.J. and Pouwels, P.H. (1991a) Complementation of the inability of *Lactobacillus* strains to utilise D-xylose with D-xylose catabolism – encoding genes of *Lactobacillus pentosus*. *Appl. Environ, Microbiol.* **57**, 2764 – 2766.

Posno, M., Leer, R.J., van Luijik, N., van Giezen, M.J.F. and Heuvelmans, P.T.M.H. (1991b). Incompatibility of *Lactobacillus* vectors with replicons derived from small cryptic *Lactobacillus* plasmids and segregational instability of the introduced vectors. *Appl. Environ. Microbiol.* **57**: 1822-1828.

Pouwels P.H., Leer R.J. and Boersma W.J.A. (1995) The potential of *Lactobacillus* as a carrier for oral immunization: Development and preliminary characterization of vectors systems for targeted delivery of antigens. *J. Biotechnol.* **44**, 183-192.

Pouwels P.H., Leer R.J., Shaw M., Heijne den Bak Glashouwer M-J., Tielen F.J., Smit E., Martinez. B., Jore J. and Conway P.L. (1998) Lactic Acid Bacteria as antigen delivery vehicles for oral immunisation purposes. *Int. J. Food. Microbiol.*. **41**, 155-167.

Pozzi G., Oggioni M.R., Manganelli R. and Fischetti V.A. (1992a) Expression of M6 protein gene of *Streptococcus pyogenes* in *Streptococcus gordonii* after chromosomal integration and transcriptional fusion. *Res. Microbiol.* **143**, 449-457.

Pozzi G., Contorni M., Oggioni M.R., Manganelli R., Tommasino M., Cavalieri F. and Fischetti V.A. (1992b) Delivery and expression of a heterologous antigen on the surface of streptococci. *Infect. Immun.* **60**, 1902-1907.

Pozzi G., Oggioni M.R., Manganelli R., Medaglini D., Fischetti V.A., Fenoglio D., Valle M.T., Kunkl A. and Manca F. (1994) Human T-helper cell recognition of an immunodominant epitope of HIV-1 gp120 expressed on the surface of *Streptococcus gordonii*. *Vaccine* **12**:1071-1077.

Puren A.J., Fantuzzi G., Gu Y., Su S.S. and Dinarello C.A. (1998) Interleuking 18 (IFN-gamma inducing factor) induces IL-8 and IL-1-β *via* TNF-α prodcution from non CD14+ human blood mononuclear cells. *J.Clin.Invest.* **101**, 711-721.

Raghupathy R. (1997) Thl type immunity is incompatible with successful pregnancy. *Immunol. Today* **18**, 478-482.

Reinkemeier M., Rocken W. and Leitzmann C. (1996) A rapid mechanical lysing procedure for routine analysis of plasmids from lactobacilli, isolated from sourdoughs. *Int. J. Food. Microbiol.* **29**, 93-104

Rescigno M., Citterio S., Thery C., Rittig M., Medaglini D., Pozzi G., Amigorena S. and Ricciardi-Castagnoli P. (1998) Bacteria-induced neo-biosynthesis, stabilization, and surface expression of functional class I molecules in mouse dendritic cells. *Proc. Natl. Acad. Sci. USA* **95**, 5229-5234.

Rojas M. and Conway P.L. (1996) Colonization by lactobacilli of piglet small intestinal mucus. *J. Appl. Bacteriol.* **81**, 474-480.

Rook G.A.W. and Stanford J.L. (1998) Give us this day our daily germs. *Immunol. Today* **19**, 113-117.

Robinson K., Chamberlain L., Schofield K.M., Wells J.M. and Le-Page R.W. (1997) Oral vaccination against tetanus with recombinant *Lactococus lactis*. *Nature Biotechnol.* **15**, 653-657.

Rush C.M., Hafner L.M., Timms P. (1995) Lactobacilli: vehicles for antigen delivery to the female urogenital tract. *Adv. Exp. Med. Biol.* **371B**, 1547-52 .

Solis-Pereyra B., Aattouri N. and Lemonnier D. (1997) Role of food in the stimulation of cytokine production. *Am. J. Clin. Nutr.* **66**, S521-525.

Steidler L., Robinson K., Chamberlain L., Schofield K.M., Remaut E., Le-Page R.W. and Wells J.M .(1998) Mucosal delivery of murine interleukin-2 (IL-2) and IL-6 by recombinant strains of *Lactococcus lactis* coexpressing antigen and cytokine. *Infect. Immun.* **66**, 3183-3189.

Steidler L., Wells J.M., Raeymakers A., VandeKerckhove J., Fiers W. and Remaut E. (1995) Secretion of biologically active murine interleukin-2 by *Lactococcus lactis* subsp. lactis. *Appl. Environ. Microbiol.* **61**, 1627-1629.

Stotzer P.O., Blomberg L., Conway P.L., Henriksson A. and Abrahamsson H. (1996) Probiotic treatment of small intestinal bacterial overgrowth by *Lactobacillus fermentum* KLD. *Scand. J. Infect. Dis.* **28**, 615-619.

Tannock G.W. (1997) Probiotic properties of lactic-acid bacteria: plenty of scope for fundamental R and D. *Trends in Biotechnol.* **15**, 270-274.

Tannock G.W., Klaenhammer T.R., Connolly J.F., FitzGerald R.J., Stanton C. and Ross R.P. (1998) Studies of the intestinal microflora: a prerequisite for the development of probiotics. Special Issue: Functional foods: designer foods for the future. *Int. Dairy J.* **8**, 527-533.

Tortuero F., Rioperez J., Fernandez E. and Rodriguez M.L. (1995) Response of piglets to oral administration of lactic acid bacteria. *J. Food Protection* **58**, 1369-1374.

Van Regenmortel M. (1997) Searching for safer, more potent, better-targeted adjuvants. *ASM News* **63**, 136-139.

Waterfield N.R., Le-Page R.W. and Wells J.M. (1995) The isolation of lactococcal promoters and their use in investigating bacterial luciferase synthesis in *Lactococcus lactis*. *Gene* **165**, 9-15.

Wells J.M., Nilson P.W., Norton P.M., Gasson M.J.and Le-Page R.W. (1993) *Lactococcus lactis*: high level expression of tetanus toxin fragment C and protection against lethal challenge *Mol. Microbiol.* **8**, 1155-1162.

Wells, J.M.,. Robinson K, Chamberlain L.M., Schofield K.M. and Le-Page R.W.F. (1996) Lactic acid bacteria as vaccine delivery vehicles.In: Lactic Acid Bacteria: Genetics, Metabolism and Applications. *Anton. Van Leeuwen.* **70**, 317 –330.

Wu, H-Y., Nikolova, E.B., Beagley, K.W., Eldridge, J.H. and Russel, M.W.(1997) Development of antibody secreting cells and antigen specific T cells in cervical lymph nodes after intranasal immunisation. *Infect. Immun.* **65**:227 –235.

CONCLUSIONS

G Perdigón and R Fuller

Originally it was thought that probiotics operated solely by modifying the composition or activity of the gut microflora. More recent research has shown that there is also an effect on the immune system. The knowledge of the role played by the gut flora in stimulation of the secretory immune system and functioning of the immune system as a whole is essential for the successuful development of probiotics for use in farm animals and human beings.

The intestinal ecosystem is a complex network of interaction between procaryotic and eucaryotic cells. The first group contains the microorganisms which comprise the indigenous gut microflora; the eucaryotic cells are the epithelial and immune cells of the host animal. The result of the interaction is not always beneficial and health claims must always be made on the basis of sound scientific evidence supporting the claim and discounting any possible adverse response.

The foregoing chapters summarize the research work that has been done on the immune response to the gut microflora and to probiotic microorganisms which have been added to it. It highlights the positive findings against the potential problems and provides a basis for future research in this area. Much of the work reported has been done in laboratory rodents and care should be taken when extrapolating these findings to man. However, this type of research does provide a basis for the design of the human trials which are so desparately needed.

Each chapter gives a review of research in a particular area of immunomodulation exerted by the microflora, by probiotic lactic acid bacteria or by milk peptides produced during its fermentation. The contributions indicate the growing scientific evidence for health enhancement based on stimulation of mucosal immunity by the gut microflora or dietary components. From this we can deduce the importance of understanding the functioning of immune cells associated with the mucosa in determining how probiotics work and in guiding the development of new preparations.

Mucosal immunity is an important arm of the immune system because it is involved in the response to infectious agents as well as in tolerance to environmental and dietary antigens. The use of mucosal adjuvants make it possible to maximise the effect and obtain an adequate immunostimulation.

The resident bacterial flora of the colon is very active metabolically and influences the survival of organisms arriving from the small intestine. Studies with gnotobiotic and conventional animals indicate the ways in

R. Fuller and G. Perdigon (eds.), Probiotics 3, 271–273.

which mucosal, immunity develops. These fundamental studies may help in the analyses of probiotic results and in suggesting new probiotic strains with improved immunogenic activity.

While an immune response may be statistically significant it will not protect against infection unless the response is sufficiently high to be antimicrobial in some way. We must make the distinction between *statistical* significance and *biological* significance. These important chapters cover the subject of development of probiotics as possible protective agents in the prevention of infections or tumours by enhancing the immune response in normal subjects or in patients immunosuppressed by malnutrition or drug therapy.

The modulation of cytokine release by LAB is important in this context. Cytokines can be involved in up or down regulation of the immune response as well as in the defense mechanisms of the gastrointestinal tract. However, the directed release of cytokines to prevent infection or enhance oral tolerance is not yet possible. The appropiate strains required to induce these effects have not been identified.

The possibility that microbial metabolites in the fermented milk are responsible for some of the immune stimulation is also discussed. Bioactive peptides derived from milk protein may be responsible for some of the probiotic effects ascribed to fermented milks such as traditional yoghurt and the widely available bioyoghurts.

In the understanding of present products and the development of new probiotics it is important to know how they modulate the gut microflora and how that, in turn, affects the host animal. In this context it is important to know how the LAB interact with the intestine and how they are able to activate the mucosal immunity; which cells are stimulated and which cytokine is released.

The use of LAB as vaccine vectors is an exciting possibility providing a chronic stimulation from a commensal organisms permanently established in the gut. This together with the adjuvant properties of LAB open up a range of different strategies for new types of vaccine therapies.

The chapters in the book contain many points of discussion about one of the most important facts of probiotic strain selection i.e. for their immunomodulatory effects. This exciting development extends the range of probiotic effects from those occurring only in the gut to systemic effects which may control infections in sites in other parts of the body. The understanding of the indigenous microflora and the way it influences the immune response is central to the future development of probiotics.

Future trends in probiotic research will be:

1 development of methods which facilitate the performance of human clinical trials.

2 influence of probiotics and the gut microflora on DNA damage and repair in the normal mucosa. This will help to determine the modulatory role of probiotics in carcinogenesis, especially in the colon.
3 understanding the GALT function and its regulation as well as the interaction of probiotics with the digestive epithelium and immune cells.
4 development of biomarkers for immune function and establishment of the pattern of cytokines released to predict the effects of probiotics on regulation of the immune response.

The role of the gut microflora in the host animal's resistance to disease is undeniable and forms the basis for the belief that specific cultures, probiotics, can promote health. The mechanisms of this effect have yet to be fully discovered but the recent findings that LAB can stimulate the immune system are an important contribution to the ultimate understanding of the whole phenomenon of probiosis.

Acknowledgement

The editors are extremely grateful to Dr. Marta Medici for her important contribution to the successful outcome of this book; she helped turn the disparate manuscripts into a unified collection.

INDEX